▲® The American
Diabetes Association®

The American
Dietetic Association

FAMILY
COOKBOOK

Volume III

Also by the authors from Simon & Schuster:

The American Diabetes Association
The American Dietetic Association
Family Cookbook, Volume I (Revised Edition)

The American Diabetes Association
The American Dietetic Association
Family Cookbook, Volume II (Revised Edition)

American Diabetes Association
Holiday Cookbook
Betty Wedman, M.S., R.D.

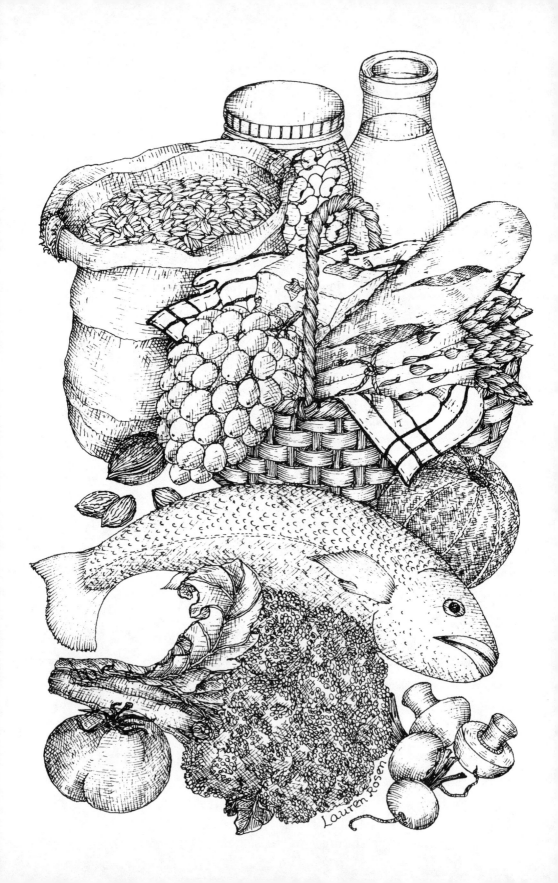

▲® The American
Diabetes Association®

The American
Dietetic Association

FAMILY COOKBOOK

Volume III

With Microwave Adaptations

Illustrated by Lauren Rosen

SIMON & SCHUSTER
NEW YORK LONDON TORONTO SYDNEY TOKYO SINGAPORE

SIMON & SCHUSTER

Rockefeller Center
1230 Avenue of the Americas
New York, New York 10020

LC No. 87-42674

ISBN 0-671-76133-1

Manufactured in the United States of America

10 9 8

Acknowledgments

The American Diabetes Association and The American Dietetic Association gratefully acknowledge the following contributors:

Recipe Development and Testing:
    Lois Levine
    Karen Levin
    Mark Steven Warnaar

Nutritional Analysis and Exchange Calculations:
    Madelyn L. Wheeler, M.S., R.D., C.D.E.
    Lawrence A. Wheeler, M.D., Ph.D.

Ethnic/Cultural Chapters:
    Madelyn L. Wheeler, M.S., R.D., C.D.E., Editor
    Susan Algert, M.S., R.D.
    Lisa Bookstein, M.S., R.D.
    Nancy Stubblefield, M.S.
    Yvonne Jackson, Ph.D., R.D.
    Brenda A. Broussard, R.D., M.P.H., M.B.A.
    Louise Loggans, R.D., D.M.Sc.
    David Marrero, Ph.D.
    Jane Erington
    Rita Rolfes, R.D.
    Ursuline Beal, R.D.
    Bridget Barrett, R.D.
    Joyce Raether, R.D.
    Beth Maddox, R.D.
    Harold Holler, R.D.
    Carolyn Templeton, R.D.

Technical Reviewers:
    Madelyn L. Wheeler, M.S., R.D., C.D.E.
    Phyllis A. Crapo, R.D.
    Harold Holler, R.D.

Text Writer/Editor:
    Dorothy H. Segal

Manuscript Production:
    Corinne Bronson-Adatto, M.S., R.D.
    Susan Hayes Coughlin
    Karen S. DelVescovo, R.D.
    Deborah McBride
    Caroline A. Stevens

Contents

Foreword

Americans today are more concerned than ever with good nutrition and healthy eating. This trend is reflected daily in newspapers and popular magazines that only a few years ago were more concerned with the cosmetic aspects of beauty and fitness than with the reality of good health. Nowadays, however, ''You are what you eat'' is fast becoming an accepted tenet of modern life.

That is why I am delighted to introduce Volume III of the *American Diabetes Association/American Dietetic Association Family Cookbook*. Like the first two volumes, this one is designed to provide delicious and nutritious recipes for everyone who cares about good nutrition—especially people with diabetes and their families.

The cookbook reflects the latest scientific findings about good nutrition. It stresses the importance of variety in the diet and emphasizes foods that are low in sugar, salt, and fat and high in complex carbohydrates. In fact, Volume III of the *Family Cookbook* is consistent with the latest nutritional guidelines developed by the American Diabetes Association and The American Dietetic Association. It also uses the newly revised *Exchange Lists for Meal Planning* to provide nutritional breakdowns per serving for each recipe.

The cookbook capitalizes on another trend by highlighting various ethnic cuisines to liven up the diet. And it is designed to fit into busy modern life-styles by offering microwave adaptations for fully half of the recipes.

If you or a member of your family has diabetes, we hope this latest volume will help you to enjoy a delicious, varied, and satisfying diet. We hope, too, that all those tempted by the prospect of a healthy life-style based on good eating will explore its pages.

JOHN A. COLWELL, M.D., PH.D.
President
American Diabetes Association

As knowledge of nutrition increases, so does the desire for healthful eating. The role of good nutrition in the treatment of diabetes also remains on the forefront as knowledge continues to expand in new directions every day.

The American Dietetic Association is pleased to collaborate again with the American Diabetes Association on this third volume of the *Family Cookbook*. Recipes in this volume incorporate the principles of good nutrition and are in accord with the latest nutrition recommendations for individuals with diabetes. A wide variety of foods is included, with an emphasis on American regional cooking. New to this volume are microwave applications of recipes for today's busy cooks.

A special section is devoted to three ethnic American cuisines: Mexican American, Native American of the northern Plains, and southern. Historical notes about foods and cooking styles are accompanied by exchange lists and recipes for each ethnic group.

Informative chapters on good nutrition basics, nutrition and diabetes, fiber, weight control, exercise, and, most important, the inclusion of the new 1986 version of the *Exchange Lists for Meal Planning* make this volume of the *Family Cookbook* more than a cookbook, but a valuable reference. An easy-to-understand explanation demystifies the new Exchange Lists, which have undergone their first revision in ten years.

The American Dietetic Association is proud to present this third volume of the *Family Cookbook* and acknowledges the contributions of our members and members of the American Diabetes Association who assisted in developing and reviewing this wonderful book.

ALICE L. SMITHERMAN, R.D.
President
The American Dietetic Association

About the Associations

The American Diabetes Association is the nation's leading voluntary health organization dedicated to improving the well-being of all people with diabetes and their families. Equally important is its unceasing support for research to find a preventive and cure for this chronic disease that affects some 11 million Americans. The ADA carries out this important mission through the efforts of thousands of volunteers working at affiliates and chapters in more than eight hundred communities across the United States.

Membership in the ADA puts you in contact with a network of more than 225,000 caring people throughout the country. Local affiliates and chapters offer support groups, educational programs, counseling, and other special services. Membership also brings twelve issues of the lively patient education magazine, *Diabetes Forecast*.

In addition, the ADA publishes an array of materials for every age group on topics important not just to the individual with diabetes, but to the entire family. Considerable effort is devoted to educating health-care professionals and building public awareness about diabetes.

The ADA also distributes a free, quarterly newsletter with practical advice and helpful hints on living with diabetes. To receive a copy, just call the toll-free number listed below. Information on ADA membership and programs is available through your local affiliate (listed in the white pages of the phone book) or through the American Diabetes Association, Inc.®, Diabetes Information Service Center, 1660 Duke Street, Alexandria, VA 22314; 800-ADA-DISC. (In Virginia and the metropolitan Washington, D.C., area, dial 703-549-1500.)

The American Dietetic Association is the nation's largest group of nutrition professionals with more than 55,000 members. Its goal is to promote optimal health and nutritional status for Americans. The ADA is dynamic as are its members—changing, adapting, and responding to new scientific findings and practical nutritional needs of the nation's people.

The ADA members with extensive scientific background apply knowledge of food, nutrition, biochemistry, physiology, management, and behavioral and social sciences to promote health, prevent disease, and speed recovery from illness.

Most members are registered dietitians (R.D.) who have completed at least a bachelor's degree and internship or equivalent experience in a qualifying examination. Continuing education is required to maintain R.D. status. This certification process encourages high standards of performance to protect the health, safety, and welfare of the public.

To find a registered dietitian (R.D.), the expert in diet, health, and nutrition, ask your physician, call your local hospital, state, or district dietetic association, or contact The American Dietetic Association, 208 South LaSalle Street, Suite 1100, Chicago, IL 60604; 312-899-0040.

Introduction

Why a "family" cookbook, you may be wondering, since only one member of my family has diabetes? That person could be Grandma, Junior, Dad, or Mom. It may be that your family has several diabetic members or that you're a family of one.

In fact, "diabetic" eating differs from healthy "regular" eating in only two ways:

- Insulin users need to keep calories and other nutrients consistent from meal to meal and day to day.
- Overweight diabetic individuals need to lose those extra pounds.

In most other respects, similarities outweigh differences. Nutritional needs of people with diabetes are pretty much the same as those for everyone else. A twelve-year-old girl who has diabetes needs the same amounts of protein, carbohydrate, and fat, the same vitamins, and the same minerals as her friend who doesn't have diabetes. The same goes for a diabetic twenty-year-old, forty-year-old, or eighty-year-old. Basically, "diabetic" eating is healthy eating. This third volume of the *Family Cookbook* provides a wide variety of healthy food choices for your family to enjoy together.

Although nutritional *needs* are comparable, the person with diabetes must take more care, spend more time, and know more to meet those needs successfully. Insulin users must have guidance about food composition, delayed meals, and sick days, while those whose diabetes is treated by diet alone, or with pills and diet, face another set of problems altogether. The *Family Cookbook, Volume III*, offers up-to-date, practical advice for managing the diabetic diet.

1

Why Volume III? New recipes, of course. But in addition a lot has changed since the appearance of the *Family Cookbook, Volume II:*

- Your supermarket shelves offer an increasingly varied selection of foods. Kiwis, mangoes, and papaya rub shoulders with old standbys like apples and oranges. Packaged products challenge your choosing power: low salt, low fat, high fiber, low cholesterol, high calcium. And ethnic specialties like moussaka and jambalaya have hopped over their borders, making their way to supermarkets across the United States. Your taste—or at least your curiosity—has broadened.
- You're almost certainly more concerned about nutrition than ever before. You're probably an intent label reader and an ever more careful cook.
- You're likely to be busier, squeezing food preparation into an ever smaller slice of your day.
- You have more and more options in food preparation and storage. Microwave ovens are in twice as many homes as they were only five years ago, and more than a third of households now own a food processor.

If you have diabetes, you need to fit these new choices, limitations, and concerns to your life-style. The *Family Cookbook, Volume III,* helps you put it all together.

RECIPES

From appetizer to dessert, the recipes are chock full of flavor. You'll find hearty main dishes such as:

> veal stew
> chicken-fried steak with gravy
> stuffed peppers with ground lamb

If your tastes run to lighter fare, sample:

fresh tuna salad
chicken nuggets with dipping sauce
quenelles of sole with shrimp sauce

Vegetarians will like:

nutty rice loaf
cheese tortellini with creamy spinach
lentils au gratin

In addition to these main dishes, there are salads, vegetables, appetizers, dips, hot and cold soups, and breads. The wide selection of desserts includes old standbys such as shortbread cookies and trifle plus:

apple-raspberry crisp
frozen blueberry crème
bittersweet chocolate sauce

And there are 215 more.

Flavor is important, but nutrition is the top priority. The recipes are designed to be lower in sodium, sugar, and fat than traditional recipes, in line with recommendations of the American Diabetes Association, The American Dietetic Association, and the *Dietary Guidelines for Americans* of the United States Department of Agriculture's Human Nutrition Information Service.

Recipes here, as in Volume II, are generally:

* reduced in total fat and saturated fat
* limited to ½ egg per serving when the recipe includes egg
* limited in salt- and sodium-rich foods; recipes containing more than 400 milligrams of sodium per serving are footnoted
* limited to about ½ teaspoon of sugar, honey, or molasses per serving when a recipe includes these ingredients

To assist you in increasing fiber in your diet, foods containing 3 grams or more of fiber per serving are indicated with a footnote. Potassium content is broken out, along with any key source nutrients—those present in amounts greater than 75 percent of the Recommended Dietary Allowance.

Note: If you've got diabetes, you need to fit these recipes into your daily meal plan. If you're taking insulin, your meal plan has already been designed to coordinate with your insulin dosage and activity patterns. Still, keep in mind that, while all of the recipes in *Family Cookbook, Volume III* have been reduced in sugar, salt, and fat, some recipes have higher amounts of these ingredients than others. It's a good idea to work with your doctor and registered dietitian to fit them into your meal plan.

NUTRITIONAL GUIDANCE

For people with diabetes, the basics of diabetes management are discussed:

> diet and insulin
> oral agents
> meal planning
> weight loss and exercise
> brand-new exchange lists
> ethnic exchanges
> handling sick days

For everyone, the basics of good nutrition are examined:

> how your body uses food
> carbohydrate, fat, and protein: the best amounts for
>   you
> vitamins, minerals, and where to find them
> diet for possible disease prevention
> reasons to increase fiber and complex carbohydrates

NUTRITION INFORMATION "LABELS"

Similar to those on packaged products, these give you specific nutrient information per serving for every recipe listed. Included are:

> calories (CAL)
> fat (FAT)
> sodium (Na)
> fiber (Fiber)
> protein (PRO)
> carbohydrate (CHO)
> potassium (K)
> cholesterol (Chol)

GENEROUS SERVINGS OF PRACTICAL ADVICE

Break out of humdrum cooking routines! Pepping up your meals is easy, fun, and can actually take you *less* time than you're spending now. Note cooking tips on how to:

- Season with herbs and spices for full-flavored, low-salt dishes.
- Introduce ethnic and regional specialties—and the special nutritional bonuses they bring.
- Combine modern technology and old-fashioned tips to cut preparation time:
  > microwave
  > food processor
  > freezer
  > bulk preparation
- Cook delicious vegetarian main dishes.
- Brighten simple meals with garnishes and condiments.
- Take advantage of no-calorie sweeteners.
- Experiment with high-fiber, high-complex-carbohydrate cooking. Don't stick to limas!
- Learn about quick-cooking methods for beans and peas.

This may be your first *Family Cookbook*. Or Volume III may be joining well-thumbed copies of Volume I, Volume II, and the *American Diabetes Association Holiday Cookbook* on your kitchen shelf. Either way, healthy eating and *bon appétit!*

1 ◇ SOUND NUTRITION FOR THE WHOLE FAMILY

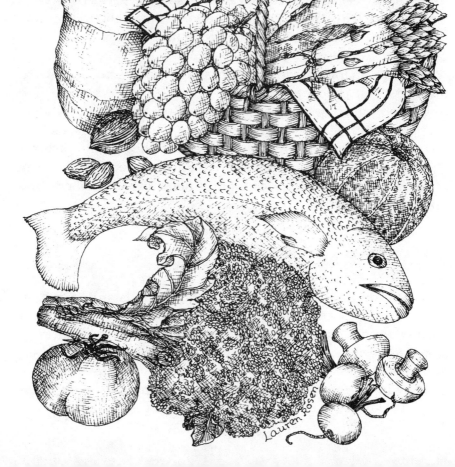

Pick up a cookbook written twenty years ago, and chances are you'll find quite a bit about *how* to cook but very little about *why* you should cook, or eat, the foods described. More and more, today we want to know about the nutritive value of the foods we eat—what our food contains. Are we eating too much of any nutrient—salt, sugar, fat, or cholesterol, for example? Are we giving our bodies enough nutrients, in the proper balance, to keep them energetic and healthy, to repair tissue damage and fight disease? It's not enough, anymore, to know that something "tastes good."

But tasting good *is* important, and thinking in terms of nutrition alone hardly begins to describe the variety of flavors, textures, and colors we enjoy when eating. Take protein, for example. Sure, it's in meat. But branch out a bit: You'll find the same protein (plus a wider range of vitamins, minerals, and fiber) in a crunchy corn tortilla stuffed with spiced beans, a silky tofu with sweet and sour sauce, or a slice of perfectly broiled fish topped with fresh herbs. Knowing more about nutrition may start you thinking about a wider variety of options in good eating.

This chapter reviews the basics of good nutrition—what nutrients your body needs, how it uses them, where to find them, and which ones you may want to cut down on. Is it only for people with diabetes? Absolutely not. Nutritional needs vary according to your age, life-style, and state of health, but diabetes does not make special *nutritional* demands on your body. So all of the information in this chapter applies to both diabetic and nondiabetic persons.

WHAT ARE NUTRIENTS?

Whether you have diabetes or not, your body is strong and resilient. It grows and maintains itself for decades. It can repair itself when damaged and detoxify many harmful substances. It stores unneeded materials for future use and can even convert nutrients it *doesn't* need into those it *does*—fat into protein or carbohydrate, for example. All this goes on automatically, as long as your body has the necessary materials—nutrients—to work with.

Nutrients are food elements that the body uses to grow, maintain itself, and repair damage. All of the fifty or so nutrients we need to stay healthy can be classified into two major groups.

The first group, called *macronutrients* (because we need them in relatively large—"macro"—quantities), includes carbohydrate, protein, and fat. The fuel they supply is converted into energy that allows muscles to contract, impulses to travel from nerve to nerve, and new cells to be created. The unit used to describe the energy-producing power of a food is called a *calorie*.

The second major group can be thought of as "helper" nutrients. They supply no energy but play key roles in all body processes. This group includes vitamins, minerals, fiber, and water. Vitamins and minerals are often called *micronutrients* because you need them in such minuscule amounts.

Each type of nutrient has a somewhat different function and ultimate destination in your body.

ENERGY-SUPPLYING NUTRIENTS

HOW YOU USE CARBOHYDRATES

Carbohydrates are the direct suppliers of energy to most of the 75 trillion cells in your body. Our cells burn glucose—a carbohydrate—much as an automobile runs on gasoline or an oil lamp burns oil. Glucose is so important that your body is equipped with backup systems to supply it. Your liver keeps glucose on hand in the form of glycogen; when you skip a meal, your liver releases glucose to ensure a steady supply. Deprived of carbohydrate for a longer time, your body would eventually break down fat and protein and reassemble them into glucose molecules.

Plants are our major source of carbohydrate. Breads, cereals, and pasta, which are made from grains, are mainly carbohydrate. So are fruits and vegetables. Many sweeteners have been extracted from plants. Sugar cane, for example, gives us table sugar; corn supplies corn syrup; and the sap of maple trees is boiled down into maple syrup.

Eggs, meat, and most other animal products contain very little carbohydrate or none at all. Milk is an interesting exception. Amounts of protein, carbohydrate, and fat are roughly equal in whole milk. (Low-fat or skim milk has less fat but the same carbohydrate and protein.) So dairy products like yogurt and cheese are good sources of carbohydrate.

For nutritional purposes, carbohydrates can be divided into two major groups—sugars (sometimes called simple carbohydrates) and starches (complex carbohydrates). Sugars include sucrose (table sugar), fructose (the sugar form found in fruits), glucose (the sugar in your blood), and lactose (milk sugar), as well as products like corn and maple syrup. Chemically, each sugar is small indeed. Starches are long chains of sugar molecules. When you digest a slice of bread, its starch molecules are broken down into glucose so they are small enough to be absorbed and used as fuel. Glucose (the type of sugar in your blood) travels in the bloodstream to individual cells, which, with the help of insulin, take it in and use it for fuel.

Most sugars taste sweet. Plant foods that do *not* taste sweet—flours, vegetables, beans, rice, and potatoes—are likely to contain predominantly starch rather than sugar.

People all over the world derive most of their calories from carbohydrates. Americans are no exception, but we eat a diet high in sugars and relatively low in starches. A current recommendation for people with diabetes is that up to 60 percent of total calories should come from carbohydrate foods, including as many unrefined, starchy, fiber-containing products as is acceptable to each individual. This recommendation, which is similar to that of the American Heart Association and the American Cancer Society, is suitable for most nondiabetic Americans as well. Sugars should come mostly from natural sugar sources like fruits.

HOW YOU USE PROTEIN

If carbohydrates are fuels, protein can be thought of as the construction materials of body tissues. Bones, muscle, and skin are largely protein. Blood components like hemoglobin, genetic structures like chromosomes, and hormones like insulin could not exist without protein. The protein in your body is being reformed constantly, as hormones and enzymes, bone and muscle cells age and need to be replaced.

What we refer to by a single name—"protein"—is in fact a long, coiled chain of smaller units called *amino acids;* it is the particular combination of amino acids that distinguishes one protein from another. Insulin protein, for example, is constructed of a different sequence of amino acids from hair protein. The protein we eat is broken down into amino acids during digestion, then recombined into various tissue proteins.

Dietary protein comes from both animal and plant sources. Meat from animals, poultry, and fish contains protein, as do milk and eggs, which are produced by animals. Grains, dried beans and peas, and nuts are good sources of plant protein.

Human beings need twenty-two different amino acids. Of these, we can manufacture twelve, but we are unable to synthesize the rest. The twelve our bodies can synthesize are not absolutely essential in our diet. We do need, though, the amino acids that we can't make ourselves. These are called "essential" amino acids (EAA) because we *must* obtain them from our diet.

Protein from animal sources *always* contains the EAA. Pork chops, hamburgers, and drumsticks are valuable protein sources because they are so dependable; you can count on them to supply all the amino acids you need. Proteins that contain all the EAA are often referred to as "complete" or "high-quality" protein.

Plant protein, on the other hand, is referred to as "incomplete" protein because the protein found in any one plant contains some but not all of the EAA. However, properly combining protein from different nonmeat sources, in the right proportion, can supply the EAA. (If you are interested in nonmeat protein sources, see "Building a Protein" on pages 87–88.)

People in the United States tend to overestimate the need for protein. In fact, most Americans eat too much protein—well over the top limit of 20 percent of the day's calories recommended by most health-care organizations, including the American Diabetes Association. Our actual protein needs are even lower—about 9 to 10 percent of total recommended calories. And eating more protein than your body can use for construction simply means the excess will be burned for energy or stored as fat.

HOW YOU USE FAT

Fat is the third nutrient that your body can break down for energy. Although attention has recently focused on the dangers of eating too much fat, it is important that a diet include some fat. Fat is an essential component of cell membranes. It cushions and protects internal organs like the heart and lungs; it helps keep the body warm in cold weather, stores certain vitamins, and provides some fatty acids that the body cannot manufacture.

Fat's most unique function is as a store of energy for future needs. It is ideally suited for this role, being both compact (fat has more than twice as many calories as protein or carbohydrate) and adaptable (fat can be broken down and reassembled into glucose or protein).

Eating too much fat is unhealthy—and most Americans eat too much fat. On average, Americans consume about 40 to 50 percent of total calories as fat. Health agencies such as the American Diabetes Association and the American Heart Association currently recommend a much lower figure—30 percent or less.

What are the health consequences of a diet that is too high in fat? One is that it makes weight gain easier. The more fat a food contains, the more calories you consume. And once you weigh more than you should, your risk of diseases like non-insulin-dependent diabetes mellitus (NIDDM or type II), hypertension, and heart disease leaps upward. But high-fat diets are probably inadvisable in themselves, even if your weight is normal. They appear to promote heart and blood vessel disease and have been linked to some forms of cancer. For certain types of fat—cholesterol and saturated fatty acids, for example—the link to coronary artery disease is especially strong.

The fats we eat come from both plant and animal sources. Meats and dairy products like cheese and butter are often high in fat. As they naturally occur, most fruits and vegetables contain very little fat. But oils extracted from plants (corn, safflower, and olive, for example) are a major dietary source of fat. Many packaged foods such as potato chips, desserts, sauces, and gravies contain large amounts of fat.

As with protein, there are some characteristic differences between plant fat and animal fat. Cholesterol is found *only* in foods of animal origin—meats, milk products, and egg yolks, for example. Saturated fatty acids occur primarily in the same foods—for the most part animal fats and certain vegetable oils like palm and coconut. As a rule of thumb, fats that are hard at room temperature, like lard or the fat on a steak, are likely to contain saturated fatty acids. Unsaturated fats come from plants and are usually liquid at room temperature. Vegetable oils, such as corn, cottonseed, sunflower, safflower, soybean, olive, and peanut, are examples of unsaturated fats.

It's a good idea to limit your intake of cholesterol and saturated fatty acids, both of which have been linked to heart disease. The fatlike substance cholesterol is the major "building block" of arterial plaque—the sludgelike deposits that collect on blood vessel walls, including those of the heart. (Risk seems especially high with a combination of high blood fats and high blood glucose, a point worth remembering if you have diabetes.)

But eating fat is not the only way to become fat. Whenever you take in more calories than you need, the excess is stored as fat. Even protein and carbohydrate are converted to fat for storage. *Total* calories count most: Eat too much of anything—protein, carbohydrate, or fat—and you'll put on the pounds.

HELPER NUTRIENTS

VITAMINS AND MINERALS

Helper nutrients like vitamins and minerals are just as important for health as are calorie-supplying nutrients. Vitamins and minerals are substances the body needs in exceedingly small amounts but cannot manufacture itself. Key players in a wide variety of body processes, their importance is often recognized only at the breakdown of some process dependent on them. Vitamin C, for example, must be present for the body to synthesize two amino acids that form part of the protein collagen. Collagen, in turn, forms part of the connective tissue holding together skin, bones, and blood vessels. Without vitamin C, blood vessel walls become fragile and bleed easily, cuts heal more slowly, and weakened bones may break.

Other vitamins and minerals are intimately involved in other processes. Some work in tandem with enzymes to break down carbohydrate, fat, and protein so they can be absorbed. Others increase your ability to use nutrients; for example, without vitamin D your intestine can absorb only about one-tenth of the calcium you eat, while with vitamin D you absorb fully one-third. At present, human beings are known to need twenty-three vitamins and seventeen minerals, but there are probably hundreds of others, as yet unidentified. (A complete list of vitamins and minerals and the role each plays can be found in the *Family Cookbook, Volume I.*)

Vitamins and minerals are unevenly distributed; no food contains *all* of those you need. Milk, for example, contains little iron but is an excellent source of calcium. Whole wheat flour is very high in phosphorus but contains no vitamin A or C. Eating a varied diet, such as that described on pages 24–25, is the best and safest way to obtain all the micronutrients you are currently known to need—plus many others.

What about vitamin pills? Doctors and dietitians differ on the advisability of vitamin supplements for healthy people. (Of course, supplements are necessary for those with a medically diagnosed vitamin deficiency.) A daily vitamin pill containing no more than 100 percent of the Recommended Dietary Allowances (RDAs) for all the micronutrients you're currently known to need is viewed by some doctors as good "insurance," while others consider it a waste of money.

An overdose of vitamins or minerals can actually be harmful. Vitamins, particularly those that are stored in your body fat, can accumulate in toxic amounts. These fat-soluble vitamins include A, E, D, and K. But the water-soluble vitamins—those that dissolve in watery substances like blood and urine—can also be harmful when used to excess. Vitamins affect your body in various ways that you need to be aware of. For example, people with diabetes should keep in mind that vitamin C supplements can interfere with urine test results.

FIBER

Although for many years fiber was considered to be of minor dietary importance, today its role is being reevaluated. Currently many health-care agencies, including the American Diabetes Association, are recommending an intake of up to 40 grams of dietary fiber per day—about twice that in most American diets.

Fiber is found only in plant foods. Its role is to make up plant cell walls, form the outer protective coating of kernels and seeds, and repair injury. Human beings cannot completely digest fiber. The digestive enzymes that break apart other carbohydrates, protein, and fat are unable to split up fiber molecules. Some fiber is fermented (a process different from digestion) in your large intestine, but most of it passes through your body more or less intact.

If you can't digest fiber, why do you need it? Although fiber is not broken down and absorbed into your body, it has important functions as it passes through. Some fibers, like bran, tend to attract water, thus increasing stool bulk and promoting regular bowel movements. Others act in a strikingly different way; they help lower cholesterol and triglycerides, and, most notable in diabetes, some can help keep blood glucose levels stable. (See Chapter 6 for a more detailed discussion of fiber.)

WATER

Although we don't usually think of water as ''nutritious,'' lack of water has a quicker and more widespread negative effect than lack of any other nutrient. About half of your body is water. Water is needed for every single function that cells perform.

Deprived of water, cells are unable to move substances across membranes; tiny electrical impulses that control muscles like the heart are short-circuited; cells quickly die.

Fortunately, most other living matter also is largely water, so sources of water are widespread. It is, of course, in drinks like milk and juice; most fruits, vegetables, and even meats are largely water. In addition, your body makes some water as a byproduct of chemical reactions. So water sources are plentiful.

It is a good idea to drink about eight glasses of water each day. Making a conscious effort to drink water is especially important when you are losing more water than usual through vomiting, diarrhea, sweating, or urinating.

FOOD GROUPS: EASY WAY TO A BALANCED DIET

How can you be sure your diet is a healthy one? Is your fat consumption under 30 percent of total calories or closer to 50 percent? More? And how much cholesterol do you consume in an average day? Most foods contain such a mixture of nutrients (see pages 19–20) that it is hard to be sure exactly what you are eating and what you aren't.

Food groups are an easy way to good nutrition. They are classifications of foods according to their *general* nutritional similarity. Eating recommended amounts from among these groupings will ensure that you get the proper amounts of protein, carbohydrate, fat, fiber, vitamins, and minerals.

Below are the six groupings currently recommended by the United States Department of Agriculture's Human Nutrition Information Service and the advised number of servings per day, which vary depending on your age, sex, level of activity, and so on. Note that these categories are similar to those in the American Diabetes Association/The American Dietetic Association *Exchange Lists for Meal Planning* (Appendix). Both groupings provide a well-balanced diet, although the Exchange Lists group according to the needs of the insulin-taking diabetic person, who needs to know the macronutrient composition of the foods he or she is eating more than the person who does not take insulin.

BREADS, CEREALS, AND OTHER GRAIN PRODUCTS*

You need six to eleven servings daily, including several servings a day of whole grain products. Typical serving sizes are 1 slice bread, 1 small muffin, or ½ cup cooked cereal. This group includes foods such as crackers, rolls, breads, noodles, pancakes, rice, popcorn, and tortillas.

This food group is generally high in iron, niacin, and vitamins B_1 and B_2. Additional minerals, vitamins, and fiber are found in whole grain products. It is low in vitamin A and vitamin C.

FRUITS

You need two to four servings a day, including citrus, melon, or berries. Typical serving sizes are 1 apple, banana, or orange; ½ cup berries; ¾ cup juice. This group includes melon, raspberries, grapes, dates, fruit juices, and raisins.

This group is generally high in carbohydrate, fiber, iron, potassium, and B vitamins. Citrus, melon, and berries are especially high in vitamins A and C. It is low in fat and calcium.

VEGETABLES

You need three to five servings daily. There are significant nutrient differences among vegetables, so variety within this category is especially important. It is best to include all of the following each week: (1) dark green leafy vegetables such as spinach, kale, or collards; (2) deep yellow vegetables such as carrots, winter squash, or yams; (3) dry beans, peas, and lentils

*Each individual food in this group contains *some* of the essential amino acids you need from food sources.

(legumes); (4) starchy vegetables like corn, limas, and potatoes. A typical serving size is ½ cup of cooked or 1 cup of raw leafy vegetables like lettuce or spinach.

1. *Dark green leafy.* Generally high in vitamin A and carotene (from which your body can make vitamin A), vitamin C, riboflavin, folic acid, iron, calcium, magnesium, and potassium. Low in thiamine, niacin, and phosphorus.
2. *Deep yellow.* Generally high in vitamin A.
3. *Legumes.* Generally high in thiamine, folic acid, iron, magnesium, phosphorus, zinc, potassium, protein, starch, and fiber. Low in fat, vitamin C, and vitamin A.
4. *Starchy vegetables.* Generally high in niacin, vitamin B_6, zinc, and potassium. Low in calcium, vitamin A, thiamine, and riboflavin.

MEAT, POULTRY, FISH, AND ALTERNATES

You need two to three servings per day. Typical foods are meats, poultry, fish, eggs, dry beans, tofu, and seeds. Serving sizes will differ. In meat, poultry, or fish, a serving is 2 to 3 ounces; 1 egg, ½ cup cooked dry beans, or 2 tablespoons of peanut butter equals 1 ounce of lean meat. This group is generally high in protein, niacin, B vitamins, phosphorus, zinc, and iron. It is low in vitamins A and C and calcium.

MILK, CHEESE, AND YOGURT

You need two servings daily (three for teenagers and for women who are pregnant or breastfeeding; four for teenagers who are pregnant or breastfeeding). Typical serving sizes are 1 cup milk, 8 ounces of yogurt, or 1½ to 2 ounces of cheese. This group is generally high in protein, calcium, and vitamin B_2. It is low in iron, manganese, copper, and vitamin C.

FATS, SWEETS, AND ALCOHOL

Most Americans consume too many fats and sugars and so should try to limit consumption of foods in this group. Drink alcohol only in moderation.

These foods are often called "empty" calories. By themselves, sugars and oils contribute no vitamins or minerals to your diet. Distilled alcohol, for example, contributes no vitamins or minerals, no protein, no fat, only a trace of carbohydrate, and 1 milligram of potassium.

ANIMAL, VEGETABLE, OR MINERAL?: A QUICK GUIDE TO NUTRIENT CONTENT

Finding the full nutrient information for a food is a complex and time-consuming project. But knowing something about its original source—plant or animal—takes only a moment of thought and can in fact tell you a lot. Most foods from plant sources have the following profile:

Major nutrient: carbohydrate (If the food tastes sweet, it probably contains some sugar; if not, starch is likely to predominate.)
Fats: *un*saturated
Cholesterol: none
Protein: *some* of the eight to ten essential amino acids
Fiber: present in whole grains, legumes, fruits, vegetables

Foods from animal sources have a different profile:

Major nutrients: protein and fat
Fats: saturated
Cholesterol: present
Protein: eight to ten essential amino acids
Fiber: none

If you're curious about the nutrient composition of a dish, think about its major ingredients. This won't tell you all you need to know, nutritionally, but it's a good start. For example:

> *Dish:* Dilled Potato Salad (page 150)
> *Major ingredients:* potatoes (plant); egg (animal); sour cream (animal)

> *Dish:* Pears Filled with Strawberry Cream Cheese (page 342)
> *Major ingredients:* cream cheese (animal); pears, strawberries (plant)

> *Dish:* Tandoori Chicken (page 218)
> *Major ingredients:* chicken (animal); yogurt (animal); spices (plant)

A lead on the nutritional content of packaged foods is a bit harder. As with foods you prepare yourself, start by classifying the major ingredients. Turkey hash, for example, probably contains significant quantities of turkey and potatoes. But be sure to check the label. Manufacturers often add sugars, salt, flour, or fats in varying amounts to alter texture or flavor. Bear in mind that in a packaged food, ingredients are listed in order of the amount by weight, with first place going to the predominant ingredient.

COMMON NUTRITIONAL PROBLEMS IN THE UNITED STATES TODAY

The United States today has the most abundant and varied food supply in the world's history. Why, then, do we have any nutritional problems at all? Poor nutrition isn't limited to *under*nutrition or the starvation that plagues so many underdeveloped countries today.

In fact, Americans face a set of nutritional problems relating to *over*nutrition. Constantly surrounded by food that's cheap, fast, and tasty, we eat too much, and many of us are too fat. Being overweight contributes directly to your chances of having non-insulin-dependent (type II) diabetes (and losing that weight is the best way to control it). Extra pounds aggravate high blood pressure, heart conditions, and arthritis. Although we may think of such illnesses as characteristic of aging, in fact they're linked to life-style. In underdeveloped nations, such illnesses are far less common.

Another American problem is that we don't always eat a variety of foods. So many foods are available that we can eat all we want while limiting our choices to a few food categories. Vitamin C, for example, simply doesn't occur in animal foods; if you eat few fruits and vegetables, you may be getting too little vitamin C. A diet low in calcium is also not uncommon. This nutrient occurs in dairy products and deep green leafy vegetables. But few Americans eat mustard greens, dandelion leaves, or kale on a regular basis and many skip dairy products.

How often would you eat potato chips if you had to make them instead of buying them in a bag? Americans eat a lot of ready-to-eat and prepared foods. Designed for easy eating, they require little or no preparation time and are available year-round.

But a diet high in prepared foods has drawbacks. One is that you tend to eat too much. Another is that no calories are spent in preparation—shopping, carrying the potatoes home, peeling and cooking them, and washing the pan. Most prepared foods contain more sugar, sodium, and fat than unprocessed foods, and less complex carbohydrate and fiber. A diet high in salt can contribute to high blood pressure and stroke; too much sugar makes tooth decay more likely; and heart disease and certain cancers have been linked to high-fat diets. The fact that fiber is removed from most processed foods means that you're not getting its health-giving benefits.

The *Dietary Guidelines for Americans* (sponsored jointly by the U.S. Departments of Agriculture and Health and Human Services) summarizes the points above.

DIETARY GUIDELINES FOR AMERICANS

1. Eat a variety of foods.
2. Maintain desirable weight.

3. Avoid too much fat, saturated fat, and cholesterol.
4. Eat foods with adequate starch and fiber.
5. Avoid too much sugar.
6. Avoid too much sodium.
7. If you drink alcoholic beverages, do so in moderation.

A NUTRITION CHECKLIST

Sometimes people wonder if their diet is adequate in one nutrient or another. Although deficiencies are not common, you may want to check with your physician if you score low in any of the following categories.

AM I GETTING ENOUGH . . .

Protein? You may not be if your diet is low in meat or dairy products (or if you are not properly combining protein from other sources).

Complex Carbohydrate and Fiber? You may not be if your diet is low in whole grain products, fruits, vegetables, and legumes.

Calcium? You may not be if your diet is low in dairy products and leafy green vegetables.

Iron? You may not be if your diet is low in legumes, whole grain products, red meat, and dried fruits. (Other foods high in iron, such as liver and egg yolks, are also high in cholesterol and should be limited.)

Vitamin D? You may not be if your diet is low in dairy products (especially fortified ones).

Vitamin E? You may not be if your diet is low in vegetable oils and whole grains.

Vitamin A? You may not be if your diet is low in dark green leafy and deep yellow vegetables.

Vitamin C? You may not be if your diet is low in citrus fruits, tomatoes, melon, and broccoli.

Vitamin B₁ (thiamine)? You may not be if your diet is low in meats, poultry, fish, whole grains, legumes, and green vegetables.

Vitamin B₂ (riboflavin)? You may not be if your diet is low in lean meat, whole grains, organ meats, milk, eggs, and green leafy vegetables.

Niacin? You may not be if your diet is low in whole grains, liver, poultry, fish and meat, legumes, and peanuts.

Vitamin B₁₂? You may not be if your diet is low in organ meats, other meats, eggs, and most dairy products.

HOW MANY CALORIES

Carbohydrate	4 per gram
Protein	4 per gram
Fat	9 per gram

THE TYPICAL AMERICAN DIET: WHAT WE EAT NOW VERSUS WHAT WE SHOULD BE EATING

	Now	Aim
Fat	40–50% of calories	30% of calories
Refined and processed sugars (e.g., table sugar)	15%	For nondiabetic Americans, up to 10%
Complex carbohydrates and naturally occurring sugars (e.g., fruits)	28%	50–60%
Protein	20% +	10–20%

AMERICAN DIABETES ASSOCIATION
NUTRITIONAL RECOMMENDATIONS FOR INDIVIDUALS
WITH DIABETES MELLITUS: 1986

Food Group	Nutritional Recommendations
Carbohydrate	Up to 60% of total calories (all or nearly all complex carbohydrate and naturally occurring sugars, e.g., milk and fruits)
Protein	.8 gms/kg body weight
Fat	Under 30%
Fiber	Up to 40 gms
Cholesterol	Under 300 mg
Refined and processed sugars	Modest intake within the meal setting, with the amount to be determined in consultation with your doctor and dietitian

What might your meals be like if you made these changes? These "improved" menus are especially appropriate for people with diabetes. Take a look:

	Menu Now	Improved Menu
Breakfast	High-salt, high-sugar cereal with whole milk and sugar; glazed doughnut or danish pastry; coffee with nondairy creamer	Oatmeal or shredded wheat with noncaloric sweetener and skim milk; corn or bran muffin; coffee with skim milk
Lunch	Double cheeseburger; potato chips; soft drink	Broiled hamburger, boiled ham sandwich, or choices from the salad bar; popcorn, breadsticks, or crunchy raw vegetables; diet soda or fruit juice; fruit

	Menu Now	Improved Menu
Dinner	Cut of prime beef or fried chicken with mashed potatoes; salad with thousand-island dressing; ice cream	Cut of "good" quality beef, well trimmed of fat, or oven-fried or broiled chicken or fish; baked potato with margarine or mashed potatoes with skim milk and small amount of margarine; salad with low-calorie thousand-island dressing or oil-and-vinegar dressing; ice milk, sherbet, or fresh fruit

2 ◇ THE DIETARY SIDE OF DIABETES CARE

*C*enturies before "diabetes" even got its name, and several thousand years before the discovery of insulin, physicians realized that there was a link between diabetes and diet. Today, diet remains a cornerstone of diabetes care. Good diabetes management means balancing three factors: food, activity, and, sometimes, medication. In this chapter we will focus on the role of diet in diabetes management.

WHAT IS DIABETES?

Diabetes is not one but several different disorders that have high blood sugar levels in common. About 10 percent of people with diabetes have insulin-dependent diabetes (IDDM), also called type I diabetes. People with type I diabetes often become diabetic when young and they *always* need to take insulin—without it, they cannot survive. The dramatic discovery of insulin in 1921 saved the lives of many people with insulin-dependent diabetes.

Non-insulin-dependent diabetes (NIDDM), also called type II diabetes, is far more common, accounting for nearly 90 percent of cases. Typically (although not necessarily), people with type II diabetes are "over forty and overweight," reflected in the previous names "adult-onset" or "maturity-onset" diabetes. The primary treatment for type II diabetes is weight loss, but treatment can also include diet and exercise, pills, insulin injections, or some combination of these therapies. Although sometimes type II diabetes is treated with insulin, life does not literally *depend* on injections as it does in insulin-dependent diabetes.

There are other types of diabetes, although they are far more rare than type I and type II. More important, treatment is likely to be similar to that for one of the first two types.

WHAT GOES WRONG IN DIABETES?

Diabetes impairs the body's ability to use carbohydrates. As we've seen in Chapter 1, dietary carbohydrates are fuels. They are broken down in the digestive system, absorbed into the bloodstream, and ultimately taken into individual cells, where they are burned for energy.

A key player in this fueling process is *insulin*, which is produced by the pancreas and secreted into the bloodstream. Insulin's function is to move glucose out of the bloodstream and into cells. It is sometimes compared to a "key" that unlocks the cell "door," allowing the glucose molecule to pass from outside the cell to its interior.

Another key player is *the cell itself*, which must be receptive to insulin, able to take up glucose, and then to use it in a normal fashion. To return to the analogy, the cell must have normal "locks" into which the insulin "key" can fit. In addition, the cell must be able to use glucose properly once it enters the cell interior.

The hallmark of diabetes is *too much glucose in the bloodstream*. Normally, when you haven't eaten for a while, there are about 60 to 110 milligrams (mg) of glucose per deciliter (dl) of blood. After meals, the amounts rise to 140 to 160 mg/dl, then return to normal in about two hours. In diabetes, though, glucose may rise much higher—to 200 mg/dl, 300 mg/dl, or more. Blood glucose levels that are too high can cause serious short- and long-term consequences.

Type I and type II diabetes raise blood glucose levels in different ways. People with type I diabetes do not secrete insulin at all. Their body cells are starving while more and more glucose accumulates in the blood outside the cell. Eventually, muscle and fat are broken down and converted to glucose, but without insulin, hyperglycemia (high blood sugar) simply gets worse.

In people with type II diabetes, high blood glucose levels occur for different reasons. Some insulin is secreted, but not enough to keep blood sugar normal. In addition, cells may not take up glucose readily or use it appropriately so, again, more glucose than normal remains outside cells. Treatment attempts to overcome the resistance to insulin. It may involve weight loss, which makes cells more sensitive to the insulin "key"; blood glucose–lowering pills (oral hypoglycemic agents), which also seem to make cells more sensitive to glucose; or insulin.

GOALS OF TREATMENT FOR ALL DIABETIC PERSONS

Whatever your kind of diabetes, the goals you'll be aiming toward are the same.

1. To keep blood glucose levels as near to normal

as possible and to maintain blood fats at optimal
levels.
2. To provide adequate nutrition for proper growth
and development or maintenance.
3. To achieve and maintain appropriate weight.

Keeping blood glucose near normal will help prevent symptoms
of hyperglycemia or hypoglycemia (low blood sugar); it may help
prevent the heart disease, stroke, kidney, eye, and neurologic
problems that can result from diabetes.

MANAGING INSULIN-DEPENDENT DIABETES

If you have insulin-dependent diabetes, a prime goal is nutritional consistency: eating about the same number of calories at
each meal, divided into about the same proportions of protein,
carbohydrate, and fat. Several snacks may be scheduled each
day as well. Using the *Exchange Lists for Meal Planning* (pages 69
and 406–426), a registered dietitian can help you plan a meal
pattern that suits your preference and life-style. The number of
meals and snacks and just when you choose to eat them are
largely up to you.

Nutritional consistency is crucial to ensuring a good
insulin–glucose match-up, that is, to keep blood glucose near
normal. Following your meal plan as closely as possible helps
offset many factors that can destabilize blood glucose. Minor
variations in timing or depth of the insulin injection, unantici-
pated exercise, or emotional stress can alter blood glucose levels.

If you have type I diabetes, you need information on
treating insulin reactions, on exercise, and on sick days. If you
drink alcohol, you need to know how to do so safely.

YOUR INSULIN REGIMEN

Different insulin preparations have different "time schedules."
Understanding your particular insulin schedule—when you can
expect insulin to act—can help you keep blood glucose normal,

plan for changes (unexpected activity, for example, or a delayed meal), and ''diagnose'' the possible causes of high or low blood glucose.

The amount of insulin and the preparation prescribed for you will depend on your age, activity, weight, life-style, and nature of the diabetes. A common plan is a combination of a quick-acting insulin and an intermediate-acting insulin. Usually injected about half an hour before a meal, the rapid-acting insulin acts on the glucose that enters the bloodstream after the meal; the intermediate-acting insulin keeps blood glucose in the normal range between meals.

There are many other possible injection patterns, some relying on rapid-acting insulin injected more frequently, in combination with long-acting insulin. Whichever one your doctor thinks is best for you, you will be working with a dietitian to be sure you ''cover'' times of peak insulin action with adequate food.

INSULIN PREPARATIONS

Short-acting insulins begin to act fifteen to thirty minutes after injection. Their peak action—the time they are moving the most blood glucose into cells—occurs two to four hours after injection; action then tapers off and ceases five to seven hours after injection.

Intermediate-acting insulins (NPH or Lente) begin to act from one to two and one-half hours after injection; they peak at six to twelve hours, and are used up in eighteen to twenty-four hours.

Long-acting insulins begin to act in four to six hours, peak in eighteen to twenty-four hours, and last until thirty-two to thirty-six hours after injection.

INSULIN REACTIONS

If you've taken insulin for any length of time, you've probably experienced an insulin reaction. An insulin reaction, also called a hypoglycemic reaction, occurs when there is too little glucose in your blood. Meal delays are a common cause: The insulin you injected previously continues to work but the glucose you thought would be entering your system doesn't. Unexpected exercise can also bring about an insulin reaction. Exercising muscles use up more glucose than you anticipated, insulin continues to work, and blood glucose drops too low. Taking too much insulin or drinking alcohol on an empty stomach can bring about the same result.

Mild insulin reactions are fairly common, especially among diabetic people whose blood glucose is kept near normal, and are easily treated. The symptoms of a mild insulin reaction may include hunger, weakness, nausea, lightheadedness, headache, or blurred vision. Sometimes, judgment is impaired; for example, you may insist that you are *not* having an insulin reaction. Although you may experience any of these symptoms, each person usually has his or her own typical set of symptoms—early warnings of low blood sugar. Moderate hypoglycemia may include any of the previous symptoms plus sleepiness, shakiness, or rapid pulse.

Before treating an insulin reaction, it's best to test blood glucose to see if you are really having one; these symptoms are easy to confuse with symptoms of anxiety. If sugar levels are low, you'll want to get sugar into your blood *quickly*. A standard treatment is to eat about 15 grams of carbohydrate, such as:

> 1 tablespoon of honey or corn syrup
> 2 tablespoons of raisins
> ½ cup fruit juice or a *non*dietetic soft drink
> indicated portion of a packaged product for insulin
>   reactions (for example, three glucose tablets)

Usually, symptoms will go away within twenty minutes. Retest blood glucose at that point. If symptoms persist, treat again.

If blood glucose drops even lower, you may become very confused, have convulsions, or become comatose. For severe insulin reactions, you will not be able to treat yourself. Family or friends should give you honey, cake-decorating gel, or any syrup that can be gently rubbed inside your cheek or placed under your tongue (no liquids or solids, which may cause choking). If this fails to bring you around within fifteen minutes, an injection of glucagon (a hormone that raises blood sugar immediately) may be necessary.

The carbohydrate used to treat an insulin reaction that happens because of a meal delay can be subtracted from the carbohydrate allowance for that meal. Carbohydrate eaten to treat insulin reactions that occur at other times generally does not need to be subtracted.

If you have more than one or two moderate insulin reactions in a week, or one severe reaction, or a great many mild reactions, let your doctor know. He or she will want to find out if your insulin dose is too high or your food intake inadequate.

Anyone who takes insulin should always have some "quick sugar" on hand. Keep a roll of Lifesavers, some glucose tablets, or a tube of cake-decorating gel in your pocket or purse, in your automobile, at work, and at home.

ALCOHOL

If you drink alcohol and use insulin, you need some special guidance. Alcohol can prevent the liver—ordinarily a supplier of emergency glucose—from making it. The result? A situation in which you might expect a mild insulin reaction, say, a delayed snack, can produce rapid, severe hypoglycemia.

When you use alcohol, follow these guidelines:

- Drink only with meals or a little while after them— when your stomach is full and the danger of severe hypoglycemia is lessened.

- Drink only if your diabetes is well controlled.

- Drink in moderation. To keep diabetes in control, you need your wits about you. One reason some physicians are reluctant to allow alcohol is its tendency to impair judgment.

- Drink only with your physician's consent. Alcohol may interact with a number of drugs other than insulin so be sure to check with your doctor first.

- Never drink and drive.

SICK DAYS

Even a minor illness can cause a major disruption in diabetes control. Illness causes your body to pour out stress hormones that raise blood glucose and increase the output of ketones, a toxic acid produced when insulin levels are low. Your blood glucose control may also be more tricky if you are nauseated, vomiting, or have diarrhea and aren't eating or absorbing the calories you usually do.

When an illness begins, start testing blood glucose and urine ketones every four hours around the clock. And write down the results. That way, you'll have a sense of what's going on in terms of diabetes control. If you haven't done so already, be sure that you can reach your doctor during the night as well as in the daytime.

Don't stop taking insulin. Your instincts may tell you to cut back since you're not eating as much as usual, but more often than not, insulin needs to be increased during sick days—even when you eat little. (Check with your doctor about how to do so.)

Try to eat your usual number of calories and drink plenty of fluids. The latter are needed to replace those lost if you are vomiting or have diarrhea. In addition, high blood glucose draws water from body tissues into the bloodstream, so you are likely to be losing more than usual in urine.

Good sick-day foods include oatmeal, cottage cheese, yogurt, broth, or eggs. If you are nauseated, eat several small portions every few hours rather than sticking to your usual meal spacing. Keep track of what you eat so you know if you are getting your usual carbohydrate allowance.

Foods like *non*diet Jell-O, Popsicles, sherbet, and ice cream are easy to eat and high in easily absorbed sugar—your digestive tract doesn't have to be in top-notch condition to take them in. If you have trouble keeping anything down, try a diet of sugar-containing liquids like apple juice or *non*diet ginger ale, taking small sips as often as you can.

EXERCISE

Your meal plan and insulin regimen are planned to take normal daily activities into consideration. Walking to catch a bus, vacuuming the rug, or activities that are part of your job should be covered in this way.

Engaging in a sport or vigorous exercise may need to be handled differently. To exercise safely, follow these guidelines:

1. Exercise only when diabetes is well controlled; blood glucose should be in the 100 to 200 mg/dl range. At lower levels, an insulin reaction is a real possibility; on the other hand, high blood glucose in the absence of insulin may signal your body to pour even more glucose into your system, resulting in even higher blood glucose.

2. Take extra carbohydrate snacks before exercise and during prolonged activity to make up for energy expended. Since the effect of exercise may last for up to twenty-four hours, during that period you may need additional carbohydrate to prevent hypoglycemia. The amount of such snacks is best determined by self-monitoring of blood glucose and your individual experience. Decreasing your insulin dose also may help keep blood glucose levels normal during exercise. However, unless you are already adjusting your insulin dose in response to self-monitoring, any change needs to be discussed with your doctor.

3. Before beginning an exercise program, get a check-up. Your doctor will want to be sure you are up to the exercise you plan and will advise you on the best exercise for you. This is especially important if you have had diabetes for many years or have experienced diabetic eye, nerve, or kidney problems.

4. Do not inject insulin into an arm or leg that you're planning to exercise. The energetic activity can move insulin into your bloodstream faster than usual.

For tips on coping with holiday eating and advice on good nutrition for different age groups, see the *Family Cookbook, Volume II.*

NON-INSULIN-DEPENDENT DIABETES

Less well known, less understood, non-insulin-dependent (type II) diabetes is more common, more complex, and just as worthy of being taken seriously as insulin-dependent diabetes. If you have type II diabetes, you may be controlling glucose with the aid of insulin injections or oral agents, you may be losing weight, or you may be simply cutting out high-calorie desserts. Don't make the mistake, though, of judging the seriousness of the problem by the extent of the treatment. Often termed "mild," type II diabetes can bring about the same long-term complications as insulin-dependent diabetes, including heart disease, stroke, and eye, nerve, and kidney damage. However simple your treatment plan seems, it's important to follow it closely.

TREATING TYPE II DIABETES

While people with type I diabetes put much effort into balancing insulin, activity, and food intake, this juggling act is not quite so difficult for those with type II diabetes, who always secrete *some* insulin, although not enough for their needs. Having this insulin "cushion," they don't ordinarily experience quickly changing extremes of blood glucose. Instead, personal effort is more likely to go into weight loss or dietary care—the mainstays of treatment for type II diabetes.

The meal plan for people with type II diabetes, like that for type I, emphasizes avoiding concentrated sources of simple carbohydrates, such as candy, cakes, and cookies. These desserts also usually have lots of fat and calories. Substitute diet soft drinks for those that contain sugar, and be on the alert for sugars in packaged foods. Read labels carefully. "Ose" at the end of a word means "sugar," as in glucose, fructose, maltose, and dextrose. And look out for products containing sweeteners like brown sugar, corn syrup, honey, and maple syrup. Limiting sugars can help keep your blood glucose in the normal range, especially after meals, and can also help keep or bring weight toward normal. Make desserts with a noncaloric sweetener, which won't raise blood glucose. And fruits are generally fine. Eating a sweet dessert for a special occasion won't be a problem, as long as you count the calories. But don't make such goodies a routine part of your diet.

Your doctor may have given you a list of foods to eat and those to avoid. While helpful, such handouts are not tailored to your *individual* food preferences and so may be unnecessarily hard to follow. An individualized meal plan works best—one that includes your special favorites, gives you a wide variety of food choices, and is nutritionally balanced. If you find a handout sheet hard to follow, a registered dietitian may be able to help prepare a plan for more flexible choices. Your doctor will probably be able to give you the name of a registered dietitian in your city.

A registered dietitian may also be able to provide useful tips. Meal spacing, for example, may aid in keeping blood glucose levels normal. Some people find that leaving four to five hours between meals is beneficial; others, especially those who are of normal weight, find that frequent small meals are best. He or she may recommend an increase in fiber-rich foods or self-monitoring of blood glucose as an adjunct to dietary treatment.

WEIGHT LOSS

The vast majority of individuals with type II diabetes are over-weight; if you fall into this category, much of your work to control blood sugar will go into the important task of weight loss. Losing even a few pounds may by itself bring blood glucose under control even if your weight is "high normal" rather than in the frankly "overweight" range.

The benefits of weight loss are far more than cosmetic. Not only can it control diabetes but attaining normal weight may help you avoid complications like heart disease and stroke, which are far more common and likely to be more serious among diabetic people than others.

For most of us, losing weight and keeping it off is a formidable task made to seem even more insurmountable by previous unsuccessful efforts. Don't let pessimism prevent you from giving weight loss another try—it can be done! Here are some tips for safe, successful weight loss:

- Get help! Weight loss shouldn't be a do-it-yourself affair. You're likely to need lots of encouragement, support, and information. If your doctor doesn't have the time or temperament, have him or her refer you to a registered dietitian.
- Don't give up! Try different techniques until you find the one that's best for *you*. If behavior modification methods haven't worked, try a group like Weight Watchers or Overeaters Anonymous. The variety offered by *Exchange Lists for Meal Planning* appeals to some people.
- Go slow. At the beginning of a diet, when your will-power is strong and your expectations high, you may be tempted to cut back calories too much. Resist the temptation. Gradual weight loss is far safer, although it is more difficult at first.
- Be realistic. At the rate of one or two pounds per week, and calculating in those plateau periods when

you don't even lose that much, estimate how long you'll be dieting. Three months? Four? More? Settle in for the long haul.

• Be sure to focus on successes. Pat yourself on the back for *anything* you accomplish. Be especially kind to yourself if you *don't* lose weight; congratulate yourself for the pounds you previously lost, for trying, and for continuing to diet despite difficulty.

For a full discussion of both physical and emotional aspects of weight loss, see the *Family Cookbook, Volume II.*

ORAL AGENTS AND INSULIN

Sometimes diet and exercise alone aren't enough to lower blood glucose. Then your doctor may add an oral agent (blood glucose–lowering pill) or insulin to your treatment plan.

Oral agents seem to work by making body cells more sensitive to insulin. (They are not effective in type I diabetes, however, since there is no insulin present.) Pills are no substitute for diet and/or weight loss, though; those therapies must be continued while you are on the medication.

While you're on an oral agent, be sure to eat fairly regularly. It's especially important not to skip meals. Although hypoglycemia is quite uncommon for people on oral agents, it is more likely to occur if you eat irregularly.

It is not uncommon for people with type II diabetes to try diet alone, then one or more oral agents, and finally insulin. Even oral agents that lower blood sugar initially may cease doing so after a period of months or years. If you are taking insulin, you will need to be reasonably consistent with regard to meal timing, and may find the *Exchange Lists for Meal Planning* helpful.

SICK DAYS

Illness—even a minor one—may cause your blood glucose to rise much higher than it ordinarily does. In addition, as your body fights infection, ketones (toxic acid byproducts of burning fat) are released that can be dangerous if they build up to high levels. The burden of illness on your blood glucose–controlling mechanisms may make temporary insulin treatment advisable, even if you ordinarily control diabetes without it. If you already take insulin, your dose may need to increase. It is best to monitor your blood glucose and urine ketone levels more frequently than usual when you're ill.

ALCOHOL

For most people whose diabetes is controlled by diet, an occasional drink of beer, wine, or hard liquor is okay. In itself, alcohol doesn't raise blood glucose (the body uses it like a fat), although the carbohydrate in beer, wine, or liqueurs may do so, as may any sugary mixers you add. If you are attempting to lose weight, remember that alcohol has calories that must be included in your total caloric intake. And if you are taking insulin or an oral agent, be sure not to drink on an empty stomach.

EXERCISE

Regular physical activity brings a host of bonuses for people with type II diabetes. In addition to burning off unwanted calories, it increases your energy—almost like adding several hours to your day. It enhances your sense of well-being and reinforces your body's ability to cope with physical stresses like illness or infection. And it may help control diabetes by lowering blood glucose and making your body's cells more sensitive to glucose.

If you think the only way you'll benefit from an exercise program is to work out strenuously, you're wrong. Increasing your exercise level only a little—walking a few extra blocks a day, bowling a few evenings a week, climbing stairs instead of taking the elevator—may be a benefit in conjunction with diet.

If you do want to significantly increase your exercise levels by starting a more regular, formal program, check with your doctor first to be sure vigorous exercise is advisable. Also ask about special advice if you take insulin or an oral agent. As with any change in life-style, be sure to start slowly and increase activity gradually.

THE GLYCEMIC INDEX

Glycemic indexing is a ranking of foods according to their power to raise blood glucose. Previous thinking had held that sugars raised blood glucose quickly and dramatically, whereas starches caused a slower, smaller rise, presumably due to the time it took a starch to be broken down and absorbed into the bloodstream.

But ongoing research has uncovered a good deal more variability than had been anticipated. Chickpeas, dried green peas, and apples all raised blood glucose to about the same level; however, whole grain bread, a baked potato, and honey had a glycemic index fully twice as high! Yogurt and ice cream ranked identically, and rather low, while a banana ranked twice as high as a plum.

As investigation proceeded, different values were found for these foods as well as many others. Even the form of the food seemed to be important—apple juice causes a bigger leap than apple sauce, which, in turn, seems more potent than sliced apples. Another relevant factor seemed to be whether the food was eaten all alone—as a snack, for example—or as part of a meal.

In the future, it's possible that the glycemic index might mean wiser food choices, better blood glucose control, and another option to check when blood glucose is erratic. It might even mean—way down the road—a new system of meal planning and exchanges. Currently, only a few general observations can be made:

- Whole, raw foods seem to cause less of a glycemic response than do their chopped, ground, mashed, or cooked counterparts.
- Generally, lentils, beans, and peas cause less of a glycemic response than white potatoes or breads.

- Foods eaten as part of a meal tend to cause less of a glycemic rise than the same foods eaten by themselves.

Since the glycemic index has brought a good many surprises already, your own individual response to a food may be worth checking. If your glucose control has been erratic, try testing your blood glucose one to three hours after eating a preplanned meal or snack. Repeat on several different days. Then alter one food at a time, including any foods you feel may be causing your blood glucose to rise. If a certain food consistently causes a large rise in blood glucose, you may want to discuss it with your dietitian, who can help you interpret results.

SWEETENERS

The sugar bowl used to contain one thing and one thing only—sucrose, or "table sugar." Extracted from beets or sugar cane, sucrose once dominated the sweetener market in the United States, and people with diabetes had few sweetener options.

Fortunately, sweetness without sucrose is commonplace today. At present there are many products to choose for your "sugar" bowl and an abundance of low-calorie sodas, chewing gums, jellies, and candies.

Most tabletop sweeteners use one of three sweeteners: aspartame, saccharin, or fructose. There are important differences among these three. When comparing sweeteners, remember that sucrose contains 16 calories per teaspoon.

Aspartame is the newcomer to the sweetener market. First marketed in 1981 as NutraSweet, aspartame is a protein that is nearly two hundred times as sweet as sugar. Although aspartame itself is noncaloric, it is marketed in dry form (Equal) with a filler, which does contain calories. (Without the filler, each packet would contain so few grains they would be difficult to find!) So each packet of Equal has the sweetening power of 2 teaspoons of sugar and contains 4 calories. Aspartame's chief drawback at present is that it breaks down when heated and is therefore unsuitable in baked goods, puddings, and other cooked products, unless added after cooking.

Saccharin, even sweeter than aspartame, packs up to three hundred times the sweetening power of sucrose. It has been around for more than one hundred years now and comes packaged in liquid, free-pouring, and tablet form. Although some people experience an unpleasant metallic aftertaste, saccharin in its liquid or tablet form has absolutely zero calories. Free-pouring or in packets, it is packaged with a buffer and contributes about 2 calories per teaspoon.

Fructose, the type of sugar found in fruits, is the third major sweetener. Although it has the same number of calories as sucrose (16 per teaspoon), the body uses it differently, and it causes only a slight rise in blood glucose. Fructose is only slightly sweeter than sucrose, so you'll need about the same amount. If a main goal is cutting calories, a noncaloric sweetener is probably a better choice.

Whatever sweetener you choose, it's best not to depend entirely on just one. Each has advantages and disadvantages. Use each for those dishes where it will do the best job.

3 ◇ ACCENT ON VARIETY: A FEAST OF FLAVORS

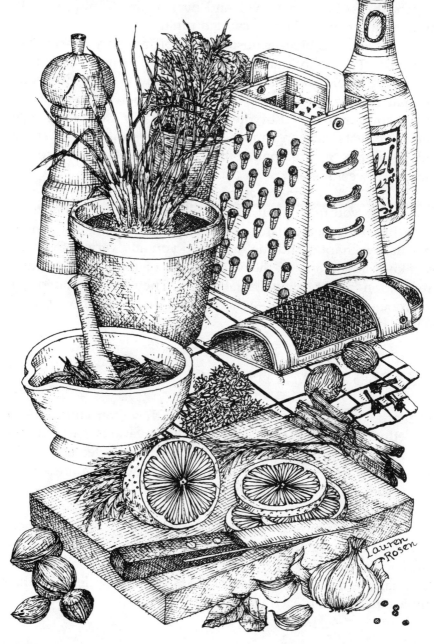

It's easy to fall into patterns. And, for the most part, we're fairly comfortable in them. But they have a downside too: the tendency to slide from the truly comfortable to the boring, from homey to humdrum. Have you cut down on salt (or sugar, or fat) only to find your meals are bland and tasteless? Perhaps you prepare the same dishes over and over again, leaning heavily on hamburger or chicken or canned tuna.

What's the biggest obstacle to spicing up your cooking repertoire? Time? Not really—new dishes don't necessarily take any longer to prepare than old ones. Family frowns? Everyone has had the experience of laboring over a new recipe only to have it soundly rejected by the entire crew. Or are you a single who never eats chicken simply because you can't face cleaning and disjointing a three-pound bird, then having it as a roommate for a week?

The biggest roadblock to varying your cooking style is *habit*. Once you're in a rut, it can be all too easy to stay right there. But jumping out isn't as hard as it may seem. The guidelines in this chapter and the next help you add variety to meals by taking advantage of the wide range of foods and cooking preparation methods available today. They are intended for everyone—diabetic or not—who wants to keep healthy and eat well and interestingly.

LESSONS FROM ETHNIC CUISINES

What are ethnic cuisines and what might they offer you? Simply put, ethnic foods are the typical foods of various parts of the world or regions of the United States. A New Orleans favorite is red beans and rice. Chow mein, chile, and pizza are ethnic dishes that originated in other countries and have been avidly adopted here.

Often, ethnic eating is tastier, healthier, and cheaper than ''mainstream'' American food. And modern technology provides a shortcut around the long preparation and cooking time that many ethnic dishes require. Here are a few lessons that ethnic cuisines can teach us.

Focus on a starch like rice, pasta, or beans as the meal's centerpiece. Meals based on a starch are likely to be low in cost, low in saturated fat, and higher in fiber than meat-based meals. We tend to think of the starch-vegetable combination as an accompaniment to the main meat course or, at best, a "poor person's meal," but millions of people all over the world make elegant, tasty, "company" meals out of just this combination. There's toasted bean curd with mushrooms and peanuts; light rice pancakes stuffed with a spicy potato-onion mixture; sweet and sour eggplant over rice.

Thomas Jefferson viewed meat as a "condiment," as do people in many other nations of the world. Italians often begin the meal with a hearty pasta dish. Then, when hunger has been largely satisfied, they continue with a far smaller serving of meat than would be customary in the United States. In the Far East, rice is the staple starch, and there, too, meat flavors and offsets the grain.

Use a larger variety of herbs and spices. Each country or region has its own special herbs and spices. Salt and sugar are favorites in the United States. In other countries, other flavors and flavor combinations take precedence: ginger, cumin, cardamom, and any of the hundreds of varieties of sweet and hot peppers. Thai lemon grass adds a lemony flavor quite different from lemon juice or zest, and a sprinkle of fresh coriander instead of parsley can transform boiled potatoes from mundane to exciting. Check the list of herbs and spices on pages 50–51 for more suggestions.

Experiment with different ingredients. U.S. Southern cooking makes far more use of various types of greens, for example, than does cuisine in the rest of the United States. Favorites include collards, mustard greens, and kale—not just spinach. The pork-greens combination is a good one, with the richness of pork contrasting well with the tangy freshness of greens. And there's a lot more to do with fish than broil and serve with a lemon wedge. The theme of fish plus a tangy, sharp flavor has variations all over the world. From seviche (scallops marinated in lime juice) to sushi (raw fish with horseradish and soy sauce) to Scandinavian herring (with dill and onions), most fish is excellent with a more pungent foil. On a worldwide scale, the variations on any theme are virtually endless.

Take advantage of contrasts. Americans depend heavily on two flavors—sweet and salty. Other cuisines make extensive use of contrasting flavors, textures, and colors. A fiery Indian curry contrasts well with a cool minted yogurt or a sweet-sour chutney. The blandness of refried beans is the perfect base for a pungent pepper and tomato sauce. A Chinese hot-and-sour soup, sweet-and-sour chicken, or a pilaf dotted with nuts, beans, and apples are other examples.

Visual contrast can be used as well. Try stir-fried yellow and green peppers, brussels sprouts and carrots, or corn and peas—whatever you fancy. Or arrange bright tangerine slices with rounds of emerald kiwi fruit.

And remember, you're free to pick and choose. You don't have to prepare an all-Mexican dinner to use a tortilla. You can use Chinese stir-fry techniques to cook the vegetables *you* prefer; there's no need to stick to snow peas and water chestnuts.

An exchange list of ethnic foods and sample recipes can be found in Chapter 8. (Additional exchanges for ethnic dishes appear in *Family Cookbook, Volume II.*) Also see Chapter 6 for suggestions on using high-carbohydrate–high-fiber foods like beans, whole grains, and legumes.

LOW SALT . . . HIGH FLAVOR

We're all being advised to cut down on salt, sugar, and fat, but salt and sugar are the cornerstones of American flavoring, and fat is an excellent carrier of flavor. Thus, cutting out these favorites means cutting way down on flavor.

If your tastes run to the bland, leaving out salt may trouble you very little. But if you're a flavor craver, omitting it may leave you miserable. There are plenty of ways to add flavor without salt. In fact, most people find that when they stop relying on salt, their cooking is more lively, more varied, and more interesting than it was before (and, of course, more healthful). In addition, you'll be reeducating your palate to be sensitive to a wider variety of flavors, including salt. Since foods that contain salt will seem "salty" to you, you'll be able to get by comfortably at far lower salt levels. You can also expect that foods you presently find salty will later seem much too salty.

Here are some tips for first cutting back on salt, then sprinkling on flavor without touching the salt shaker.

- Avoid salted foods like cured, smoked meats (bacon, luncheon meat, and hot dogs, for example), and snack foods like chips, pretzels, and salted nuts.
- Read labels carefully. You'll find salt in unlikely places. Many canned vegetables and juices, packaged meals, fast foods, breakfast cereals, and even desserts contain high levels of sodium. (If your diet is ordinarily high in sodium, however, you may not be able to taste the salt in such products.)
- Substitute fresh, unprocessed foods for processed versions: "old-fashioned" oatmeal instead of oatmeal-based cereals; fresh beans for canned. You'll be reducing sugar and fat as well.
- Reduce salt in cooking. Cookbooks written before there was so much concern about sodium often recommend much more salt than you're accustomed to. Try cutting amounts in half and see how the dish tastes.
- At the table, taste foods before adding salt.
- Make use of foods that are naturally flavorful. Some foods are more highly flavored than others. Eggplant, mushrooms, and green peppers, for example, are stronger in taste than lettuce. Flat-podded beans taste more distinctive than most round-podded green beans, and snap peas are sweeter than most green peas. Celery is another naturally tasty vegetable (although it's higher in sodium than others). And practically any vegetable tastes better the fresher it is.
- Heating is an obvious but overlooked way to vary flavor. Cooking changes the flavor of most foods. Toasted nuts and seeds can lend a very different ac-

cent to food from their untoasted versions. Heat sesame, cumin, caraway, or pumpkin seeds briefly over medium-high heat (no shortening is needed). Jiggle the pan frequently; when you smell a toasted aroma, remove from the heat. Then use them in the dishes you ordinarily do. The same goes for a wide variety of nuts—experiment with your favorites!

• Prepare your own "bouillon" cubes using cooking and natural meat juices. Don't throw away the juices from roast meats. Instead, refrigerate, then remove the fat that will congeal at the surface. Stock from chicken, meat, or fish can be treated similarly. If desired, reduce the stock until it is full flavored; the more water you boil away, the more concentrated and tasty it will be. Freeze in ice-cube trays. Then, use a cube or two instead of water to cook vegetables, to stir-fry them, or as a light, fat-free base for sauces.

• Dry wines or dry vermouths are excellent flavorers. Boil a small amount briefly to remove the alcohol (and most of the calories). Then use instead of oil to cook meat or fish.

• Make full use of the wide range of low-salt and/or low-sugar products now available in the supermarket. There are low-salt or no-salt pickles, mustards, ketchups, bouillon cubes, and soups. Although they vary in quality they are certainly worth a try. Some can be used in cooking. Use low-salt, no-sugar pickle juice to marinate meats or to make your own pickled vegetables.

• Use high-flavor foods in very small pieces. Whenever you mince a clove of garlic, you're distributing that garlicky flavor throughout a dish; you'd never just add a whole clove. Try this trick with other foods. If you like the flavor of salami, for example, but want to avoid its salt and fat, shred it and scatter a single slice over a salad or rice. You'll still have to count the calories, fat, and salt, of course, but you'll get that salami flavor at a lower nutritional cost.

- Cook with dried mushrooms. Dried mushrooms are packed with mushroomy flavor. Best use for flavor: Grind to a powder using a mini food processor. Then add a teaspoonful or so to sauces and stews, or combine with fresh mushrooms for a more full-bodied flavor.
- Taste with your *whole* tongue. Your tongue isn't uniformly supplied with taste buds. Those for sweet and salty flavors are located at the tip, for sour flavors on either side, and for bitter at the back. When tasting a new food, particularly an ethnic one, don't depend on just the tip of your tongue—you won't taste much.
- Vary texture, color, and temperature—not just taste. Add nuts or raisins to rice. Compose a salad of bright red peppers and sliced fennel rather than sticking to lettuce. With a hot curry, serve a cool yogurt dish.
- Use herbs and spices to brighten up your standard repertoire. Venture beyond lemon juice and garlic to add flavor. If you don't usually cook with spices, think of the foreign cuisines that appeal to you—each has its own repertory of flavoring agents. Many Indian dishes, for example, depend upon coriander, cumin, or turmeric; Chinese cuisines use anise and ginger; Mexican cooking includes peppers in many forms. Knowing what cuisines you already like can give you a lead on spices with which to experiment. See the spice chart on pages 50–51 for suggestions on how to dress up foods.

    Spices vary considerably in their flavor power. One-sixteenth of a teaspoon of cloves packs triple the punch of a tablespoon of refreshing herb like dill. So don't dump herbs on without tasting first. On the other hand, if your dish doesn't have much flavor, do add more.

Keep your spices and herbs in tightly sealed, moisture-proof containers, preferably away from sunlight. As spices and herbs age, their flavor diminishes, so try to use them within a year.

FOOD AND SPICES

Beef	Coriander, thyme, oregano, minced garlic	Add about 1 tsp. of a combination of any or all to a portion of hamburger and broil
	Low-sodium soy sauce, minced ginger, and garlic	Marinade for stir-fried meat
Lamb	Curry powder	Add about 1½ tsp. per lb. of stew
	Rosemary	Roasts, stew
	Garlic	Insert slivers prior to roasting
Fish	Curry powder	Sprinkle surface lightly, broil
	Dill	Fresh or dry in poaching liquid
	Paprika	Sprinkle surface lightly, broil
	Ginger	1 tbsp. to stuffing
	Cloves, cinnamon, cardamom	Marinate in a mixture of equal parts of the ground spices and broil
Chicken	Bay	Place 2–3 leaves with a lemon in cavity and roast
	Tarragon	Add ½ tsp. fresh or dry per cup of sauce
	Rosemary	With lemon and garlic as marinade
Pasta (noodles)	Caraway seeds	Add 1 tsp. to a cup of cooked pasta
	Coriander	Add 1 tbsp. chopped fresh to 2 cups cooked pasta

FOOD AND SPICES *(continued)*

Vegetables	Basil	Generously sprinkle chopped fresh basil on sliced ripe tomatoes and moisten with olive oil
	Oregano	1 tbsp. to soup or sauce, cook
	Sesame	Toast seeds; combine 1 tsp. with a portion of spinach, kale, asparagus, or broccoli
	Ginger	1 tsp., minced, per portion of stir-fried adds an Oriental note
	Caraway or poppy seeds	Add 1 tsp. per serving of cooked cabbage or coleslaw
	Dill, dried	1 tsp. mixed with 1 cup yogurt as a topping for baked or boiled potatoes
	Mint, fresh	Add 1 tbsp., minced, to a pint of yogurt and combine with cubed cucumber; chill
	Lemon zest	Add zest of ¼ lemon to 1 qt. tomato sauce, cook
	Thyme, dried	Add a pinch to cooked lima beans
Yogurt	Cumin	Add ½ tsp. whole roasted per cup for a deep smokey flavor
	Ginger, ground	1 tsp. per pint makes a zesty topping for fruit
Dried beans and peas	Cumin	2 tsp./lb. dried beans, mix with cooking liquid
	Garlic, parsley, lemon zest	Chop finely, mix, and add to cooked beans just before serving (strongly flavored)
Lentils	Cinnamon stick, lemon	Add 1 cinnamon stick and the juice and zest of a lemon to 1 cup dried lentils, cook together
Rice	Curry powder	½ tsp./cup of cooked rice before serving

4 ◇ ACCENT ON VARIETY: TOOLS OF THE TRADE

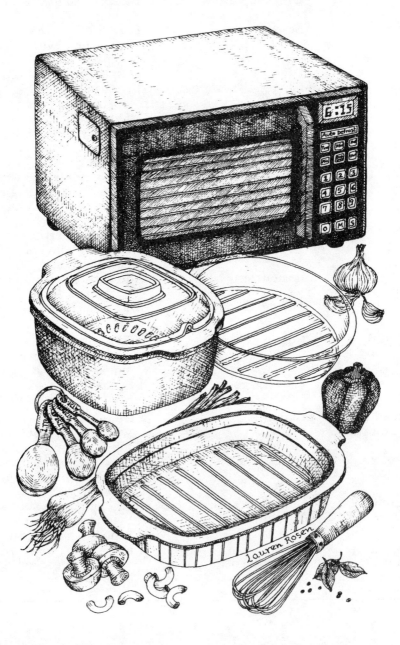

Lauren Rosen

Time is of the essence. Unless you love to cook and have the luxury to spend time on food preparation, you'll want meals that can be prepared quickly. But quick meals tend to rely heavily on fast-cooking but expensive meats like chicken breast, shrimp, or veal.

Try teaming up modern technology—freezer, food processor, microwave—with old-fashioned know-how and the ever-widening array of ingredients you'll find on supermarket shelves. The result? Easy-to-prepare, interesting dishes, including long-simmered favorites like soups, stews, and sauces. Here's how to do it.

BULK PREPARATION

Our ancestors had a day for washing, one for baking, one for ironing. Why? Because doing a task in bulk saves time. Think about it: Doubling a recipe cuts cooking time in half!

Bulk preparation gives the maximum advantage for one-pot, one-step dishes like stews, soups, and many casseroles. For dishes that require individual browning of small pieces of meat, or individual cooking of vegetables, less time is saved. Generally, it's fine to double or triple recipes for casseroles, stews, and soups. The long-cooking cuts of meat used in such dishes bring important bonuses: They are packed with flavor and they are economical.

The following cuts are excellent for stews and braising:

Beef: Chuck pot roast or rump pot roast, sirloin tip, and all types of round roasts (top, bottom, or eye of round) can be cooked whole or cut into pieces for stews. Generally, these cuts take three to four hours to cook fully.

Lamb: Older leg of lamb (or mutton) and shoulder of lamb braised in one piece take between two and one-half and four hours over a very low heat. For stews, choose neck, breast, shoulder, or short ribs; cooking time is two and one-half hours.

Veal: Round, rump, sirloin, or shoulder takes about two hours for braising whole. For stews, cuts like breast, short ribs, round, shoulder, neck, and shank cook in about one and one-half hours.

Chicken: Older chickens (stewing chickens, roasters, and fryers), disjointed, cook in about one and one-half hours.

Many such long-cooking meats can cook nearly untended. (With a crockpot or dutch oven, it's even possible to cook on very low temperatures overnight or during the day while you're at work.)

A good solution to the long time involved is making a "stew base" in advance. Cook meat in stock, tomatoes, water, or whatever your recipe calls for, until tender. Do not add vegetables at this time and do not coat the meat with flour (since fat cannot be removed easily). When the meat is tender, remove it from the cooking liquid and trim off any remaining fat clinging to the meat. Refrigerate the liquid and remove the fat. Combine the meat and liquid again, then freeze in the portions you plan to use. Generally, smaller is better since it's easier to combine two packages than to cut frozen items in half. When ready to prepare, season, add vegetables, cook briefly to warm and blend flavors, and serve.

GETTING THE MOST FROM YOUR FREEZER

Most of us underutilize our refrigerator's freezing compartment. If yours contains only orange juice and a few spare loaves of bread or cartons of milk, you aren't making full use of it. Knowing which foods freeze well and which are less successful can help you get the most from your freezer.

Ideal freezing conditions require an initial twenty-four hours in temperatures lower than −20 degrees Fahrenheit (°F), followed by temperatures that rise no higher than 0°F. Although they lack the quick-freeze capability, many home refrigerator freezing compartments are adequate for routine storage of cooked products or meats. But don't try to freeze most raw vegetables or fruits, and don't keep goods too long (see below). Nor should you freeze in small "ice-cube compartments" found on some older models. The closer your own freezing conditions approximate the "ideal" temperatures, the better. Remember that both quality and storage life are affected by temperature.

Anything to be frozen should be carefully wrapped to keep moisture inside. (The whitish "freezer burn" sometimes seen on poorly wrapped meats and vegetables results from drying.) Your best bets are materials—plastic storage bags, containers, wrap, markers, and tape—intended for freezer use. They withstand very low temperatures in ways that used yogurt containers, cellophane tape, aluminum foil, and ordinary plastic wrap do not. And even when using the proper materials, it's a good idea to double wrap anything you plan to store. Finally, be sure to mark clearly the date your package went into the freezer and what it contains. Distinguishing between frozen chile and frozen meat sauce can be nearly impossible!

Under the ideal conditions described above, blanched fresh vegetables will keep from eight months to a year; meats (other than lunch meats), six months to a year; most fish two to four months. Precooked foods like casseroles and soups keep four to eight months, and most baked goods, four to six months. *Important:* As a general rule, each ten-degree rise in temperature halves the storage life. It is better to underestimate safe freezing time than to overestimate it.

Not everything freezes well. Do not freeze gelatin desserts or salads, fried foods, or cooked potatoes. Hardboiled egg whites become rubbery, cream- or milk-based sauces separate, and hard cheeses become dry and crumbly. Note too that many herb flavors disappear when frozen and don't come back.

HOW TO FREEZE

Vegetables. To freeze fresh vegetables, blanch or undercook before freezing (the microwave is excellent for this). Cooked vegetables such as those in casseroles may be frozen but texture often changes. On the other hand, freezing small amounts of cooked or uncooked chopped mushrooms, onions, celery, or green pepper for use in later cooking is a fine time saver.

Breads. Cooked or store-bought breads freeze well. Cold tends to slow down chemical reactions. You can let dough rise in the refrigerator; it will do so more slowly than it would at room temperature. It's even possible to freeze uncooked bread with satisfactory results. Just double the amount of yeast you usually add. When you're ready to bake, let the loaves rise at room temperature until they are ready for the oven.

Beans. Cooked, dried beans and peas keep well in the freezer. Since beans take a while to soak and cook, they're ideal for freezing in quantity. Pack some for garnishes and others for soups and main dishes.

If you plan to use only a few at a time, try this manner of freezing: Drain cooked beans well, then spread them out on a cookie sheet. Put the sheet in the freezer until the beans are just frozen (don't wait too long, or they will dry out). Remove the beans, pour them into containers, and wrap well. Remove as many beans as needed for salads or garnishes. Beans for soups and stews may be frozen in larger quantities, in cooking liquid, if desired.

Rice and Pasta. Cooked rice freezes well, while pasta texture changes somewhat. Plan to prepare more than you need of these starches, then warm up for a second use. Both keep well for a week or so in the refrigerator. Warm the rice or pasta with a few spoonfuls of water, to soften any hardened grains. Pastas sometimes become sticky when not eaten immediately. A very small amount of oil (1 teaspoon per pound of uncooked pasta) can help prevent this, as can a quick wash immediately after cooking. Rewarm in sauce in a double boiler.

Meats and poultry. Meats freeze well. Most frozen raw meats will need thawing before cooking. Generally, allow about an hour per pound to thaw meat at room temperature. (Thawing under cold running water shortens thaw time somewhat.) Thawing in the refrigerator takes three to five times as long, depending on size. Some meats can be cooked frozen (no thawing required). These include individual portion–size meats such as hamburgers, minute steaks, and chops. Stews and other cooked meats may also be reheated, preferably in a double boiler, without previous defrosting. But once a meat is thawed, use it, since refreezing thawed meat is a dangerous practice.

Consider buying boneless cuts of meat (chicken, pork, beef), trim them well of all visible fat, then freeze them in well-wrapped individual portions. You can prepare a quick meal by removing the frozen block and shaving off thin slices (they may actually be easier to cut than when they're in a slightly defrosted state). Stir-fry briefly. Surprisingly, even some tougher cuts of meat, such as chuck, take well to this treatment. Marinating before can help to tenderize them, and be sure you slice them razor thin.

QUICK COOKING AT HOME

Make maximum use of quick-cooking methods like sautéing, stir-frying, and poaching in addition to that old standby, broiling. Each is a highly flavorful form of cooking that does not rely on thick sauces or gravies for flavor. The variations on each are endless, so innovate and experiment with the basic recipe.

SAUTÉING

Sautéing is an excellent way to prepare chicken parts, veal, or other fairly tender meats in serving-size pieces. Use a very small amount of shortening or a shortening spray in a frying pan. To sauté:

1. Brown the meat on both sides over fairly high heat. Then reduce the heat to low, cover the pan, and cook until done. Check occasionally to be sure the meat is not browning too much; if necessary, add a *small* amount of water or stock to prevent burning. Pour off any accumulated fat. Put the meat on a separate platter.

2. Add a small quantity of liquid—just enough to cover the bottom of the pan. Water, wine or vermouth, tomatoes (including the juice), and stock are possibilities.

3. Add flavorings: garlic, lemon, vinegar, shallots, tarragon, rosemary, mustard—whatever appeals to you. (For suggestions, see the herb chart on pages 50–51.)

4. On high heat, scrape up the tasty cooking bits that cling to the pan. (High heat also evaporates the alcohol, if you're cooking with wine.) Taste the sauce. Add more seasoning or salt if desired. Return the meat to the pan, warm briefly, and serve. There should be very little, but highly flavored sauce— barely enough to go around.

5. Optional at this stage would be to add a contrasting garnish such as scallions, fresh herbs, capers, diced ham or salami, sesame seeds, or cooked beans.

STIR-FRYING

A Chinese cooking method, stir-frying relies on quick cooking of small pieces of meat or vegetable over a very hot flame. Oil is required, making stir-frying more caloric than broiling, for example. However, very little oil is used. To stir-fry:

1. Assemble all ingredients. Once you begin to cook, you won't have time even to peel a clove of garlic! Cut the meat into bite-size pieces; slice the vegetables very thin, or into julienne strips. Meats should be boneless and as thin as possible.

2. Heat a wok or frying pan over very high heat. Add a small quantity of oil—a teaspoon per person is usually enough—a clove of garlic, or a slice of fresh ginger, diced.

3. Add the main ingredient. Vegetables like asparagus, celery, peas, or spinach cook in under a minute. Larger or tougher vegetables like broccoli,

cauliflower, corn, or brussels sprouts may be cooked
for three to four minutes; stir and mix frequently or
cover and cook with ½ cup of stock or water. Meats
in very thin strips generally cook in only a minute
or two.
4. Add garnishes, if desired, or a dash of low-sodium
   soy sauce. Serve over rice.

POACHING

Poaching is an excellent, easy method of preparation for fish. To
poach:

1. In a pan large enough to hold the fish—whole or
   fillets—bring to just under a boil a small quantity of
   water (flavored with herbs, an onion, or whatever
   you prefer). Wine or stock could be used alterna-
   tively. If desired, reduce the liquid to bring out the
   flavor.
2. Add the fish, and, keeping the liquid on very low
   heat so it doesn't boil, cook until done. The fish
   juices and poaching liquid can be boiled down further, if desired, and poured over the fish.

To perk up meat, poultry, and fish that you plan to cook
quickly, marinate for half an hour to a day in seasoned mixtures
based on lemon juice, onion, yogurt, wine, or other low-fat
choices. Removing the skin from chicken helps a marinade or
other flavoring penetrate the meat more quickly and thoroughly.

FOOD PROCESSOR

It's mortar and pestle, food mill, grater, mixer, and blender. It's
the food processor, and it's more than a time saver. Used properly, it should spark your imagination to try dishes you'd never
before have attempted and to allow you to make many dishes
regularly that have previously been once-in-a-while favorites.

The food processor cuts from hours to seconds the time of processes like chopping, grating, and puréeing.

The chopping for six portions of vegetable soup or stir-fried vegetables takes only a couple of minutes. The time for kneading breads and other doughs is similarly shortened. Any puréed dish like chickpea spread, guacamole, or gazpacho is only a press of the finger away. Fresh bread crumbs are a snap.

Other tasks that become easy include:

whipping egg whites
making nut butters
shredding—especially in large quantities
preparing fresh fruit sherbets
freezing fruit bars
grating cheese
cutting julienned vegetables

If you have a mini-processor (a small gadget that holds only a cup or so) you can chop a spoonful of a fresh herb or mince a garlic clove in a matter of seconds. Only two or three peanuts, finely chopped, can completely alter the flavor of a vegetable dish. Other foods that work well in the food processor or mini-processor include coconut, chives, parsley, garlic, fresh chervil, and dill. For a sweet treat try puréed fresh raspberries or strawberries or other fresh fruit.

AN INTRODUCTION TO MICROWAVE COOKING

Microwave cooking is a natural for any health-conscious individual. It's fast, can be virtually fat- and salt-free, and cleanup is a snap. Little or no margarine or oil is required because utensils remain relatively cool during the cooking process, preventing the sticking that occurs at higher temperatures. Salt—from the shaker or in salted margarine or butter—is actually *inadvisable* in microwave cooking because of its tendency to draw moisture out of food. Because the microwave cooks so quickly, foods are naturally flavorful, juicy, and tender.

Because of these advantages and the increasing popularity of microwave cooking, the *Family Cookbook, Volume III,* offers a microwave adaptation of every recipe suitable for microwave cooking. To get the best results from your microwave, follow these guidelines.

Know your oven. Read the manual that comes with your oven before preparing food. Ovens vary significantly by manufacturer and model. Check your oven wattage. The recipes in this book were tested in ovens with power ranging between 650 and 700 watts. The following percentages were used: 100 percent power (high), 70 percent power (medium-high), 50 percent power (medium), 30 percent power (medium-low).

Metal utensils and cookware cannot be used in a microwave oven. Plastic microwave cookware is your best choice, since it stays relatively cool and cooks most evenly. Most oven-proof glass, ceramic, and pottery dishes may be used as well, as long as they have no metal trim. Cooking bags and frozen food pouches are fine, but remember not to close with wire twist-ties. Paper dishes, unless they are made specifically for the microwave, should be restricted to brief cooking times. In all cases, cook in round containers for the most even cooking results.

If you aren't sure whether or not a dish is safe to use in the microwave, here is a simple test: Place 1 cup of cool water next to the dish you are testing. Microwave on high power for one minute. If the empty dish is warm, it is absorbing microwave energy and so is not suitable for use in the microwave.

The type of lid or cover that is best depends on the kind of cooking you're doing. When steaming, always cover the container with its own lid or with plastic wrap to keep foods from drying out and help to cook them faster. For less moist results, use waxed paper instead; roasts and chickens adapt well to this method. Bacon, hamburgers, and bakery products should be covered with paper towels, which absorb grease and prevent bread from becoming soggy.

Cooking times may vary. Try to begin with foods at room temperature rather than chilled for quickest cooking. Always begin by cooking a dish for the minimum amount of time a recipe calls for. Then allow for "standing time." Microwaved dishes continue to cook for a while after they are removed from the oven, so before cooking further, wait. "Standing time" for small items is approximately one to three minutes; vegetables and similar foods take five minutes, main dishes ten minutes, and roasts about fifteen minutes. If your dish still seems underdone, microwave a bit longer.

For even cooking, use round containers and be sure to stir the food or rotate the dish halfway around at least once during the cooking time. It's best to place denser foods on the outside of the dish since microwave ovens cook from the outside in. And avoid using nonstick sprays, which tend to coat the dish in such a way that uneven cooking results.

While some ovens have browning elements, others do not. The surface of meats cooked in the microwave may not become as brown as you'd like. If browning is desired, coat the meat before cooking with paprika, Worcestershire sauce, or salt-reduced soy sauce. Or you might undercook the meat slightly, and then place it under the broiler or in a hot oven to brown the surface.

The microwave is excellent for skinning fruits or tomatoes. Boil 1 cup of water in a 2-cup glass measure for two minutes on high power. Plunge the fruit or vegetable into the water for thirty to forty-five seconds until the skin splits; then dip in cold water and peel.

To convert conventional recipes to microwave, cut the cooking time by one-quarter and check often for doneness. Or follow the cooking instructions for a similar microwave recipe.

Keep your oven clean. The more food there is in it, the slower cooking time will be, and even crumbs lying on the bottom of the oven may mean you're taking longer to cook than you need to. To freshen a stale oven, simply place 1 cup of water in a 2-cup glass measure along with 2 tablespoons of lemon juice, and then boil for two or three minutes.

BASIC COOKING TIMES*

Vegetables	6–7 minutes per pound	High power	Requires little or no water. Cover with plastic wrap or waxed paper.
Fish	4–5 minutes per pound	High power	Cook on a microwave roast rack. Cover with plastic wrap or waxed paper.
Ground beef	4–5 minutes per pound	High power	Place ground beef in a colander. Set into a microwave casserole.
Chicken breasts	6–7 minutes per pound	High power	Cook on a microwave roast rack. Cover with plastic wrap.
Whole chicken	6–7 minutes per pound	Medium-high power	Cook on a microwave roast rack. Cover with waxed paper.
Bacon 2 slices	1½–2 minutes	High power	Cook on a microwave roast rack. Cover with paper towel.
4 slices	2½–3½ minutes	High power	

*All food should be weighed for the most accurate cooking time. Trim meats before weighing.

5 ◇ 1986 *EXCHANGE LISTS FOR MEAL PLANNING:* AN EASY WAY TO VARIED EATING

*A*t first glance they may seem intimidating. But their popularity is good evidence that, once you get to know them, Exchange Lists are "user friendly." The *Exchange Lists for Meal Planning* have been published by the American Diabetes Association and The American Dietetic Association for nearly forty years. During that time they have become the most common meal planning system for people with diabetes, offering a relatively easy way to achieve important goals of therapy. Newly revised 1986 lists are presented here.

Although the large majority of people who use the Exchange Lists take insulin, the lists may benefit non-insulin users as well. They may aid in weight loss, for example, by helping individuals achieve the right caloric levels. And the wide range of choices they offer may make sticking to a weight-loss plan easier.

The lists—there are six of them—are simply groupings of nutritionally similar foods. In the specific amounts listed, each food on a list is equivalent, in terms of calories, protein, fat, and carbohydrate, to every other item on that list. For example, on the Starch/Bread List, 1 slice of bread = 3 tablespoons of wheat germ = 8 animal crackers. Any item can be used in place of, that is, exchanged or traded for, any other item on the same list.

Nutritional consistency is an important treatment goal for insulin users: Each meal should contain approximately the same proportion of protein, fat, and carbohydrate and the same number of calories as every other meal. Yet to be appetizing—and maximally nutritious—food choices should also be varied. The "tradeoffs" on the Exchange Lists offer a means to achieve nutritional similarity while offering a variety of choices.

Monotonous they're not. The Exchange Lists provide plenty of variety. From bagels and water chestnuts to peanut butter and pumpkin seeds, you're likely to find your special favorites. Or you might want to experiment with new foods. If you were to try, one by one, every item in the Starch/Bread List with every fruit on the Fruit List, you'd have 2,784 combinations. At the rate of one taste-test a day, you'd need seven and one-half years to sample them all!

A MEAL PLAN BUILT AROUND YOU

A "meal plan" is a personalized eating pattern worked out with you by your doctor and registered dietitian. Don't think of it as a "diet." If you are of normal weight, it won't be low in calories. And, rather than stressing foods not to eat, it shows you how to eat, combine, and enjoy a large variety of foods. In fact, a good meal plan should actually broaden your eating choices.

Your meal plan will take into account both your nutritional needs and your personal preferences. Your doctor and dietitian will assess your general health and determine the number of calories you'll need based on your sex, age, weight, and life-style. The more energy you expend in growing or exercising, the more calories are allotted. An active eighteen-year-old boy usually needs more calories than a girl the same age. The larger you are, the more calories you'll need to maintain that weight, and women who are pregnant or breastfeeding should consume extra calories. By the time you reach seventy-five or eighty years old, you may need only half as many calories as you did when you were six or seven. Occupation is another factor: A thirty-five-year-old, 153-pound man who sits at a desk all day may need only half the calories he would if he had an active physical job like construction work, lumbering, or deep-sea diving.

The American Diabetes Association currently recommends that up to 60 percent of your daily calories come from carbohydrate, less than 30 percent from fat, and the rest from protein. Although adequate for most people, this macronutrient distribution may vary. If blood fats are high (hyperlipidemia), your doctor may recommend a diet with a fat content closer to 20 percent than 30 percent of total calories. And if you have kidney disease, lower protein levels may be advisable. Of course, the calories subtracted from one area must be made up in another. Cutting back on fats, for example, will probably mean eating more carbohydrate.

If you have food allergies or other diseases requiring diet modification, your meal plan must be tailored to avoid one food or another while providing adequate nutrition. And, of course, it must supply the proper amounts of vitamins, minerals, and fiber.

Using this information, plus knowledge about the type of insulin schedule you are on, the dietitian helps you to map out a meal plan. A common plan is three meals and two or three snacks daily, timed to coincide with peak insulin action. But yours may be different, depending on factors such as your insulin regimen, the rate at which your body absorbs and uses insulin, your life-style, and your preferences. If you're trying to lose weight to control non-insulin-dependent diabetes, just three small meals a day will do nicely.

YOUR PREFERENCES COUNT: A REGISTERED DIETITIAN CAN HELP

The better a meal plan suits you, the more likely you are to follow it. So the dietitian will have *you* in mind as much as nutrition. She or he will take your food preferences into account. If you don't like milk, for example, your dietitian can substitute cheese or yogurt. But if you prefer that even these be minimal in your diet, she or he will suggest alternatives or combinations of other foods that provide the same nutrients but are more palatable to you. Meats, leafy green vegetables, and whole grains can provide much of the protein, calcium, and vitamins that milk would supply in someone else's meal plan.

Although concentrated carbohydrate sources must be restricted, your dietitian can help you work an occasional favorite sugar-containing treat into your meal plan. She or he may suggest that you reduce portion size or modify a recipe, or may help you find a brand that is low in sugar. Ethnic preferences are important, too. To prepare a favorite family dish—Greek *stifatho,* Mexican *menudo,* or Indian *biryani*—your dietitian can provide nutrient information and suggestions in modifying recipes, if necessary.

CHANGING THE MEAL PLAN

Expect your meal plan to change. As a child grows, the meal plan must be modified to include more calories. During adolescence, when the temptation to ''go along with the crowd'' is strong, unscheduled snacking is common and ''fast food'' meals with friends occur often. The dietitian can suggest wise "fast food" and snacking options. If alcohol use begins, the dietitian with the physician can explain the rules of safe drinking to the young adult.

Adult meal plans need modification as well. An avid skier may need more calories during the ski season than in the summer months. A promotion from assembly line to supervisor may mean you're settling a dispute during lunch hour or reviewing safety regulations at snack time. Trying to stick to your former, more regular, meal regimen will be difficult, and diabetes control may suffer. Anyone who is in an "emergency" profession will need extra advice. Firefighters or surgical nurses, for example, have such unpredictable schedules that they'll need special help in meal scheduling and dealing with delays.

GETTING TO KNOW THE EXCHANGE LISTS

The Exchange Lists offer an ingenious solution to a complex problem. The problem is this: As an insulin user you need nutritional *sameness*, but as an eater you want *variety*. Nondiabetic people and many people with type II diabetes have the whole day—or several days—to "balance out" their nutrients. A lunch that's too high in fat can be made up for by eating less fat at dinner. The insulin user doesn't have that luxury.

Constructing a meal that contains the proper proportion of carbohydrate, protein, and fat is difficult indeed. Each food contains a *mixture* of nutrients, in different proportions. Moreover, nutrients vary in the calories they contain. (Carbohydrate and protein have 4 calories per gram and fat has 9.) By grouping together nutritionally similar foods, the Exchange Lists do most of the calculating for you, allowing you to focus on foods, not grams, calories, and proportions.

Take a look at the Exchange Lists themselves—you'll find them in the Appendix. Notice that foods are grouped into six categories similar to those mentioned on pages 17–19. The six groups are:

Exchange List	Carbohydrate (grams)	Protein (grams)	Fat (grams)	Calories
Starch/Bread	15	3	trace	80
Meat				
Lean	—	7	3	55
Medium-Fat	—	7	5	75
High-Fat	—	7	8	100
Vegetable	5	2	—	25
Fruit	15	—	—	60
Milk				
Skim	12	8	trace	90
Low-fat	12	8	5	120
Whole	12	8	8	150
Fat	—	—	5	45

Source: From *Exchange Lists for Meal Planning.* Copyright © 1986 American Diabetes Association, Inc., The American Dietetic Association.

Most of the foods listed in any particular group will make sense to you. Spinach, lettuce, and green beans, for example, appear in the vegetable group, while hamburger, shrimp, and chicken are grouped with other meats. There may be a few surprises, however. The trick to understanding them is to remember that the groups are based on *nutritional* similarity. Take the avocado, for example. It's green, it grows on a tree, and you'll find it in the produce section of your supermarket. To all appearances, it's a vegetable, but, at nearly 70 percent fat per gram, its nutrient profile is close to that of margarine, mayonnaise, olive oil, and other foods on the fat list. It bears little resemblance to a typical vegetable like asparagus, which contains less than 1 percent fat. Nuts, edible seeds, and nondairy coffee "creamer" also appear on the fat list because of their high oil content.

All foods in the Starch/Bread List contain 15 grams of carbohydrate, 3 grams of protein, a trace of fat, and 80 calories. Most breads, rolls, and English muffins have this nutritional profile. But so do dried beans, peas, and lentils. Corn, lima beans, and yams fall into this category, too. Nutritionally, these vegetables have more in common with grains than they do with spinach or zucchini. For similar reasons, cheeses, peanut butter, and tofu are found in the Meat and Substitutes List.

FREE FOODS, COMBINATION FOODS, AND FOODS FOR OCCASIONAL USE

Important additions to the 1986 *Exchange Lists for Meal Planning* are three new or greatly enlarged categories that allow easy, more flexible use of the lists: Free Foods, Combination Foods, and Foods for Occasional Use.

"Free Foods" are foods or drinks with fewer than 20 calories per serving. These may be eaten in either unlimited quantities or very freely. You may eat all you like of foods such as spinach; dill pickles; sugar-free hard candy, gum, and gelatin; coffee; tea; and diet sodas. Green peppers, sugar-free jams and jellies, low-calorie salad dressings, and ketchup may be enjoyed two or three times a day in reasonable quantities. Herbs, spices, "lite" soy sauce, and ¼ cup of cooking wine to enhance flavor may also be used liberally.

Average exchange values are listed for "Combination Foods" like homemade casseroles and macaroni and cheese. Such food mixtures do not fit well into any one Exchange List, although most are prepared in similar enough ways to be classified here. Exchanges for some popular packaged products like "chunky" soups, spaghetti and meatballs, and sugar-free puddings have also been calculated.

Finally, there's the "Foods for Occasional Use" section, containing ice cream, granola, cookies, and (un-iced) cakes. Most people can enjoy these high-sugar treats in small portions every once in a while, although you'll want to talk to your registered dietitian about the best way to fit them into your meal plan and how frequently you can have them.

HOW EXCHANGE LISTS WORK

When a registered dietitian devises a meal plan with you, several combinations of exchanges, all satisfying your nutritional needs, are available. For example, for a meal containing about

60 grams of carbohydrate, 25 grams of protein, and 16 grams of fat (the approximately 60 percent–20 percent–30 percent distribution), any of the following combinations, plus many more, would be possible. NOTE: This is only a SAMPLE. It is not a meal plan, which must be developed for you by a registered dietitian.

CHOICE A: 2 Starch/Bread exchanges
2 Meat (lean)
3 Vegetable
1 Fruit
0 Milk
1 Fat

CHOICE B: 3 Starch/Bread
1 Meat (medium-fat)
0 Vegetable
1 Fruit
1 Milk (low-fat)
1 Fat

CHOICE C: 2 Starch/Bread
0 Meat
1 Vegetable
0 Fruit
2 Milk (low-fat)
0 Fat

As you can see, there are many possibilities. Depending on your preferences and nutrient needs, your meal plan might be designed to include many choices from the Starch/Bread List, or the Milk List, or the Vegetable List and fewer from a list whose choices appeal to you less. (In theory, one could even have a meal identical in *macro*nutrients to those above by choosing from only two categories: 3 Low-Fat Milk exchanges and 1½ Fruit exchanges, although such a meal would not provide a wide enough range of micronutrients.)

HOW THE NEW LISTS ARE DIFFERENT

If you've been using the Exchange Lists for some time, you'll notice that those printed here are somewhat different from those you're accustomed to. The new lists reflect the most up-to-date information on dietary management of diabetes and on nutrient composition of foods.

Expansion of the Free Foods, Combination Foods, and Foods for Occasional Use categories has already been mentioned. Among the other changes are:

1. The Bread List is now the Starch/Bread List as a reminder of the legumes, beans, and starchy vegetables it contains. It now holds the place of honor as List 1, to reflect a greater stress on a high-complex-carbohydrate diet. Nutritional values for foods on this list are somewhat different, too; each exchange now has 3 grams of protein instead of 2, and 80 instead of 70 calories.

2. The Meat List has become the Meat and Substitutes List—all high in protein and containing varying quantities of fat. Tofu, eggs, and peanut butter can be found here, for example. (The high-fat foods on this list should be limited to three times per week.)

3. Fruit exchanges now contain 15 grams of carbohydrate and 60 calories (instead of 10 grams of carbohydrate and 40 calories).

4. Milk exchanges continue to be broken down by fat content: Skim contains a trace; low-fat, 5 grams per exchange; and whole, 8 grams per exchange. (Choose from the first two categories, if possible.)

5. Items that contain 400 milligrams of sodium or more per serving, making them especially high in sodium, have been footnoted to alert people who are trying to cut down on salt.

6. Items that are especially high in fiber (3 or more grams per serving) are indicated with a footnote. You'll want to include more of these in your diet.

PRACTICE USING EXCHANGE LISTS

Once you and your registered dietitian have worked out a meal plan, the next step is to "fill in the blanks" with the foods you have chosen. At first this takes some practice. You'll want to be in touch with your dietitian since adjustments to the meal plan are often made as you're getting used to it. At first, it's a good idea to measure portions carefully, both to ensure accuracy and as a way to learn to estimate portions correctly (a skill that's invaluable when you're eating in restaurants).

The Exchange Lists have been designed to use common measures you'll have around the house, such as teaspoons, tablespoons, and cups. Pretzels and french fried potatoes, certain fruits, and pancakes and breadsticks, for example, are measured in inches, so you'll want to be sure you have a ruler. A postage scale or simple balance is good for weighing meat portions. Although all this may sound difficult, getting the "feel" of a portion size will come easily. Soon, you'll be estimating by eye, and only referring to rulers and scales as a periodic check on accuracy.

The meal plan designed for you will have a certain number of exchanges from various categories at each meal. For lunch, your meal plan might specify:

2 *Starch*/Bread
2 *Meat* (lean)
1 *Vegetable*
1 *Fruit*
0 *Milk*
1 *Fat*

Using this particular combination of exchanges you might come up with menus as varied as these:

2 slices bread (2S) in a sandwich with
1 teaspoon of mayonnaise (1F) and
2 ounces of turkey (2M)
½ cup of cooked green beans (1V)
Large green salad (free) and low-calorie dressing
    (free)
1 apple (1Fr)

OR

1 cup of spaghetti (2S) topped with
¼ cup of cottage cheese (1M) and
2 tablespoons of Parmesan cheese (1M)
Salad of 1 large fresh tomato (1V) with ⅛ avocado,
    cubed (1F), and low-calorie dressing (free)
½ mango (1Fr)

OR

1 cup of bean soup (1S, 1V, 1M)
1 ounce of diet cheese (1M)
Large green salad (free) with 1 cup of low-fat
    croutons (1S) and low-calorie dressing (free)
Raisin-peanut mix (2 tablespoons of raisins, 20 small
    peanuts: 1Fr, 1F)

Breakfast? Choices need not be limited to toast and margarine, fruit juice, and coffee. Using the exchanges and some help from a registered dietitian, a person of Japanese background might plan a breakfast of tea, rice, and pickled vegetables; a Swede might choose black bread, cheese, and coffee; or an Italian might prefer Foccacia (pages 179–181) and *caffè latte.*

You could even get your starch and fat exchanges from chow mein noodles left over from last night's Chinese dinner!

FITTING IN YOUR FAVORITE RECIPES

Your registered dietitian can help you plan menus around a special recipe or food you want to try. Doing so requires some advice because the exchanges called for in the recipe may not be exactly those that your meal plan specifies. Say, for example, that you are using the meal plan above, which calls for 2 Starch/ Bread exchanges, 3 Lean Meat exchanges, and 1 Vegetable exchange. The recipe you'd like to prepare, Veal Stew (pages 207– 208), has 2 Vegetable exchanges and 2 Lean Meat exchanges. Your dietitian can give you advice on "borrowing" the carbohydrate you need from some other category. If you cut your fruit portion by one-third, for example, you could have the veal stew. Serve over rice with a large green salad. Dessert? Dip a few strawberries, grapes, or other small fruits into Bittersweet Chocolate Sauce (page 360). Used in the appropriate portion sizes, all of this will fit well into the meal plan given above.

You'll find your "menu file" will build quickly if you jot down and keep your favorite combinations. In general, you'll start with the dish you're interested in making, then build around it. Say the Strawberry and Rhubarb Compote (page 343) appeals to you. You'd like to combine a large portion of the compote with a slice of Old-Fashioned Lemon Cake (page 347). Subtract the Starch/Bread, Fruit, and Fat exchanges used up by this combination from your total for the meal, and then plan the rest of the meal with the remaining exchanges. A good choice might be Fillet of Sole Italiano with Cucumber Sauce (pages 245 and 332), a baked potato, and a green salad.

Let exchanges stimulate your imagination and tempt you to experiment with new foods. This chapter, along with the Ethnic Exchange Lists in Volume II of the *Family Cookbook*, and the information on ethnic eating in Chapter 8, should keep you out of the eating doldrums for a long time to come.

6 ◇ A SIMPLE GUIDE TO STARCH AND FIBER

*A*mericans sometimes tend toward nutritional snobbery—we look down on beans and peas, and dismiss potatoes and pasta as too fattening. In other countries, these nutritious staples are given their due. Italy boasts a Museum of Pasta and Ireland a statue honoring the potato. But the United States is beginning to wise up.

The latest *Dietary Guidelines for Americans* encourages everyone to eat foods with adequate starch and fiber. Why the recommendation? At present, compared to those of most of the rest of the world, our diets are low in whole grains, fruits, vegetables, and beans. We may be missing out on some of the benefits of high-starch, high-fiber eating. In addition to the well-known beneficial effects on bowel function, such foods seem to help lower blood fats and cholesterol, may aid in colon cancer prevention, and, especially for people with diabetes, have a stabilizing effect on blood glucose.

Unrefined high-carbohydrate foods have a lot going for them. They are naturally "packaged" with a wide variety of vitamins and minerals—some protein, too. They're inexpensive compared to some meats, milk products, and fats, and they store far better than these "perishables." Fiber aids digestion, and starch has less than half the calories of fat: 4 per gram, compared to 9 per gram for fat. The variety available is astonishing. There are thousands of edible plants, they come in a wide range of colors, textures, and flavors, and they can be adapted to forms of cooking and shaping limited only by the imagination.

THE PLANTS THEY COME FROM

Fiber foods are plant foods. Fruits and vegetables, grains, legumes, and nuts are our chief sources of carbohydrate and fiber. Knowing a little about the plants they come from can help make sense of the confusing vocabulary of high-carbohydrate, high-fiber eating. What exactly is a legume? Wheat germ? Roughage? Bran? Refined flours?

The next time you're at a bad movie, sneak a peek at your popcorn. Each light puff is a kernel of corn turned inside out, and it gives you a good idea of the anatomy of grains (oats, rice, and barley, for example) and legumes (beans, lentils, and peas). All are seeds, and as such they have a similar basic structure consisting of an outer protective coat, the beginnings of a new plant, and a food store.

The tough, brownish part of your popcorn kernel is its

outer protective coat. These are the *bran* layers, and they contain most of the fiber the kernel has. Bran cereals are often made of wheat bran, although, of course, there are as many other brans as there are grains.

The white, puffy, "exploded" part is the *starch;* it makes up nearly all of the kernel and, if the seed were allowed to grow, would form its food supply. You're familiar with starch in its "pure" form as cornstarch, for example—the starch completely refined and purified of bran and germ.

A third element of a seed is the embryo, or *germ.* So small it is difficult to see with the naked eye, it makes up only about 2 percent of the seed. The germ consists of the root and shoot of the young plant and contains nearly all of the seed's protein, vitamins, and minerals. Nutty, nutrient-rich wheat germ is marketed for home use, while corn germ is ordinarily processed into corn oil.

Although the thin bran coating and the tiny germ make up only a fraction of the whole, they pack a big nutritional wallop, containing:

> all the fat
> nearly all of the protein and fiber
> more than twenty vitamins and minerals

Refining grains is the process of separating starch from bran and germ. From the miller's standpoint, refining is a good thing, since milling (the grinding process) is easier with the bran and germ removed. Another plus is that refined flour can be stored longer and more easily than whole grain flour because the fat in the grain's germ can turn rancid.

The 1942 Enrichment Act requires that refined flour be enriched with thiamine, niacin, iron, and riboflavin—four of the nutrients lost in the refining process. Nevertheless, refined flours are still missing nearly all the micronutrients and all the fiber of a whole grain product.

Botanically, *legumes* are simply pod-bearing plants. Green beans, lima beans, lentils, kidney beans, chickpeas (garbanzo beans), soybeans, and even peanuts are legumes. However, in cooking, the word "legume" is used in a more limited sense to apply to fully mature, dried members of this family. Nutritionally, the maturing process is an important one. Left on the vine to ripen throughout the summer, legumes build a supply of vitamins, minerals, protein, and fiber, and they lose water. By harvest time, the dried legumes are a much richer store of nutrients than their immature counterparts.

Traditionally, pinto beans, chickpeas (garbanzo beans), kidney beans, and white beans are eaten *after* drying and are thus considered legumes. String beans, on the other hand, are usually eaten young and green (that is, immature), and so are called vegetables. Peas, lima beans, black-eyed peas, and fava beans, among others, are popular both fresh and dried.

WHAT FIBER DOES FOR THE PLANT . . . AND WHAT IT CAN DO FOR YOU

Call it fiber, roughage, or bulk, it is found only in plant foods and generally refers to the parts of a plant that human beings cannot readily digest. In plants, fibers make up cell walls, form the outer protective coating of kernels and seeds, repair injury, and store some plant nutrients.

Tough and woody, structural fibers help to give plants shape. The bran layers that encase the soft starch and germ parts inside a seed are made up of structural fibers. A second type of fiber is the gums and mucilages. They swell in the presence of water (are "water soluble") and thus help seal plant wounds. Familiar gumlike substances include chicle (the base of chewing gum) and the sticky resin found on pine and spruce trees. A third type of fiber is an indigestible starch that is similar to the digestible starch in a grain or legume. It stores energy for the plant to use as it grows.

What can fiber do for you? Fiber's effects have only recently begun to be thoroughly investigated, so there's still a lot we *don't* know about fiber. We don't know exactly how much and which types of fiber a person should eat each day. But it is clear that the U.S. diet is low in fiber and that eating more fiber-rich foods can bring big payoffs. In terms of their effect on your body, fibers can be divided into two different types: those that dissolve in water and those that do not. Interestingly, the two types of fiber act very differently.

The first, known as soluble fibers, include pectin, gums, and indigestible starches. Small amounts of soluble fibers are found in most plant foods. They tend to form gels when they come into contact with water. In your stomach, they swell, giving you a sense of fullness, and they tend to make food remain in your stomach longer and pass more slowly through the rest of your gastrointestinal tract. The gels formed act as filters, possibly delaying absorption of nutrients and binding some harmful substances. A diet high in soluble fibers works to lower blood fats and blood sugars.

Found mostly in whole grains, insoluble fibers tend to move food *quickly* through your stomach and intestines, taking up water along the way and thus increasing the bulkiness of stools. Bran's well-known laxative effect is largely due to its content of insoluble fiber.

It's advisable to get fiber from natural food sources, not supplements. Since different types of fiber have different effects and since soluble and insoluble fibers occur together in different foods, it's best to consume a *variety* of fruits, vegetables, grains, and legumes to get a full fiber effect. Interestingly, a high-fiber diet tends to reduce *both* constipation and diarrhea.

SPECIAL BENEFITS FOR PEOPLE WITH DIABETES

In addition to the benefits above, fiber brings special bonuses for people with diabetes. Eating a high-fiber meal seems to delay digestion and absorption and thus slows the entrance of glucose into the circulation. Blood glucose levels don't shoot up as quickly or as high as they otherwise do. And eating more fiber on a regular basis seems to lead to a *general* reduction in blood glucose so that the need for insulin or an oral hypoglycemic agent may be lessened.

If you are considering adding fiber to your diet, do so gradually and communicate with your doctor or dietitian, especially if you are taking insulin or an oral hypoglycemic agent. The blood glucose–lowering properties of fiber may be so effective that, especially for type I patients, hypoglycemia results unless insulin is adjusted simultaneously.

FINDING FIBER

Good high-fiber foods are:

- *Fresh fruits (preferably with skins on).* Generally whole fruit contains more fiber than fruit juice. Especially high in fiber: dried apricots, figs, and prunes, and fresh blackberries, blueberries, nectarines, pomegranates, raspberries, and strawberries.
- *Whole grains and whole grain products.* Whole grain breads, whole grain cereals like oatmeal or Wheatena. Especially good sources are wheat germ, bran cereals, corn, and rye bread.
- *Legumes:* Especially good sources are all dried beans and peas, lentils, baked beans, and lima beans.
- *Vegetables:* Most fresh, raw vegetables, especially zucchini and celery.
- *Nuts and seeds.* Because of their high fat content, these won't be a major source of fiber. However, for variety, try using them more as a fat source and cutting back on margarines and oils, which contain no fiber.

BEYOND LIMAS

"I was determined to know beans," wrote Henry David Thoreau during his stay at Walden Pond. Most of us think we already *do* know beans—or at least all we want to know about them. If your associations with beans run to an army mess hall, Boston, or beanbags, think again. Legumes and whole grains are among the most underrated of edibles.

Beans' virtues are many. They are storable, nutritious, and cheap. They have fed the world's population for thousands of years. They come in an astounding variety of colors, textures, sizes, and shapes. Ever heard of the Dalmatian bean (white with maroon splashes), the Paul Bunyan bean (pods reach a foot in length), or the Rattlesnake bean?

Of course, legumes do carry with them some genuine disadvantages. They tend to take a long time to cook, and beans give some people gas. Both of these problems, however, can be surmounted. What follows are tips to get the most from legumes and whole grains.

AT THEIR BEST: STORAGE AND PREPARATION

Legumes are "keepers." Dried peas and beans keep almost indefinitely if stored in a dry, preferably cool, place. Whole grains, because of their higher fat content, may not last quite as long but should be good for up to a year if kept in well-sealed containers. They'll last even longer in the refrigerator.

Many dried beans need soaking before they can be cooked; however, beans developed today in the United States generally need less soaking and less cooking than those of years ago. Try this technique: After rinsing the beans briefly, pour boiling water over them, and then let stand for four hours or more. Throw away the soaking water and proceed with cooking. The boiling water is important. A cold-water soak, even an overnight one, won't get rid of the "hardshell" that affects an occasional bean. And do throw away the soaking water—in it are complex sugars that, like fiber, are fermented in the large intestine and cause gas.

After soaking, as a test of "doneness," break open a bean. If the bean is easy to break and the color uniform throughout, it's ready to cook. If tiny bubbles cling to the sides of the soaking bowl, you've soaked too long: The beans are beginning to ferment. They are still fine to eat, though.

What to do if you have a bowl of soaked beans and a last-minute invitation to go out to dinner? If you have no time at all, stick the beans in the refrigerator to slow down any fermentation that may take place, and then cook them the next day. If you have the time, simmer the beans until they are done, cool them in the refrigerator, and freeze until you can use them. If you're planning to make soup, keep the bean broth, too.

Canned beans, of course, need no soaking or cooking. Because they're speedy, it's a good idea to keep a can or two on hand. But remember to wash them under cold running water for about a minute before proceeding with your recipe. You'll remove much of the salt and the "tinny" flavor some people find objectionable.

Follow package directions for cooking times, but you can be somewhat flexible. Both bean soaking and cooking times are only rules of thumb. Cooking times differ significantly from season to season and batch to batch. Hardness of water in which you cook them and bean age also affect length of cooking time. A high-quality bean, grown and stored under ideal conditions, may need no soaking at all! Cooking time should also be influenced by the use to which you're putting them. Beans for a purée or spread are best cooked until nearly mushy, while those for use whole in a bean salad or as a garnish should be slightly firmer and so would need less cooking time.

Your best check is to taste a few beans. When they're doubled to tripled in size, of the texture you like all the way through, and tasty . . . they're ready.

A GRAIN AND LEGUME SAMPLER

NO-SOAK LEGUMES AND GRAINS

Like white rice, these legumes and grains need no presoaking at all. In fact, you can prepare these in less time than it takes to bake a potato. Just cook and enjoy.

Cracked wheat. Tastes nutty and sweet; slightly chewy texture. Blend half-and-half with white rice, for variety, or use as an "extender" for meatloaves or stuffed peppers.

Buckwheat groats. Vaguely smoky taste. Use as side dish plain or cooked with mushrooms or carrots.

Cornmeal. Typical corn taste. Cook as polenta (pages 284–285) and serve as starch accompaniment to a meal or make into muffins.

Bulgur (parboiled, cracked wheat). Tastes like cracked wheat. Excellent for tabbouleh salad combined with tomatoes, cucumber, scallions, and fresh mint or parsley. Serve cold with a simple oil-and-vinegar dressing.

Lentils (brown or red). Lentils have a slightly peppery flavor and can be used in a limitless variety of ways. Thoroughly cooked, puréed, and spiced with ginger, turmeric, and cumin, they form the basis of *dal,* an Indian staple served over rice. Lentils are also good for soups, as salads prepared similarly to tabbouleh salad, or as a side dish.

Black-eyed peas. Cooked dried beans have a "raw" taste similar to their immature counterparts. A staple of Southern cooking, they combine well with pork or greens. Good as a side dish lightly sprinkled with marjoram.

Split peas (green, yellow). Peas have a unique flavor and creamy texture. Unlike most other legumes, they soften quickly, making them good for soups and less good for salads and stews.

Soy granules (partly cooked, cracked soy beans). Mild in flavor and rich in protein, this quick-cooking soy product is used as an addition to soups, as an extender in meatloaves, or (combined with grains) as a filler for stuffed vegetables such as zucchini, tomatoes, and cabbage leaves.

Pearl barley (has outer husk removed; Scotch barley does need soaking). Its distinctive flavor makes it a good addition to vegetable soups and stews. Combine with mushrooms as a side dish.

SOAKING REQUIRED

Lima beans. Taste somewhat blander than fresh limas. Add to soups or combine with rice and herbs as a side dish.

Adzuki beans. Tiny, red, slightly sweet beans are good added to salads or, if precooked, combined with rice as a color contrast. Flavor combines well with garlic and ginger.

Black beans. Unlike many other beans, these highly flavored, slightly tangy beans add their own distinctive flavor rather than absorbing flavors of the foods cooked with them. Also called turtle beans, they are the basis of black bean soup. A fine contrast with brown or white rice.

Brown rice. More assertive in flavor than white rice, it is slightly stickier in texture. Uses are the same.

Fava beans. These very large beans taste and look somewhat like large, mild-flavored lima beans. Dressed with fresh dill, thyme, or parsley, they are an excellent starchy accompaniment to roasts or poultry. Cold, they make a good "starchy" salad variation in place of potato or macaroni salad.

White beans (navy, great northern, and pea beans). All have a typical "beany" taste, although they are not strongly flavored. These are the standard beans for bean soups, and may also be added to vegetable soups. Combine cooked or partially cooked beans with a defatted stew base for a hearty main course. Puréed and seasoned as you like, these beans can be used for sandwich spreads.

Pinto beans. Taste typically "beany" and can be used similarly to white beans.

Chickpeas (garbanzo beans). With a nutty and chestnutlike taste, chickpeas are excellent in a wide variety of uses. Puréed, they are good as a sandwich spread (see page 371). Shredded, they form the usual base for *falafel*, spicy Middle Eastern chickpea balls. Or roast cooked chickpeas and toss lightly with curry powder or salt as a munchie. Add to soups and stews.

Kidney beans. Kidney beans have a fairly strong bean flavor and are the basis for many chile recipes. They are also fine in salads with other beans.

Mung beans. These "sprout" beans can be added to stir-fry dishes, or given an Italian flavor by cooking for an additional thirty minutes or so in tomatoes, onions, and garlic.

WORKING THEM IN

Introduce whole grains and legumes gradually, both to let your digestive system become used to them and to give yourself the best chance to enjoy and experiment. Resist the temptation to make a huge quantity of an all-bean or mainly grain main dish at first.

Instead, you might want to soak and cook a half-pound of beans, and then freeze them in small portions. Marinate some—they'll keep for a week or so in the refrigerator—and put a few in salads now and then. Substitute chopped beans for breadcrumbs as a meatloaf binder. Add a few beans to your favorite recipes for vegetable soups, casseroles, and stews. Cooked beans are a delicious, if untraditional, addition to Chinese stir-fry dishes. When the first batch of beans is used up, try another kind. Once you know the beans and grains you like, you can try dishes like Hearty Lentil Stew (page 272), Hot Brown Rice with Chiles (pages 291–292), Frijoles Cocidos (page 385), or North African Couscous (pages 328–329).

If possible, buy a small quantity of a grain you're experimenting with, and try mixing it with one that already appeals to you. Most grains pick up the flavor of cooking liquids well, so cook with broth, onion, or other seasonings. Or try toasting any grain before cooking. It lends a nutty flavor and shortens cooking time somewhat. Just put grain in a frying pan (no fat is needed) over medium-high heat, moving constantly for a minute or two, until you can smell the toasting grains. Remove and proceed. Most grains can be cooked as you would cook rice, using twice as much water or other liquid as dry grain.

BUILDING A PROTEIN

Many cuisines combine grains and legumes to nutritional as well as culinary advantage. This combination, plus milk, if available, has been a chief protein source for many nations of the world. For flavor, attractiveness, and nutrition, the combination is unequaled. A classic Italian dish is pasta and beans—a thick, main-dish soup. Other variations include rice and beans and rice and peas.

Grains and legumes are good sources of amino acids (the components of protein), but, except in the case of soybeans, they don't contain every amino acid we need to make a complete protein.

To construct a complete protein using vegetables only, try these combinations:

> grain + legume
> grain + milk
> legumes + seeds

Generally, these amino acid sources are considered complementary. That is, the amino acids missing in grain are contained in many legumes or milk products. Those missing in legumes are contained in many seeds. So combining foods from these groups gives you all the amino acids to make a complete protein. Eating them at the same meal or combining with even very small amounts of meat can supply most of the amino acids you need.

If you're interested in eating low- or no-meat meals frequently, it's best to consult a registered dietitian. He or she can be sure your combinations will give you all the amino aids you need, and that you are including the micronutrients you need without too many calories.

We've come a long way from the days when all carbohydrates—sugars and starches alike—were considered "forbidden foods" for individuals with diabetes. Today's eating, abundant in starch and fiber, offers a panorama of food choices unheard of not so long ago. Take advantage of them!

A FAMILY OF COOKBOOKS

The American Diabetes Association/The American Dietetic Association Family Cookbook series is more than a fantastic collection of recipes.

In addition to diabetes basics, each volume offers something special and unique. In the first *Family Cookbook,* now newly revised and updated, you'll find information on canning and freezing fruits, calculating exchanges from food labels and recipes, and fast food exchanges. The *Family Cookbook, Volume II,* has also been newly revised. It covers topics such as different nutritional needs through life's stages, boasts three chapters on weight loss, including coping with feelings, bingeing, and information on exercise, and provides still more information about fast foods. Volume III focuses on variety, providing brand-new exchange values, guidance on ethnic eating, sections on microwave, food processor, and freezer, and lots of practical cooking advice.

Taken together, our family of cookbooks offers you a complete nutrition manual—a source to turn to for tasty, healthy eating, authoritative information, and the friendly guidance and support you need while living well with diabetes.

7 ◇ RECIPES

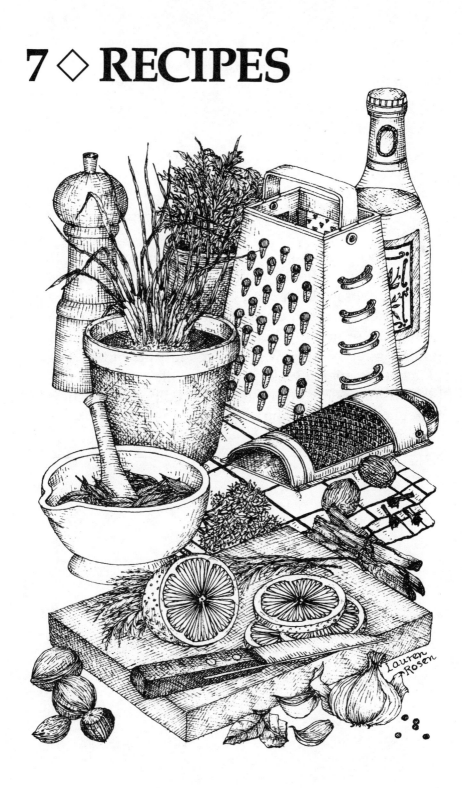

*R*ecipes have to fit into your day, your mood, and, often, the ingredients you have on hand. The recipes you'll choose will depend on your food budget, the season of the year, and whether, on any particular day, you're in the mood for pots, pans, slicing and mincing, or simply want to get in and out of the kitchen as speedily as possible, while serving a nutritious meal. The suggestions preceding each section should help direct you toward recipes that fit your needs.

The recipes in this cookbook were specially developed to complement and expand on the collections in Volumes I and II of the *Family Cookbook*. What's more, the recipes reflect the latest scientific thinking on good nutrition and healthy eating.

The United States Department of Agriculture's *Dietary Guidelines for Americans* recommends eating a wide variety of foods with an emphasis on increasing starch and fiber in the diet while reducing sugar, salt, fat, and alcohol. In 1986, an American Diabetes Association task force supported these recommendations in its report, *Nutritional Recommendations and Principles for Individuals with Diabetes Mellitus.*

The recipes in this cookbook should help you follow these guidelines. As with the recipes in Volumes I and II of the *Family Cookbook* the recipes in Volume III are:

Reduced in total fat and saturated fat.

Limited to ½ egg per serving when a recipe includes egg.

Limited in salt- and sodium-rich ingredients. Recipes with 400 milligrams or more of sodium are footnoted.

Limited to about ½ teaspoon sugar, honey, or molasses per serving when a recipe includes these ingredients. Foods containing 3 grams or more of fiber per serving are noted by a footnote.

Potassium is broken out for those who must watch their potassium levels.

Even within these limits, the recipes still maintain their individuality, taste, and heritage. These principles can also be used to adapt your own favorite recipes.

If you've got diabetes, you need to fit these recipes—or your own adapted favorites—into your daily meal plan. If you're taking insulin, your meal plan has already been designed to coordinate with your insulin dosage. And, while all the recipes here have been reduced in sugar, fat, and salt, some have higher amounts of these ingredients than others. You'll want to work with your doctor and registered dietitian to fit them into your meal plan.

RECIPE ANALYSIS

Recipes were analyzed with a completely revised and updated version of the computer software program used for the *Family Cookbook, Volume II*. The data base for the recipe analysis program contains more than seven hundred foods, including all of the ingredients in this cookbook. For each food, the data base includes twenty-eight different nutrients. Of those, the amount per serving of protein, fat, carbohydrate, sodium, potassium, cholesterol, and total dietary fiber appears for each recipe. Nutrient analysis information for calories and the first six nutrients is from the United States Department of Agriculture, Handbook 8 and Handbooks 8-1 through 8-14. Nutrient information for foods not available in these sources was obtained from provisional information or from the producers of the products. Total dietary fiber analysis is from a published source.

The recipe analysis program, developed by Lawrence A. Wheeler, M.D., Ph.D., was written in Pascal and runs on IBM type computers. The program not only analyzes recipes for individual nutrients per serving (as described above) but also:

1. Provides "exchanges" for an individual serving based on the 1986 edition of *Exchange Lists for Meal Planning*, so that the exchange value of the serving is close to the actual nutrient content.
2. "Flags" key nutrients. A "key nutrient" is defined as a nutrient in a single serving that will provide more than 75 percent of the Recommended Daily Allowance (USRDA).

For some recipes, there were several possible combinations of exchanges that yielded good nutritional approximations. Combinations that might have been "best" in terms of reflecting the actual nutrient content of the recipe, but that seemed inappropriate (for example, a milk exchange in a recipe that did not contain a milk product) were eliminated. Full exchanges were used instead of fractional exchanges, whenever possible.

REFERENCES

American Diabetes Association. 1987. Nutritional Recommendations and Principles for Individuals with Diabetes Mellitus: 1986. *Diabetes Care* 10: 126–132.

Anderson, J. W. 1986. *Plant Fiber in Foods*. Lexington, KY: HCF Diabetes Research Foundation, Inc.

United States Department of Agriculture and Health and Human Services. 1985. *Dietary Guidelines for Americans*. Washington, DC: HHS.

United States Department of Agriculture Handbook. 1976–86. *8-1: Dairy and Egg Products; 8-2: Spices & Herbs; 8-4: Fats & Oils; 8-5: Poultry Products; 8-6: Soups, Sauces & Gravies; 8-7: Sausages & Luncheon Meats; 8-8: Breakfast Cereals; 8-9: Fruits and Fruit Juices; 8-10: Pork Products; 8-11: Vegetables and Vegetable Products; 8-12: Nut and Seed Products; 8-13: Beef Products; 8-14: Beverages*. Washington, DC: HHS.

Watt, B. K., and A. C. P. Merrill. 1984. *Composition of Foods: Raw, Processed, Prepared. USDA Agriculture Handbook No. 8*. Washington, DC: Government Printing Office.

Wheeler, L. A., M. L. Wheeler, and P. Ours. 1985. Computer Selected Exchange Lists Approximations for Recipes. *J. Am. Diet. Assn.* 85:700–703.

Appetizers

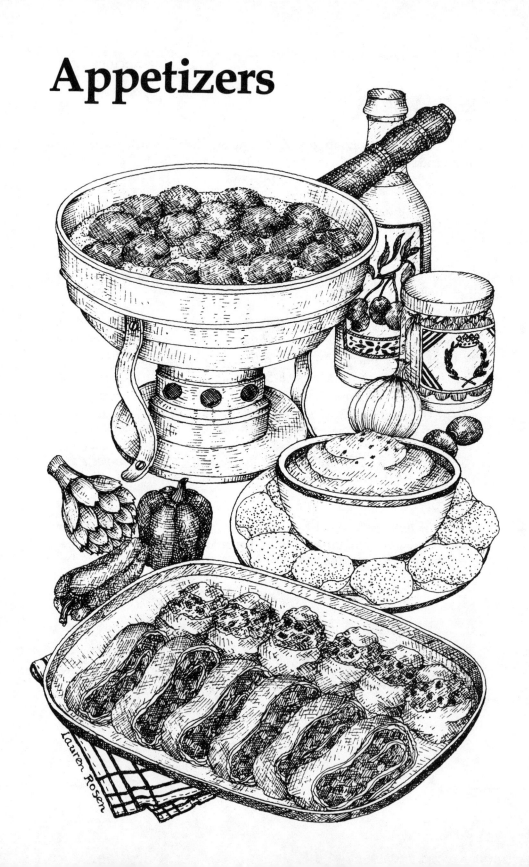

*A*ppetizers are for fun and festivity. Less functional than any other part of your meal except perhaps dessert, appetizers can be exactly what you want them to be—stick-to-the-ribs or airy and elegant, quick or elaborate.

For example, if you're in the mood to cook you might want to try Meat Strudel, served whole with its attractive shiny crust, or sliced into spirals of meat and flaky pastry. On the other hand, if you've only got a minute or two, try a quick appetizer like Smørrebrød—thin slices of black bread topped with ham and cheese, roast beef, or salmon, and garnished with capers, cornichons, or a twirl of lemon peel. There are many others you'll want to try.

Mushroom Paté

Yield: 1 cup (8 servings)		Nutrient Content per Serving:		
Serving Size: 2 tablespoons		CAL 35	PRO	1 (gm)
Exchanges:		FAT 3 (gm)	CHO	3 (gm)
Vegetable	½	Na 96 (mg)	K	129 (mg)
Fat	½	Fiber 1 (gm)	Chol	2 (mg)

Ingredients

   1 TABLESPOON UNSALTED MARGARINE
   ½ POUND FRESH MUSHROOMS, CLEANED AND
      FINELY CHOPPED
   1 MEDIUM ONION, FINELY CHOPPED
   1 TEASPOON WORCESTERSHIRE SAUCE
   1 TEASPOON LEMON JUICE
   ¼ TEASPOON SALT
   ⅛ TEASPOON BLACK PEPPER
   2 TABLESPOONS REDUCED-CALORIE
      MAYONNAISE

Method

1. In medium skillet over medium heat, melt margarine. Cook mushrooms and onion.
2. Stir in Worcestershire sauce, lemon juice, salt, and pepper. Cook until all juices have evaporated, about 15 minutes, stirring occasionally.
3. Cool; then stir in mayonnaise. Chill. Serve with low-salt crackers or vegetables.

Method–Microwave

1. Melt margarine in 2-quart microwave-safe saucepan.
2. Cook onions for 2 minutes on high power. Add mushrooms, Worcestershire sauce, lemon juice, salt, and pepper. Cook for 5–7 minutes on high power, or until all juices have evaporated, stirring once.
3. Cool; then stir in mayonnaise. Chill. Serve with low-salt crackers or vegetables.

Sesame-Orange Beef Bites

Yield: 6 servings
Serving Size: 5 pieces
Exchanges:
Meat, lean   1

Nutrient Content per Serving:

CAL	58	PRO	7 (gm)
FAT	3 (gm)	CHO	2 (gm)
Na	104 (mg)	K	122 (mg)
Fiber	0 (gm)	Chol	20 (mg)

Ingredients

½ POUND BEEF TENDERLOIN
¼ CUP CANNED BEEF BROTH*
¼ CUP ORANGE JUICE
½ TEASPOON FRESH GINGER, CHOPPED, OR
    ¼ TEASPOON GROUND GINGER
¼ TEASPOON ORANGE PEEL
¼ TEASPOON SALT
    NONSTICK VEGETABLE SPRAY
½ TEASPOON CORNSTARCH
1 TEASPOON SESAME SEEDS
    FRESH ORANGE SLICES FOR GARNISH

Method

1. Trim fat from beef. Cut into 30 cubes. Place beef in noncor-
   rodible dish.
2. Combine broth with orange juice, ginger, orange peel, salt,
   and cornstarch. Pour over beef. Cover and refrigerate for 1½
   hours. Turn beef frequently. Drain marinade; reserve.
3. Cook beef in well-sprayed skillet for about 5 minutes, turning
   to brown all sides. Remove to warm platter.
4. Stir ¼ cup marinade into skillet. Cook over high heat until
   slightly thickened.
5. Stir cornstarch into remaining marinade; stir into sauce. Cook
   and stir until thickened. Stir in sesame seeds.
6. To serve: Place beef in chafing dish on serving platter. Pour
   sauce over beef. Garnish with orange slices. Serve with
   toothpicks.

*For reduced salt and fat, use homemade beef broth.

Mini-Pita Reubens*

Yield: 2 servings**

Serving Size: 1 mini-pita

Exchanges:

Starch/Bread   1

Meat, medium-fat 1

Fat   1

Nutrient Content per Serving:

CAL	195	PRO	11 (gm)
FAT	10 (gm)	CHO	13 (gm)
Na	797 (mg)	K	103 (mg)
Fiber	1 (gm)	Chol	30 (mg)

Ingredients

> 2 MINI-PITAS OR 1 REGULAR PITA, CUT IN HALF
> 1 TABLESPOON LOW-CALORIE THOUSAND
>   ISLAND DRESSING OR LOUIS DRESSING (SEE
>   PAGE 148)
> 2 OUNCES LEAN, COOKED CORNED BEEF, SLICED
> 1 TABLESPOON SAUERKRAUT, DRAINED
> 1 TABLESPOON SWISS CHEESE, SHREDDED
>   PINCH OF PAPRIKA

Method

1. Preheat oven to 350°F.
2. Spread pitas with dressing. Top with corned beef, sauer-kraut, and cheese, and sprinkle with paprika. Place on cookie sheet.
3. Bake 8–10 minutes or until cheese is melted and bubbly.

   *400 milligrams or more of sodium per serving.
   **To make 4 servings, double the recipe.

Italian Pita Triangles

Yield: 8 appetizers

Serving Size: ¼ pita round

Exchanges:

Starch/Bread   ½

Nutrient Content per Serving:

CAL	39	PRO	2 (gm)
FAT	1 (gm)	CHO	6 (gm)
Na	98 (mg)	K	18 (mg)
Fiber	0 (gm)	Chol	0 (mg)

Ingredients

2 PITAS, ABOUT 6 INCHES IN DIAMETER

2 TEASPOONS MARGARINE, MELTED

¼ TEASPOON GARLIC POWDER

¼ TEASPOON BASIL OR OREGANO

1 TEASPOON GRATED PARMESAN CHEESE

Method

1. Preheat oven to 350°F.
2. Brush pitas with margarine.
3. Sprinkle with garlic powder, basil, and cheese.
4. Bake 8–10 minutes or until lightly browned. Cut into wedges; serve immediately.

Buffalo Style Chicken Wings

Yield: 28 individual wings
(7 appetizers or 4 main
courses)
Serving Size: 4 individual
wings
Exchanges:
Meat, medium-fat 3
Fat   2

Nutrient Content per Serving:

CAL	315	PRO	18 (gm)
FAT	26 (gm)	CHO	0 (gm)
Na	208 (mg)	K	124 (mg)
Fiber	0 (gm)	Chol	58 (mg)

Ingredients

NONSTICK VEGETABLE SPRAY
2½ POUNDS CHICKEN OR 14 WHOLE WINGS
4 TABLESPOONS UNSALTED MARGARINE, MELTED
5–6 TEASPOONS HOT PEPPER SAUCE
¼ TEASPOON SALT
⅛ TEASPOON CAYENNE PEPPER

Method

1. Preheat oven to 325°F. Spray cookie sheet.
2. Split wings at each joint and discard tips; pat dry.
3. Place on prepared pan and bake for 30 minutes.
4. Combine margarine, hot pepper sauce, salt, and cayenne pepper.
5. Place wings in covered container. Pour margarine mixture over wings, reserving some marinade. Cover and refrigerate at least 3 hours or overnight. Turn several times.
6. Before serving, broil wings 3–4 inches from heat for 5–6 minutes on each side, turning until brown and crisp; brush often with reserved marinade. Brush with any remaining marinade before serving.

Note: If spicier wings are desired, increase amount of hot pepper sauce.

Chile Con Queso

Yield: 1 cup (8 servings) Nutrient Content per Serving:

Serving Size: 2 tablespoons	CAL	94	PRO	6 (gm)
Exchanges:	FAT	7 (gm)	CHO	3 (gm)
Meat, medium-fat 1	Na	198 (mg)	K	79 (mg)
Vegetable 1	Fiber	1 (gm)	Chol	21 (mg)

Ingredients

NONSTICK VEGETABLE SPRAY
½ CUP ONION, CHOPPED
1 LARGE CLOVE GARLIC, MINCED
1 4-OUNCE CAN CHOPPED GREEN CHILES, DRAINED
1 8-OUNCE CAN STEWED TOMATOES, DRAINED
⅛ TEASPOON SALT
1½ CUPS MONTEREY JACK OR CHEDDAR OR COMBINATION OF CHEESES, SHREDDED

Method

1. Spray 2-quart saucepan with nonstick vegetable spray. Sauté onion and garlic until soft, about 3–4 minutes.
2. Stir in chiles, tomatoes, and salt; simmer 10 minutes.
3. Add cheese, stirring until melted. Serve with nacho chips, if desired.

Method–Microwave

1. Place onion and garlic in microwave-safe 2-quart saucepan (do not spray). Cook on high power, uncovered, 2–3 minutes or until softened.
2. Stir in chiles, tomatoes, and salt. Cook for 4 minutes on medium-high power, stirring once.
3. Stir in cheese until almost melted. Cook for 30 seconds on high power; serve with nacho chips*, if desired.

*Chips not included in exchange calculations.

Meat Strudel*

Yield: 10 slices

Serving Size: ½-inch slice

Exchanges:

Starch/Bread	1½
Meat, lean	1
Fat	3½

Nutrient Content per Serving:

CAL	336	PRO	12 (gm)
FAT	22 (gm)	CHO	23 (gm)
Na	443 (mg)	K	228 (mg)
Fiber	2 (gm)	Chol	55 (mg)

Ingredients

NONSTICK VEGETABLE SPRAY

1 SMALL ONION, CHOPPED FINE

1 POUND LEAN GROUND BEEF

1 MEDIUM GREEN PEPPER, SEEDED, CORED, AND CHOPPED FINE

1 MEDIUM TOMATO, PEELED, SEEDED, AND CHOPPED FINE

2 TABLESPOONS TOMATO PASTE

¼ CUP DRY RED WINE

1 TEASPOON WORCESTERSHIRE SAUCE

½ TEASPOON GARLIC POWDER

½ TEASPOON ONION POWDER

½ TEASPOON SALT

¼ TEASPOON BLACK PEPPER

1 PACKAGE (17¼ OUNCE) FROZEN PUFF PASTRY, THAWED AND WARMED TO ROOM TEMPERATURE

1 EGG YOLK MIXED WITH 1 TABLESPOON WATER

Method

1. Preheat oven to 425°F. Spray cookie sheet.
2. Heat vegetable spray in large skillet. Sauté onion until golden. Add ground beef and green pepper. Cook for 5 minutes. Stir in tomato and cook for 5 more minutes. Drain fat.
3. Stir in tomato paste, wine, Worcestershire sauce, and seasonings. Simmer for 5 more minutes.

4. Place two pieces of puff pastry together lengthwise to make a 15-by-10-inch rectangle. Spread beef mixture over dough, leaving a ½-inch border all around. Roll up widthwise, pinch ends and seam together, and place seam side down on prepared cookie sheet.
5. Brush with egg mixture. Bake for 20 minutes. Reduce heat to 350°F and bake for 30 more minutes.
6. Cut into slices and serve.

Method–Microwave (filling only)

1. Cook onion in 2-quart microwave saucepan for 4–5 minutes on high power or until golden. Set aside.
2. Put ground beef and pepper in plastic colander set in 2-quart microwave casserole. Stir in onion. Cook for 4–5 minutes. Drain fat. Put beef mixture in casserole.
3. Stir in tomatoes, tomato paste, wine, Worcestershire sauce, and seasonings. Cook for 6–7 minutes on medium-high power. Stir once.
4. Prepare dough following conventional directions. It is not recommended that the pastry be baked in the microwave.

*400 milligrams or more of sodium per serving.

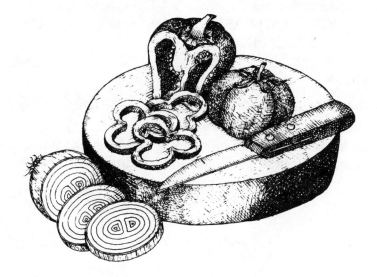

Caponata

Yield: 3 cups (12 servings)*	Nutrient Content per Serving:		
Serving Size: ¼ cup	CAL	35	PRO	1 (gm)
Exchanges:	FAT	2 (gm)	CHO	6 (gm)
Vegetable ½	Na	230 (mg)	K	168 (mg)
Fat ½	Fiber	2 (gm)	Chol	0 (mg)

Ingredients

  1 POUND EGGPLANT, PEELED AND CUBED
  1 TEASPOON COARSE SALT
    NONSTICK VEGETABLE SPRAY
  1 TABLESPOON OLIVE OIL
  1 MEDIUM ONION, THINLY SLICED
  1 LARGE CLOVE GARLIC, MINCED
  1 8¼-OUNCE CAN WHOLE TOMATOES, COARSELY
    CHOPPED AND UNDRAINED
  1 RIB CELERY, THINLY SLICED
  ½ YELLOW OR GREEN BELL PEPPER, DICED
  2 TABLESPOONS STUFFED GREEN OLIVES, SLICED
  1 TEASPOON CAPERS, DRAINED
  2 TEASPOONS SUGAR
  2 TABLESPOONS RED WINE VINEGAR
  2 LARGE FRESH BASIL LEAVES, SHREDDED, OR
    ½ TEASPOON DRIED BASIL

Method

1. Sprinkle eggplant with salt and place in colander to drain for
   1 hour. Pat dry with paper towels.
2. Spray large skillet with nonstick vegetable spray and add half
   the olive oil. Sauté eggplant over medium heat until tender,
   about 5 minutes; drain on paper towels.

3. Heat remaining oil in same skillet. Sauté onion and garlic until tender, about 5 minutes.
4. Stir in tomatoes with liquid, celery, peppers, olives, capers, sugar, vinegar, and basil. Cover; simmer for 30 minutes, stirring occasionally.
5. Stir in eggplant and cook uncovered for 5–10 minutes or until most of liquid is absorbed. Serve as an appetizer on toasted Italian bread, if desired.

*To make 6 cups (24 servings), double the recipe.

Deviled Meatballs

Yield: 24 meatballs

Serving Size: 4 meatballs plus sauce

Exchanges:

Meat, medium-fat 2

Fruit 1

Nutrient Content per Serving:

CAL	204	PRO	15 (gm)
FAT	11 (gm)	CHO	14 (gm)
Na	302 (mg)	K	208 (mg)
Fiber	0 (gm)	Chol	93 (mg)

Ingredients

NONSTICK VEGETABLE SPRAY

1 POUND LEAN GROUND BEEF

1 EGG

2 TABLESPOONS DRY BREAD CRUMBS

1 TEASPOON WORCESTERSHIRE SAUCE

1 TEASPOON DEHYDRATED MINCED ONION

1 TEASPOON DRIED PARSLEY

1/4 TEASPOON GARLIC POWDER

1/4 TEASPOON ONION POWDER

1/8 TEASPOON BLACK PEPPER

Sauce

1 10-OUNCE JAR UNSWEETENED GRAPE CONSERVE OR DIET GRAPE JELLY

2 TABLESPOONS PREPARED MUSTARD

2 TABLESPOONS CHILE SAUCE

4 TEASPOONS CORNSTARCH

2 TABLESPOONS WATER

Method

1. Preheat oven to 350°F. Spray a 2-quart baking dish with a nonstick vegetable spray.
2. Combine the second through tenth ingredients. Shape into 24 (¾-inch) meatballs. Bake for 15–20 minutes. Drain.
3. In a 2-quart saucepan, heat grape conserve, mustard, and chile sauce until melted.
4. Stir in cornstarch mixed with water. Cook until thickened, stirring constantly.
5. Stir in meatballs and coat with sauce. Heat for 5–10 minutes or until heated thoroughly.

Method–Microwave

1. Place meatballs in an 11-by-17-inch microwave-safe baking dish. Cover with waxed paper and cook for 4–5 minutes on high power. Drain.
2. In a 2-quart microwave-safe saucepan, combine conserve, mustard, and chile sauce. Cook for 3–4 minutes on high power or until melted. Stir once.
3. Stir in cornstarch mixed with water. Cook for 2 minutes on high power or until thickened. Stir in meatballs and coat with sauce.
4. Cover and cook for 4–5 minutes on high power or until heated thoroughly.

Note: Use a conserve that is naturally sweetened with no added sugar.

Miniature Cream Puff Hors D'oeuvres

Yield: 16 puffs (8 appetizer servings)

Serving Size: 2 puffs

Exchanges:

Starch/Bread ½
Meat, lean ½
Fat 1½

Nutrient Content per Serving:

CAL	137	PRO	6 (gm)
FAT	9 (gm)	CHO	8 (gm)
Na	287 (mg)	K	52 (mg)
Fiber	0 (gm)	Chol	91 (mg)

Ingredients

Paté à Choux

½ CUP WATER
4 TABLESPOONS UNSALTED MARGARINE
⅛ TEASPOON SALT
½ CUP FLOUR
2 EGGS

Filling

1 6½-OUNCE CAN CRAB MEAT, DRAINED AND FLAKED, OR 6 OUNCES CRAB MEAT, FLAKED
1 GREEN ONION, THINLY SLICED, OR 2 TABLESPOONS CHIVES, CHOPPED
2 TABLESPOONS PIMIENTO OR RED BELL PEPPER, CHOPPED
2 TABLESPOONS REDUCED-CALORIE MAYONNAISE
⅛ TEASPOON GARLIC POWDER

Method

1. Preheat oven to 425°F.
2. In 1-quart saucepan, bring water, margarine, and salt to a boil. Add the flour all at once. Vigorously stir over medium heat until dough leaves sides of pan and forms a ball.
3. Remove from heat; allow to cool for 5 minutes. Beat in eggs one at a time.
4. Drop by rounded teaspoonfuls onto an ungreased cookie sheet. Bake for 10 minutes; reduce heat to 350°F. Continue baking for 17–20 minutes or until golden brown. Cool on wire rack.
5. Slice a thin cap off top of puffs; remove doughy filaments. (May be kept several days in a tightly covered container.)
6. Combine all filling ingredients and mix well. Fill puffs and replace caps.

Tex-Mex Hot 'n' Spicy Artichoke Dip

Yield: 1 cup

Serving Size: 2 tablespoons

Exchanges:

		Nutrient Content per Serving:			
		CAL	38	PRO	1 (gm)
		FAT	3 (gm)	CHO	3 (gm)
Vegetable	½	Na	32 (mg)	K	55 (mg)
Fat	½	Fiber	0 (gm)	Chol	2 (mg)

Ingredients

> 1 14-OUNCE CAN ARTICHOKE HEARTS, DRAINED
> 1 4-OUNCE CAN CHOPPED CHILES
> 2 TABLESPOONS REDUCED-CALORIE MAYONNAISE
> 1 TABLESPOON LEMON JUICE
> 1 TABLESPOON OLIVE OIL
> ¼ TEASPOON HOT SAUCE

Method

1. Combine all ingredients in food processor or blender. Blend until smooth.
2. Heat in 1-quart saucepan for 5 minutes or until hot on low heat.
3. You can also serve dip cold. Serve with nacho chips, crackers, or cut-up vegetables.*

Method–Microwave

1. Heat dip in 2-quart microwave-safe saucepan for 3–5 minutes on medium-high power or until hot. Stir once.

*Chips or crackers not included in exchange calculations.

Quesadillas

Yield: 12 appetizers
Serving Size: 1 appetizer

Exchanges:
Starch/Bread ½
Meat, lean 1

Nutrient Content per Serving:

CAL	94	PRO	6 (gm)
FAT	4 (gm)	CHO	9 (gm)
Na	42 (mg)	K	40 (mg)
Fiber	0 (gm)	Chol	15 (mg)

Ingredients

    NONSTICK VEGETABLE SPRAY
1 WHOLE CHICKEN BREAST, COOKED, SKINNED, DEBONED, AND CUT INTO THIN STRIPS
1 TABLESPOON CHOPPED GREEN CHILES, DRAINED
⅓ CUP MONTEREY JACK CHEESE, SHREDDED
4 TEASPOONS MARGARINE, MELTED
6 (6-INCH) FLOUR TORTILLAS

Method

1. Preheat oven to 400°F. Spray cookie sheet with nonstick vegetable spray.
2. Combine chicken, chiles, and cheese. Place 2 heaping teaspoonfuls mixture on ½ of each tortilla. Brush edges with margarine; fold over and brush top with margarine.
3. Place on prepared cookie sheet. Bake for 10–15 minutes or until brown and crisp. Cut each tortilla in half; serve with salsa (page 384), if desired.

Salmon Mousse

Yield: 6 appetizers
Serving Size: 6 appetizers
Exchanges:
Meat, lean   2
Milk, skim   ½

Nutrient Content per Serving:

CAL	163	PRO	23 (gm)
FAT	5 (gm)	CHO	5 (gm)
Na	329 (mg)	K	459 (mg)
Fiber	0 (gm)	Chol	32 (mg)

Ingredients

NONSTICK VEGETABLE SPRAY
1 POUND SALMON FILLET, SKINNED AND DEBONED
3 EGG WHITES
1 TEASPOON DRIED DILL OR 1 TABLESPOON FRESH DILL
½ TEASPOON SALT
⅛ TEASPOON WHITE PEPPER
1 CUP EVAPORATED SKIM MILK, VERY COLD

Method

1. Preheat oven to 350°F. Spray 3-cup ring mold with nonstick vegetable spray.
2. Purée fish in food processor or food grinder. If using food processor, add egg whites, dill, salt, and pepper. With machine running, pour in milk through feed tube. Process just until blended. If using food grinder, grind fish into bowl. Combine with remaining ingredients. Blend until smooth.
3. Pour into prepared mold. Cover with waxed paper. Set into pan with about 1-inch hot water. Bake for 20–25 minutes or until firm to touch. May serve hot, at room temperature, or cold.

Calzone and Company* **

Yield: 8 appetizers
Serving Size: ½ calzone

	CHICKEN	SUN-DRIED TOMATOES	PINE NUTS	MUSHROOMS
CAL	334	355	297	271
FAT (gm)	8	12	7	5
Na (mg)	316	585	335	285
Fiber (gm)	2	3	2	3
PRO (gm)	18	11	10	8
CHO (gm)	47	51	48	48
K (mg)	165	209	102	123
Chol (mg)	33	25	8	2

	Exchanges			Exchanges	
Chicken	Starch/ Bread	3	Sun-dried Tomatoes	Starch/Bread	3
	Meat, lean	1½		Vegetable	1
				Fat	2
Pine Nuts	Starch/ Bread	3	Mushrooms	Starch/Bread	3
	Meat, medium- fat	½		Fat	½
	Fat	½			

Ingredients

Dough

    1 ENVELOPE YEAST
  1⅓ CUPS WARM WATER (105–115° F)
 3–4 CUPS ALL-PURPOSE FLOUR
    2 TABLESPOONS VEGETABLE OIL
    1 TEASPOON SALT
    1 TABLESPOON CORNMEAL
      NONSTICK VEGETABLE SPRAY
    1 TABLESPOON OLIVE OIL

Fillings—per 1 calzone

CHICKEN
  ½ CUP COOKED CHICKEN, CUBED
  1 TABLESPOON MOZZARELLA CHEESE,
    SHREDDED
  ¼ TEASPOON BASIL
  ¼ TEASPOON GARLIC POWDER

SUN-DRIED TOMATOES
  2 OUNCES SUN-DRIED TOMATOES PACKED IN
    OIL, DRAINED AND CHOPPED
  2 OUNCES CRUMBLED GOAT CHEESE,
    PREFERABLY MONTRACHET

PINE NUTS
  ¼ CUP MOZZARELLA CHEESE, SHREDDED
  1 TABLESPOON FRESH TOMATO, CHOPPED
  1 TABLESPOON FRESH BASIL OR 1 TEASPOON
    DRIED BASIL
  ¼ TEASPOON PINE NUTS, TOASTED

MUSHROOMS
2 TABLESPOONS RED PEPPER, CHOPPED
3 FRESH MUSHROOMS, SLICED
   NONSTICK VEGETABLE SPRAY
6 GRINDS BLACK PEPPER
1 TABLESPOON MOZZARELLA CHEESE, SHREDDED

Method

1. Dissolve yeast in warm water.
2. Mix together yeast and remaining ingredients (except non-stick vegetable spray and olive oil) either in food processor or by hand. If doing by hand, turn well-mixed dough out on floured board and knead about 10 minutes or until it is smooth and elastic.
3. Place dough in a well-sprayed bowl. Cover, put in warm place, and allow to double (1–1½ hours). Punch down. Divide dough into 4 pieces.
4. Roll each piece out to round shape about ¼-inch thick and 8–10 inches in diameter.
5. Place desired filling on half of dough, leaving a ½-inch border. Brush edges with water. Fold the other half over, pressing edges together with fingers to seal.
6. Lightly brush top with 1 tablespoon olive oil, cut 2 small slashes on top for steam vents, and place on cookie sheet lightly sprinkled with cornmeal.
7. Bake at 450°F for 15–20 minutes. Crust will be browned and puffed. Serve hot or at room temperature.
8. Fillings: Combine ingredients for each filling in a small bowl. All 4 fillings may be used, or only one, or any combination. Use your imagination. For filling 4: Sauté mushrooms and red pepper in well-sprayed skillet for about 5 minutes. Stir in pepper. Place filling on dough and sprinkle with mozzarella cheese.

Note: Calzone is an Italian pielike sandwich.

   *400 milligrams or more of sodium per serving, for Calzone with Sun-dried Tomatoes.
   **3 or more grams of fiber per serving, for Calzone with Sun-dried Tomatoes or Mushrooms.

Cottage Cheese Spread

Yield: 1½ cups
Serving Size: 1 tablespoon
for dip
Exchanges: Free food

Nutrient Content per Serving:

CAL	13	PRO	2 (gm)
FAT	0 (gm)	CHO	1 (gm)
Na	58 (mg)	K	16 (mg)
Fiber	0 (gm)	Chol	1 (mg)

Serving Size: ¼ cup, to
spread on bread
Exchanges:
Meat, lean   1

Nutrient Content per Serving:

CAL	52	PRO	8 (gm)
FAT	1 (gm)	CHO	2 (gm)
Na	230 (mg)	K	63 (mg)
Fiber	0 (gm)	Chol	5 (mg)

Ingredients

   1½ CUPS 2-PERCENT LOW-FAT COTTAGE CHEESE
    1 GREEN ONION, SLICED
    ⅛ TEASPOON PAPRIKA
    ⅛ TEASPOON WHITE PEPPER
    1 TEASPOON FRESH PARSLEY, CHOPPED

Method

1. Combine all ingredients in small bowl or food processor. Blend until smooth. Chill several hours.
2. Use as a spread; as a dip with vegetables; or as a quick take-along breakfast.

Steak Tartare

Yield: 1 cup
Serving Size: ¼ cup
Exchanges:
Meat, lean   1½

Nutrient Content per Serving:

CAL	86	PRO	11 (gm)
FAT	4 (gm)	CHO	1 (gm)
Na	182 (mg)	K	207 (mg)
Fiber	0 (gm)	Chol	94 (mg)

Ingredients

- ½ POUND TOP ROUND OR SIRLOIN STEAK, FAT REMOVED
- 1 EGG YOLK
- 1 CLOVE GARLIC, CHOPPED
- ¼ CUP ONION, CHOPPED
- ¼ TEASPOON SALT
- ⅛ TEASPOON BLACK PEPPER
- ½ TEASPOON DIJON MUSTARD
- 1 TEASPOON CAPERS, RINSED AND DRAINED
- 1 TEASPOON WORCESTERSHIRE SAUCE

Method

1. Cut meat into 1-inch cubes; discard all fat and sinews. Chop meat in food processor or meat grinder.
2. Combine meat with egg, garlic, onion, seasonings, mustard, capers, and Worcestershire sauce.
3. Mound mixture on plate; sprinkle with chopped parsley and chill. Serve with more chopped onions and capers if desired. Serve with cocktail rye, thinly sliced garlic toast, or low-salt crackers or use as part of a Danish *smørrebrød*.

Danish Smørrebrød—Open-Faced Sandwiches* **

Yield: 1 open-faced
sandwich or 4 appetizers
Serving Size: 1 sandwich

	SALMON	ROAST BEEF	STEAK TARTARE	HAM AND CHEESE
CAL	139	199	158	261
FAT (gm)	5	9	4	14
Na (mg)	331	686	800	808
Fiber (gm)	4	4	4	4
PRO (gm)	9	15	14	18
CHO (gm)	16	10	17	17
K (mg)	269	356	398	299
Chol (mg)	17	34	94	51

	Exchanges			Exchanges	
Salmon	Starch/		Roast Beef	Starch/	
	Bread	1		Bread	1
	Meat, lean	1		Meat, medium-fat	1
				Fat	1
Steak Tartare	Starch/		Ham and Cheese	Starch/	
	Bread	1		Bread	1
	Meat, lean	1½		Meat, medium-fat	2
				Fat	½

Ingredients

> GERMAN STYLE BLACK BREAD—1 SLICE PER
> SANDWICH (4-INCH SQUARE) OR CUT INTO 4
> APPETIZERS

Toppings

SALMON

½ TEASPOON SOFT MARGARINE
2 SLICES (1 OUNCE) SCOTTISH SMOKED SALMON
2 THIN SLICES ONION

ROAST BEEF

½ TEASPOON DIJON MUSTARD
1½ SLICES (1½ OUNCES) RARE ROAST BEEF
1 CORNICHON, SPLIT IN HALF AND FANNED

STEAK TARTARE

¼ CUP STEAK TARTARE (SEE PAGE 117)
1 OR 4 CAPERS OR 1 CORNICHON, SPLIT IN HALF
AND FANNED

HAM AND CHEESE

½ TEASPOON REDUCED-CALORIE MAYONNAISE
1 SLICE (1½ OUNCES) DANISH HAM
1 SLICE (1 OUNCE) SWISS OR DANISH CHEESE

Method

1. Depending on choice of topping, spread bread with desired
   spread, top with meat, and garnish. Serve 1 whole slice for
   a lunch sandwich or cut bread into 4 squares for appetizers
   or buffet. An assortment of smørrebrød cut into quarters set
   on a buffet table is pretty, delicious, and easy to make.

Note: Cornichons are small French pickles, packed in vinegar. A
small dill pickle may be substituted.

*400 milligrams or more of sodium per serving, for all variations
except salmon.
**3 grams or more of fiber per serving, for all variations.

Venison Antipasto*

Yield: 4 servings
Serving Size: ¼ of recipe
Exchanges:
Meat, medium-fat ½
Vegetable 1
Fat 3

Nutrient Content per Serving:

CAL	201	PRO	7 (gm)
FAT	18 (gm)	CHO	5 (gm)
Na	458 (mg)	K	203 (mg)
Fiber	1 (gm)	Chol	23 (mg)

Ingredients

- ¼ POUND VENISON SAUSAGE, CUT INTO CHUNKS, OR ¼-INCH STRIPS
- 1 OUNCE PROVOLONE OR LOW-FAT MOZZARELLA CHEESE, CUT INTO CUBES
- 4–5 CHERRY TOMATOES, SPLIT
- ¼ CUP FRESH MUSHROOMS, SLICED
- 1 SMALL YELLOW OR GREEN PEPPER, CUT INTO THIN STRIPS
- ⅓ CUP ONION, CUT INTO RINGS, SAUTÉED
- ¼ CUP BASIC VINAIGRETTE (SEE PAGE 165)

Method

1. Combine all ingredients except for dressing in a small bowl. Gently toss in dressing. Chill before serving.
2. Serve with low-salt crackers, or slices of French bread.

*400 milligrams or more of sodium per serving.

Seviche

Yield: 4 main-course or 8
appetizer servings
Serving Size: ¼ of recipe
for main course; ⅛ for
appetizer
Exchanges:

Meat, lean	1
Vegetable	2

Nutrient Content per Serving:

CAL	111	PRO	11 (gm)
FAT	4 (gm)	CHO	9 (gm)
Na	250 (mg)	K	340 (mg)
Fiber	1 (gm)	Chol	23 (mg)

Ingredients

    8 OUNCES SEA SCALLOPS, CUT IN HALF, OR BAY
      SCALLOPS OR FIRM WHITE FISH SUCH AS
      HALIBUT, HADDOCK, OR TURBOT
      LIME JUICE*
    1 SMALL, FIRM TOMATO, SEEDED AND CHOPPED
    1 GREEN ONION, SLICED
    1 4-OUNCE CAN CHOPPED GREEN CHILES,
      DRAINED
    1 TABLESPOON VEGETABLE OIL
    ¼ TEASPOON SALT
    4 DASHES TABASCO SAUCE
    2 TABLESPOONS FRESH CILANTRO, CHOPPED

Method

1. Place scallops in shallow dish (glass or porcelain). Cover with
   lime juice. Marinate covered in refrigerator at least 4 hours or
   overnight, stirring at least once.
2. Add remaining ingredients; mix gently. Serve chilled.

   *1 cup of lime juice was used in recipe analysis.

Chopped Eggs and Onions

Yield: 1 cup (8 servings)
Serving Size: 2 tablespoons
Exchanges:
Vegetable   ½
Fat   ½

Nutrient Content per Serving:

CAL	40	PRO	2 (gm)
FAT	3 (gm)	CHO	2 (gm)
Na	84 (mg)	K	60 (mg)
Fiber	1 (gm)	Chol	68 (mg)

Ingredients

NONSTICK VEGETABLE SPRAY
2 MEDIUM ONIONS, CUT INTO 8 WEDGES
2 HARDCOOKED EGGS
2 TEASPOONS CORN OIL
¼ TEASPOON SALT
¼ TEASPOON GARLIC POWDER
⅛ TEASPOON GROUND WHITE PEPPER

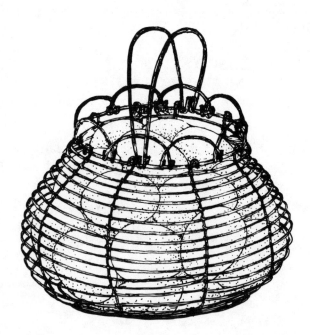

Method

1. Spray a medium skillet with nonstick vegetable spray. Sauté onions over medium heat until soft and lightly browned, about 15 minutes.
2. In food processor or by hand, finely chop eggs and onions in separate batches.
3. Combine eggs, onions, and remaining ingredients; chill. Serve with crackers or cocktail rye bread, if desired.

Method–Microwave

1. Place onions in 1½-quart microwave-safe casserole (do not spray). Cover; cook on high power for 8–10 minutes or until soft, stirring once.
2. To cook eggs, drop each egg into a custard cup. Pierce yolk with toothpick. Cover tightly with plastic wrap. Cook for 40–45 seconds on high power. Let stand, covered, for 3–4 minutes to finish cooking.
3. Proceed as in steps 2 and 3 above.

Soups

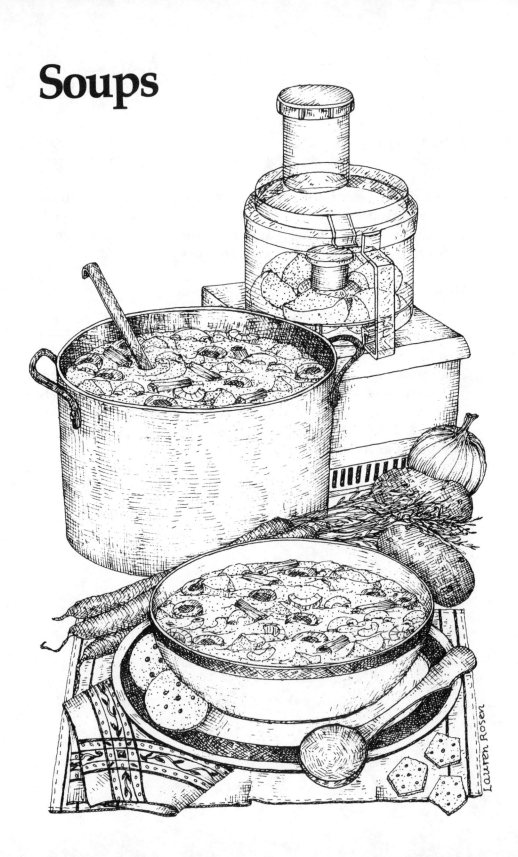

*M*ore than any solid food, soups seem to quickly permeate every nook and cranny of your body— warm and nourishing in wintertime, cool as an icy swim on a hot summer day.

Minestrone* **

Yield: 10 cups
Serving Size: 1 cup
Exchanges:
Starch/Bread 1
Vegetable 4
Fat ½

Nutrient Content per Serving:

CAL	208	PRO	13 (gm)
FAT	4 (gm)	CHO	33 (gm)
Na	883 (mg)	K	851 (mg)
Fiber	8 (gm)	Chol	3 (mg)

Ingredients

1 CUP ONION, CHOPPED
3 CLOVES GARLIC, CHOPPED
1 TABLESPOON OLIVE OIL
2 QUARTS BEEF BROTH†
1 CUP ZUCCHINI, SLICED
¾ CUP CARROT, CHOPPED
2 RIBS CELERY, CHOPPED
1 28-OUNCE CAN ITALIAN PLUM TOMATOES
   WITH JUICE, SLIGHTLY CRUSHED
2 19-OUNCE CANS CANNELLINI BEANS, DRAINED,
   OR ANY WHITE COOKED BEAN
1 CUP WHITE CABBAGE, SHREDDED
1 CUP POTATO, PEELED AND CUBED
1 TEASPOON BASIL
½ TEASPOON BLACK PEPPER
2 TABLESPOONS TOMATO PASTE
1 10-OUNCE PACKAGE FROZEN ITALIAN-CUT
   STRING BEANS
½ CUP ELBOW MACARONI
½ CUP GRATED PARMESAN CHEESE

Method

1. In large stock pot, sauté onion and garlic in olive oil until soft but not brown (about 10 minutes). Add remaining ingredients except Italian green beans, pasta, and Parmesan cheese.
2. Bring to boil; cover; reduce heat and simmer for 1 hour.
3. Stir in beans, pasta, and half the Parmesan cheese. Simmer for additional 15 minutes.
4. Taste for seasoning. Serve hot or at room temperature. Serve in bowls with remaining Parmesan cheese.

Method–Microwave

1. Combine onion, garlic, and olive oil in 4-quart microwave-safe casserole. Cook for 2 minutes on high power. Stir in potatoes; cover and cook for 3–4 minutes on high power.
2. Stir in remaining ingredients except for string beans, pasta, and Parmesan cheese. Cover. Cook for 45–50 minutes on medium power, stirring occasionally.
3. Add beans, pasta, and half of Parmesan cheese. Cook for 8–12 minutes on high power or until pasta is just tender. Allow to stand covered for 5 minutes before serving.
4. Serve with remaining Parmesan cheese.

*400 milligrams or more of sodium per serving.
**3 grams or more of fiber per serving.
†For reduced salt and fat, use homemade beef broth.

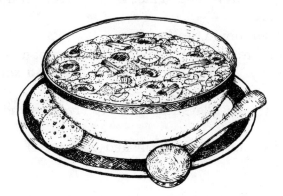

Tortilla Soup* **

Yield: 2 servings†
Serving Size: 1 cup
Exchanges:
Starch/Bread 2
Meat, lean 2

Nutrient Content per Serving:

CAL	269	PRO	18 (gm)
FAT	8 (gm)	CHO	33 (gm)
Na	1,974 (mg)	K	612 (mg)
Fiber	3 (gm)	Chol	10 (mg)

Key Source Nutrients:
Vitamin B_{12} 5 (mcg)

Ingredients

3 6-INCH FLOUR TORTILLAS, CUT INTO ½-INCH STRIPS
NONSTICK VEGETABLE SPRAY
1 4-OUNCE CAN WHOLE TOMATOES
½ SMALL ONION, CHOPPED
½ CLOVE GARLIC, CHOPPED
2 CUPS CHICKEN BROTH‡
¼ TEASPOON SALT
1 TABLESPOON CILANTRO
2 TABLESPOONS MONTEREY JACK CHEESE, SHREDDED

Method

1. Fry tortilla strips in heated skillet well sprayed with nonstick vegetable spray.
2. Purée tomatoes, onion, and garlic.
3. Bring chicken broth to a boil in 2-quart saucepan. Stir in tomato purée, salt, and cilantro. Reduce heat and simmer for 10 minutes.
4. Add half of the tortilla strips to soup; reserve the rest for garnish.
5. Serve in individual bowls, garnished with tortilla strips and cheese.

Method–Microwave

1. Heat chicken broth in a 2-quart microwave saucepan until boiling, about 5–6 minutes on high power.
2. Stir in tomato purée, salt, and cilantro. Cook for 5 minutes on medium-high power; stir once.
3. Add half of the tortilla strips; reserve the rest for garnish.
4. Serve in individual bowls, garnished with tortilla strips and cheese.

*400 milligrams or more of sodium per serving.
**3 grams or more of fiber per serving.
†To make 4 servings, double the recipe.
‡For reduced salt and fat, use homemade chicken broth.

Dutch Apple Soup*

Yield: 4 servings	Nutrient Content per Serving:			
Serving Size: 1 cup	CAL	103	PRO	0 (gm)
Exchanges:	FAT	1 (gm)	CHO	23 (gm)
Fruit 1½	Na	4 (mg)	K	194 (mg)
	Fiber	3 (gm)	Chol	0 (mg)

Ingredients

    1 POUND TART COOKING APPLES, UNPEELED,
      CORED, CUT INTO EIGHTHS
    1 QUART WATER PLUS 1½ TEASPOONS WATER
    ½ CINNAMON STICK
    6 PACKETS SUGAR SUBSTITUTE
 1½ TEASPOONS LEMON JUICE
    ¼ TEASPOON LEMON PEEL
      PINCH CARDAMOM
 1½ TEASPOONS CORNSTARCH
    ¼ CUP SAUTERNE WINE
    ⅛ CUP DARK SEEDLESS RAISINS

Method

1. Combine apples with water, cinnamon stick, sugar substitute, lemon juice, lemon peel, and cardamom.
2. Bring to boil; stir in cornstarch mixed with 1½ teaspoons water. Continue boiling until apples are fork tender. Remove cinnamon stick.
3. Purée apples without liquid in food processor or food mill and return to pot.
4. Stir in wine and raisins; cook for 3 more minutes.
5. Serve hot or cold.

Method–Microwave

1. Combine apples with hot water, cinnamon stick, sugar substitute, lemon juice, lemon peel, and cardamom in 3-quart microwave-safe casserole. Cover; cook for 6 minutes on high power.
2. Stir in cornstarch mixed with 1½ teaspoons water. Cover; cook for 6–8 minutes on high power or until apples are tender.
3. Purée apples.
4. Stir in wine and raisins. Uncover; cook for 3 more minutes on high power.

*3 grams or more of fiber per serving.

Vichyssoise*

Yield: 9 cups
Serving Size: 1 cup
Exchanges:

		Nutrient Content per Serving:		
		CAL	139	PRO	11 (gm)
		FAT	2 (gm)	CHO	20 (gm)
Starch/Bread	½	Na	1,208 (mg)	K	607 (mg)
Vegetable	3	Fiber	2 (gm)	Chol	3 (mg)
Fat	½				

Ingredients

    3 CUPS LEEKS (2 LARGE), SLICED, WHITE PART
      ONLY
    3 CUPS POTATOES (2 LARGE), PEELED AND
      SLICED
    6 CUPS CHICKEN BROTH (1 46-OUNCE CAN)**
    1 CUP EVAPORATED SKIM MILK
    ½ TEASPOON SALT
    ¼ TEASPOON WHITE PEPPER
    2 TEASPOONS FRESH CHIVES, MINCED, OR
      1 TEASPOON DRIED CHIVES

Method

1. In large saucepan, combine leeks, potatoes, and broth. Cook, covered, over medium heat until vegetables are tender, about 30 minutes.
2. Purée through food mill, food processor, or blender in batches, until smooth. Chill.
3. Stir in evaporated skim milk, salt, and pepper. Serve garnished with chives.

Method–Microwave

1. In 2-quart microwave-safe casserole, cook potatoes, covered with plastic wrap, for 8–10 minutes on high power or until soft. Stir once. Set aside.
2. In same casserole, stir in leeks. Cover with plastic wrap and cook for 4–5 minutes on high power or until soft. Stir once.
3. Stir in broth and potatoes. Cook uncovered for 6–8 minutes on high power or until heated thoroughly.
4. Purée; then chill. Stir in evaporated skim milk and seasonings. Serve garnished with chives.

Note: Vichyssoise is a delightful soup to serve in the summer. It is very cool and refreshing. May be served hot, if desired. May also be frozen before milk is added.

    *400 milligrams or more of sodium per serving.
    **For reduced salt and fat, use homemade chicken broth.

Plantation Peanut Soup* **

Yield: 5 servings
Serving Size: 1 cup
Exchanges:
Meat, medium-fat 2
Vegetable 3
Fat 2

Nutrient Content per Serving:

CAL	314	PRO	19 (gm)
FAT	21 (gm)	CHO	15 (gm)
Na	1,487 (mg)	K	730 (mg)
Fiber	4 (gm)	Chol	3 (mg)

Ingredients

- 1 SMALL ONION, CHOPPED
- 2 RIBS CELERY, CHOPPED
- 2 TABLESPOONS MARGARINE
- 3 TABLESPOONS ALL-PURPOSE FLOUR
- 4 CUPS CHICKEN BROTH†
- 1 CUP SKIM MILK
- ½ CUP PEANUT BUTTER
- 1 TEASPOON WORCESTERSHIRE SAUCE
- ¼ CUP DRY-ROASTED, UNSALTED PEANUTS, CHOPPED

Method

1. Sauté onion and celery in margarine until tender, about 5 minutes, in 5-quart saucepan.
2. Stir in flour. Gradually stir in chicken broth and milk. Cook and stir until soup slightly thickens and comes to a boil.
3. Stir in peanut butter, stirring well until blended. Reduce heat; stir in Worcestershire sauce; heat for 5 more minutes.
4. Serve hot in individual bowls; sprinkle with chopped peanuts.

Method–Microwave

1. Combine onion, celery, and margarine in 4-quart microwave-safe casserole. Cook covered for 3–5 minutes on high power; stir once.
2. Stir in flour. Gradually stir in chicken broth and milk. Cook for 8–10 minutes (or until slightly thickened), on medium-high power; stir once.
3. Add peanut butter, stirring until well blended. Stir in Worcestershire sauce. Cook 5 minutes on high power; stir once.
4. Serve hot in individual bowls; sprinkle with chopped peanuts.

    *400 milligrams or more of sodium per serving.
    **3 grams or more of fiber per serving.
    †For reduced salt and fat, use homemade chicken broth.

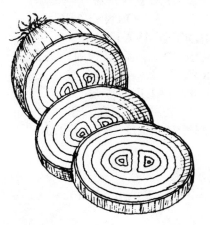

Cream of Chicken and Mushroom Soup*

Yield: 4 servings
Serving Size: 1 cup
Exchanges:
Starch/Bread   ½
Meat, medium-
   fat   3½
Vegetable   1

Nutrient Content per Serving:

CAL	334	PRO	29 (gm)
FAT	18 (gm)	CHO	12 (gm)
Na	1,905 (mg)	K	689 (mg)
Fiber	0 (gm)	Chol	54 (mg)

Key Source Nutrients:
Vitamin B_{12} 5 (mcg)

Ingredients

4 TABLESPOONS MARGARINE
1 CUP FRESH MUSHROOMS, SLICED
4 CUPS CHICKEN BROTH**
4 TABLESPOONS CORNSTARCH
3 TABLESPOONS WATER
1 CUP COOKED CHICKEN, DICED
¼ TEASPOON TARRAGON
¼ TEASPOON SALT
¼ TEASPOON WHITE PEPPER
¼ CUP EVAPORATED SKIM MILK

Method

1. Melt margarine in a 2½-quart saucepan. Sauté mushrooms for 3 minutes.
2. Pour in chicken broth, bring to boil. Whisk in cornstarch mixed with water. Whisk constantly until thickened.
3. Stir in chicken, seasonings, and evaporated skim milk. Simmer for 10 minutes.

Method–Microwave

1. Melt margarine in 3-quart microwave-safe casserole. Cook mushrooms for 2 minutes on high power.
2. Pour in chicken broth. Whisk in cornstarch mixed with water. Cook for 10–12 minutes on medium-high power or until thickened.
3. Stir in chicken, seasonings, and evaporated skim milk. Cook for 8–10 minutes on medium-high power or until heated thoroughly.

*400 milligrams or more of sodium per serving.
**For reduced salt and fat, use homemade chicken broth.

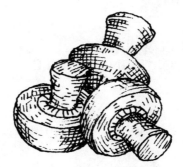

Chinese Chicken Soup with Chicken Balls*

Yield: 2 servings**
Serving Size: 1 cup
Exchanges:
Meat, lean   4

Nutrient Content per Serving:

CAL	220	PRO	33 (gm)
FAT	8 (gm)	CHO	2 (gm)
Na	1,145 (mg)	K	482 (mg)
Fiber	0 (gm)	Chol	81 (mg)

Ingredients

Chicken Balls

½ POUND RAW CHICKEN, GROUND
½ GREEN ONION, FINELY CHOPPED
1 EGG WHITE
¼ TEASPOON SALT
⅛ TEASPOON GROUND GINGER
PINCH OF WHITE PEPPER

Broth

2 CUPS CHICKEN BROTH⁺
½ GREEN ONION, THINLY SLICED

Method

1. Combine all ingredients for chicken balls. Form into 1-inch balls. Set aside.
2. Put broth with sliced green onion in 2-quart saucepan. Bring to a boil. Drop 6–8 chicken balls into boiling broth. Reduce heat to simmer and cook for 3 minutes.
3. Remove with a slotted spoon; keep warm while cooking remaining chicken balls.
4. Add all chicken balls back to broth; heat thoroughly.

Method–Microwave

1. In 2-quart microwave-safe saucepan, bring broth and onions to a boil (about 5–6 minutes on high power).
2. Drop in balls and cook for 1½ minutes on high power. Let stand for 2 minutes before serving.

*400 milligrams or more of sodium per serving.
**To make 4 servings, double the recipe.
†For reduced salt and fat, use homemade chicken broth.

Pumpkin Soup* **

Yield: 5 servings
Serving Size: 1 cup
Exchanges:
Starch/Bread 1
Fat ½

Nutrient Content per Serving:

CAL	104	PRO	7 (gm)
FAT	3 (gm)	CHO	13 (gm)
Na	183 (mg)	K	489 (mg)
Fiber	3 (gm)	Chol	2 (mg)

Key Source Nutrients:
Vitamin A   21,688 (IU)

Ingredients

    2 TEASPOONS MARGARINE
    1 MEDIUM ONION, CHOPPED
    1 16-OUNCE CAN UNSWEETENED PUMPKIN
      (2 CUPS)
    2 CUPS CHICKEN BROTH†
    ¼ TEASPOON SALT
    ½ TEASPOON SUGAR
    ⅛ TEASPOON CLOVES
    1 CUP SKIM MILK

Method

1. Melt margarine in 2-quart saucepan. Sauté onion until softened, about 10 minutes.
2. Add pumpkin, broth, salt, sugar, and cloves; mix well.
3. Bring to a boil; reduce heat and simmer for 15 minutes.
4. Purée in food mill or food processor. Return to saucepan.
5. Add milk; heat thoroughly but do not boil. Serve with rye croutons, if desired.

Method–Microwave

1. Place onions and margarine in microwave-safe 2-quart casserole. Cook for 4–6 minutes on high power or until soft, stirring once.
2. Add pumpkin, broth, salt, sugar, and cloves. Cook for 8–10 minutes on medium-high power or until heated thoroughly.
3. Purée in food mill or food processor; return to casserole.
4. Stir in milk. Cook for 8–10 minutes on medium-high power or until heated thoroughly, but not boiling.

*400 milligrams or more of sodium per serving.
**3 grams or more of fiber per serving.
†For reduced salt and fat, use homemade chicken broth.

Cold Cherry Soup

Yield: 3 cups
Serving Size: ½ cup
Exchanges:
Fruit   1

Nutrient Content per Serving:

CAL	72	PRO	2 (gm)
FAT	1 (gm)	CHO	15 (gm)
Na	19 (mg)	K	220 (mg)
Fiber	1 (gm)	Chol	2 (mg)

Ingredients

- 1 POUND FRESH OR FROZEN CHERRIES, PITTED (IF FROZEN, DEFROST AND DRAIN)
- ½ CUP SAUTERNE WINE
- 1 CUP WATER
- 2 TEASPOONS ORANGE ZEST, GRATED
- 1½ TEASPOONS HONEY
- 3 WHOLE CLOVES
- 1 CINNAMON STICK
- ¼ TEASPOON GROUND GINGER
- ⅔ CUP PLAIN LOW-FAT YOGURT
- 2 PACKETS SUGAR SUBSTITUTE

Method

1. Combine first 8 ingredients in medium saucepan. Bring to a boil; cover and simmer until fruit is soft, about 40 minutes.
2. Cool; remove cloves and cinnamon stick. Purée cherries with liquid in batches; strain.
3. Whisk in yogurt and sugar substitute; chill.

Method–Microwave

1. Combine first 8 ingredients in 2-quart microwave-safe casserole (use hot water). Cover; cook on high power for 7–8 minutes or until fruit is soft, stirring once.
2. Cool; remove cloves and cinnamon stick. Purée cherries with liquid in batches; strain.
3. Whisk in yogurt and sugar substitute; chill.

Cold Roasted Red Pepper Soup* **

Yield: 4 servings
Serving Size: ¾ cup
Exchanges:
Vegetable   1
Milk, low-fat   ½
Fat   ½

Nutrient Content per Serving:
CAL   109   PRO   11 (gm)
FAT   4 (gm) CHO   9 (gm)
Na   1,347 (mg) K   541 (mg)
Fiber   3 (gm) Chol   4 (mg)

Key Source Nutrients:
Ascorbic acid   103 (mg)

Ingredients

    1 POUND RED BELL PEPPERS
    ½ CUP ONION, CHOPPED
    1 TEASPOON MARGARINE
    3 CUPS CHICKEN BROTH†
    ½ CUP PLAIN LOW-FAT YOGURT
    ¼ TEASPOON SALT

Method

1. Broil peppers until skins are burnt on all sides. Place in a paper bag for 10 minutes to loosen skin. Peel and seed peppers. Coarsely chop.
2. Sauté onion in margarine in 2-quart saucepan.
3. Add peppers and broth; simmer for 15 minutes. Purée in blender or food processor.
4. Cool; stir in yogurt and salt; chill.

   *400 milligrams or more of sodium per serving.
   **3 grams or more of fiber per serving.
   †For reduced salt and fat, use homemade chicken broth.

Salads

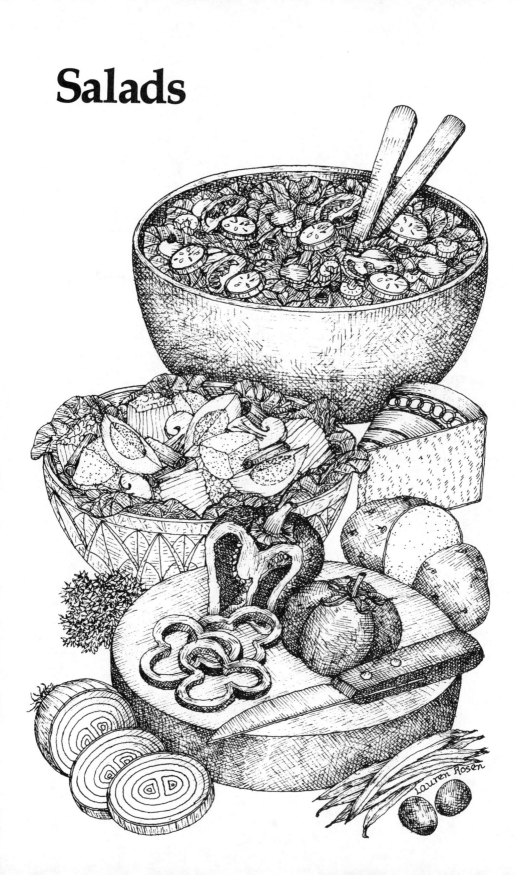

Lauren Rosen

*A*s any salad bar lover can attest, the days when "salad" meant a wedge of lettuce and a slice of tomato are long gone. Fruits, pasta, gelatin, fish, and meats are salad staples, along with crispy green vegetables. Light and refreshing, salads deserve to be enjoyed.

Try the Cobb Salad with Louis Dressing—creamy avocado and crunchy bacon team up with chicken, tomatoes, and a zesty yogurt dressing. Or try Fresh Tuna Salad Niçoise, easy to make and delicious.

Fresh California Pear Salad*

Yield: 2 cups (4 servings)
Serving Size: ½ cup
Exchanges:
Fruit   1
Milk, low-fat   ½
Fat   1½

Nutrient Content per Serving:

CAL	176	PRO	6 (gm)
FAT	10 (gm)	CHO	18 (gm)
Na	281 (mg)	K	340 (mg)
Fiber	3 (gm)	Chol	9 (mg)

Ingredients

8 OUNCES PLAIN LOW-FAT YOGURT
1 TEASPOON GROUND GINGER
1 CLOVE GARLIC, CHOPPED (ABOUT ¼ TEASPOON)
½ TEASPOON DIJON MUSTARD
¼ TEASPOON SALT
⅛ TEASPOON WHITE PEPPER
¼ TEASPOON BROWN SUGAR SUBSTITUTE
¼ CUP REDUCED-CALORIE MAYONNAISE
2 RIPE BARTLETT PEARS, CORED AND DICED
1 GREEN ONION, SLICED
1 CELERY RIB, THINLY SLICED
¼ CUP UNSALTED, DRY-ROASTED PEANUTS, CHOPPED
2 TEASPOONS LEMON JUICE

Method

1. Combine yogurt, ginger, garlic, mustard, salt, pepper, and brown sugar substitute.
2. Stir in mayonnaise and reserve.
3. Combine pears with lemon juice, onion, celery, and peanuts. Stir in yogurt mixture. Combine gently. Chill before serving.

*3 grams or more of fiber per serving.

Herring Supreme Salad*

Yield: 4 entrées or 8 appetizers

Serving Size: 1 cup

Exchanges:

Meat, lean	2
Vegetable	1
Fruit	1
Fat	1½

Nutrient Content per Serving:

CAL	269	PRO	16 (gm)
FAT	14 (gm)	CHO	21 (gm)
Na	143 (mg)	K	274 (mg)
Fiber	4 (gm)	Chol	62 (mg)

Key Source Nutrients:
Vitamin A   10,261 (IU)

Serving Size: ½ cup

Exchanges:

Meat, lean	½
Fruit	1
Fat	1

Nutrient Content per Serving:

CAL	179	PRO	11 (gm)
FAT	10 (gm)	CHO	14 (gm)
Na	95 (mg)	K	183 (mg)
Fiber	2 (gm)	Chol	41 (mg)

Key Source Nutrients:
Vitamin A   6,841 (IU)

Ingredients

 1 12-OUNCE JAR HERRING IN WINE SAUCE, RINSED AND DRAINED
 ½ CUP REDUCED-CALORIE SOUR CREAM
 ¼ CUP REDUCED-CALORIE MAYONNAISE
 2 CARROTS, PEELED AND SHREDDED
 ½ LARGE GREEN PEPPER, CORED AND DICED
 1 MEDIUM ONION, DICED
 1 PACKET SUGAR SUBSTITUTE
 1½ TEASPOONS CELERY SEED
 1 TABLESPOON LEMON JUICE
 1 GOLDEN DELICIOUS APPLE, PEELED, CORED, AND DICED

Method

1. Cut herring into very small pieces. Combine with remaining ingredients. Add additional sugar substitute if sweeter salad is desired.
2. Best when chilled several hours before serving.
3. Serve in pretty glass bowl with crackers or cocktail rye bread.

*3 grams or more of fiber per entrée serving.

Fresh Tuna Salad*

Yield: 6 servings
Serving Size: 1 cup
Exchanges:
Starch/Bread   1½
Meat, lean   1

Nutrient Content per Serving:

CAL	182	PRO	13 (gm)
FAT	4 (gm)	CHO	23 (gm)
Na	641 (mg)	K	253 (mg)
Fiber	2 (gm)	Chol	23 (mg)

Ingredients

- 3 CUPS COOKED PASTA, WAGON WHEELS OR ANY SMALL SHAPE (5 OUNCES DRY)
- ½ POUND FRESH TUNA, BROILED, COOLED, AND CUBED (OR 1 6½-OUNCE CAN WATER-PACKED TUNA, DRAINED)
- 1 CUP UNPEELED ZUCCHINI (1 MEDIUM ZUCCHINI), CUBED
- ½ CUP RED OR GREEN PEPPER, CUBED
- 1 CUP BROCCOLI FLORETS, BLANCHED
- ¼ CUP CARROT, THINLY SLICED
- ⅓ CUP RED ONION, CHOPPED
- ¼ CUP SWEET GHERKIN PICKLES, SLICED
- ¼ CUP REDUCED-CALORIE MAYONNAISE
- 1 TABLESPOON REDUCED-CALORIE SOUR CREAM
- 1½ TEASPOONS DRIED TARRAGON
- ¾ TEASPOON SALT
- ½ TEASPOON CHERVIL
- ¼ TEASPOON BLACK PEPPER

Method

1. Combine pasta, tuna, vegetables, onion, and pickles in a large bowl. Stir in mayonnaise, sour cream, and seasonings.
2. Serve at room temperature.

*400 milligrams or more of sodium per serving.

Tuna Niçoise

Yield: 6 servings
Serving Size: ¾ cup
Exchanges:
Meat, lean 1
Vegetable 2
Fat ½

Nutrient Content per Serving:

CAL	131	PRO	11 (gm)
FAT	6 (gm)	CHO	8 (gm)
Na	334 (mg)	K	264 (mg)
Fiber	2 (gm)	Chol	65 (mg)

Ingredients

1 6½-OUNCE CAN WATER-PACKED TUNA,
DRAINED AND FLAKED
1 MEDIUM POTATO, COOKED, PEELED, AND CUT
INTO WEDGES
1 HARDBOILED EGG, PEELED AND QUARTERED
1 CUP MUSHROOMS, SLICED
1 9-OUNCE PACKAGE FROZEN WHOLE GREEN
BEANS, BLANCHED
1 TEASPOON CAPERS, RINSED AND DRAINED
⅓ CUP BASIC VINAIGRETTE DRESSING (SEE PAGE
165)
LETTUCE

Method

1. Combine all ingredients except vinaigrette and lettuce.
2. Gently toss dressing with tuna mixture.
3. Chill. Before serving, taste for seasonings. Line a pretty glass
   bowl with lettuce leaves; add Tuna Niçoise and serve.

Cobb Salad with Louis Dressing*

Yield: 4 servings
Serving Size: 1 cup plus 3
tablespoons dressing plus
egg
Exchanges:
Meat, medium-
    fat   2½
Vegetable   2

Nutrient Content per Serving:

CAL	243	PRO	21 (gm)
FAT	12 (gm)	CHO	13 (gm)
Na	398 (mg)	K	772 (mg)
Fiber	3 (gm)	Chol	112 (mg)

Ingredients

- 2 CUPS EACH TORN HEAD AND RED LEAF LETTUCE
- 1 HARDCOOKED EGG, CHOPPED
- 1 WHOLE BONELESS CHICKEN BREAST, COOKED AND CUT INTO SMALL CUBES (1 CUP)
- 4 STRIPS BACON, COOKED CRISP AND CRUMBLED
- 1 SMALL RIPE AVOCADO, CUBED
- ½ CUP RED ONION, CHOPPED
- 2 FIRM SMALL TOMATOES OR PLUM TOMATOES, SEEDED AND CHOPPED

Louis Dressing (¾ cup)

- ¾ CUP PLAIN LOW-FAT YOGURT
- 4 TEASPOONS CHILE SAUCE
- 1 TEASPOON DRIED PARSLEY FLAKES
- ¼ TEASPOON SALT
- ⅛ TEASPOON GARLIC POWDER
- ⅛ TEASPOON BLACK PEPPER
- 2–4 DROPS TABASCO SAUCE

Method

1. Line a large, flat bowl with mixed lettuce.
2. Place egg, chicken, bacon, avocado, onion, and tomato in straight rows on top of lettuce.
3. Combine all ingredients for dressing and serve with salad.

*3 grams or more of fiber per serving.

Tofu "Egg" Salad

Yield: 2 servings
Serving Size: ¾ cup
Exchanges:
Meat, medium-fat 1
Vegetable 1
Fat ½

Nutrient Content per Serving:
CAL 120   PRO 10 (gm)
FAT 8 (gm)   CHO 6 (gm)
Na 250 (mg)   K 191 (mg)
Fiber 1 (gm)   Chol 3 (mg)

Ingredients

   ½ POUND FIRM TOFU, WELL DRAINED
   1 RIB CELERY, FINELY CHOPPED
   1 GREEN ONION, FINELY CHOPPED
   1 TABLESPOON REDUCED-CALORIE MAYONNAISE
   1 TEASPOON DIJON MUSTARD
   ⅛ TEASPOON SALT
     PINCH OF WHITE PEPPER
   2 TABLESPOONS RED BELL PEPPER, CHOPPED

Method

1. In food processor fitted with steel blade or by hand, finely chop the tofu.
2. Stir in remaining ingredients. Chill before serving.

Variation: Add ⅛ teaspoon curry powder.

Dilled Potato Salad

Yield: 4 servings*
Serving Size: ½ cup
Exchanges:
Starch/Bread 1
Fat ½

Nutrient Content per Serving:
CAL 102 PRO 4 (gm)
FAT 3 (gm) CHO 16 (gm)
Na 177 (mg) K 453 (mg)
Fiber 2 (gm) Chol 68 (mg)

Ingredients

3 MEDIUM OR 6 SMALL RED POTATOES,
QUARTERED AND BOILED IN JACKETS
1 HARDCOOKED EGG, FINELY CHOPPED
¼ TEASPOON SALT
PINCH OF BLACK PEPPER
1 TEASPOON FRESH DILL, CHOPPED, OR
½ TEASPOON DRIED DILL
¼ CUP REDUCED-CALORIE SOUR CREAM

Method

1. Cool potatoes, peel, and cut in chunks.
2. Toss potatoes with remaining ingredients. Chill.

*To make 8 servings, double the recipe.

Chicken Salad à la King* **

Yield: 6 servings
Serving Size: ⅙ wedge
Exchanges:
Starch/Bread ½
Meat, lean 2
Fruit 1
Fat 1

Nutrient Content per Serving:
CAL 252 PRO 14 (gm)
FAT 12 (gm) CHO 22 (gm)
Na 469 (mg) K 384 (mg)
Fiber 3 (gm) Chol 87 (mg)

Ingredients

> 1 16-OUNCE CAN CLING PEACH HALVES IN LIGHT
>   SYRUP, DRAINED (RESERVE JUICE)
> 1 CUP COOKED CHICKEN CUT INTO ¼-INCH
>   CUBES
> 1 RIB CELERY, THINLY SLICED
> ½ CUP FROZEN PEAS, THAWED
> 1 TABLESPOON PIMIENTO
> 1 PACKET (0.3 OUNCE) LOW-CALORIE LEMON-
>   FLAVORED GELATIN
> 1 TEASPOON INSTANT CHICKEN BOUILLON
> 1 CUP ICE WATER
>   NONSTICK VEGETABLE SPRAY

Garnish

> ½ CUP REDUCED-CALORIE MAYONNAISE
> ½ TEASPOON CURRY POWDER
> 2 HARDCOOKED EGGS, CUT IN THIRDS
>   SALAD GREENS

Method

1. Slice peaches, reserving 6 slices for garnish. Chill peaches, chicken, and vegetables.
2. Add enough water to reserved juice to make 1 cup. Bring juice to boil. Remove from heat. Gradually add gelatin to hot juice, stirring constantly until dissolved. Dissolve chicken bouillon in hot liquid. Add ice water; chill until slightly thickened or until mixture begins to mound on spoon.
3. Stir in chicken, celery, peas, and pimiento, and all peach slices except for garnish.
4. Pour into 9-inch pie plate well sprayed with nonstick vegetable spray. Chill until firm. Cut into 6 wedges.
5. Line individual plates with salad greens. Place slice of salad on plate. Dollop with mayonnaise mixed with curry. Garnish with peach slices and hardboiled egg.

*400 milligrams or more of sodium per serving.
**3 grams or more of fiber per serving.

Piña Colada Salad*

Yield: 4 servings
Serving Size: ¾ cup
Exchanges:
Fruit   2
Fat   1

Nutrient Content per Serving:

CAL	174	PRO	1 (gm)
FAT	5 (gm)	CHO	34 (gm)
Na	13 (mg)	K	326 (mg)
Fiber	3 (gm)	Chol	0 (mg)

Ingredients

- 1 11-OUNCE CAN MANDARIN ORANGES, DRAINED (RESERVE LIQUID)
- 1 8-OUNCE CAN PINEAPPLE CHUNKS IN OWN JUICE, DRAIN AND RESERVE JUICE
- 1 SMALL BANANA, SLICED AND SPRINKLED WITH 1 TEASPOON LEMON JUICE
- 1 ENVELOPE WHIPPED TOPPING MIX
- ½ TEASPOON VANILLA EXTRACT
- ½ TEASPOON RUM EXTRACT OR 2 TEASPOONS RUM
- 2 TABLESPOONS TOASTED COCONUT

Method

1. Combine oranges, pineapple, and banana in medium bowl.
2. Whip low-calorie topping with ½ cup fruit liquid (all of pineapple juice and enough orange liquid to make ½ cup). Whip in vanilla and rum extracts.
3. Fold into fruit mixture; sprinkle with coconut.
4. Chill several hours before serving.

*3 grams or more of fiber per serving.

Sun-Cooked Pasta Salad* **

Yield: 6 servings
Serving Size: 1½ cups
Exchanges:
Starch/Bread   4
Vegetable   1
Fat   2½

Nutrient Content per Serving:
CAL 450   PRO   15 (gm)
FAT   15 (gm)   CHO   65 (gm)
Na   552 (mg)   K   479 (mg)
Fiber 4 (gm)   Chol   5 (mg)

Ingredients

- 2 28-OUNCE CANS ITALIAN PLUM TOMATOES, DRAINED, SEEDED, AND CHOPPED
- ¼ CUP OLIVE OIL
- 2 CLOVES GARLIC, MINCED
- ¼ CUP PITTED BLACK OLIVES, SLICED
- 2 TABLESPOONS PINE NUTS, TOASTED
- 2 TEASPOONS DRIED BASIL OR 2 TABLESPOONS FRESH BASIL, CHOPPED
- ½ TEASPOON ONION POWDER
- ½ TEASPOON GARLIC POWDER
- ½ TEASPOON MARJORAM
- ¼ TEASPOON SALT
- ¼ TEASPOON BLACK PEPPER
- 1 POUND ROTINI (CORKSCREW) PASTA, COOKED AND DRAINED
- ¼ CUP GRATED PARMESAN CHEESE

Method

1. Combine all ingredients except pasta and cheese in 2-quart glass bowl or casserole. Cover with cheesecloth; place in a sunny location for 2–3 hours, or let stand at room temperature for 2–3 hours, stirring occasionally.
2. Stir in pasta and cheese; adjust seasonings. Serve at room temperature.

*400 milligrams or more of sodium per serving.
**3 grams or more of fiber per serving.

Pacific Northwest Salmon Salad* **

Yield: 4 servings
Serving Size: 1 cup
Exchanges:
Starch/Bread   1½
Meat, lean   1½
Vegetable   1

Nutrient Content per Serving:

CAL	229	PRO	16 (gm)
FAT	6 (gm)	CHO	26 (gm)
Na	572 (mg)†	K	399 (mg)
Fiber	3 (gm)	Chol	25 (mg)

Ingredients

   2 CUPS COOKED WHITE RICE
   ½ POUND FRESH COOKED SALMON OR CANNED
       SALMON, FLAKED
   ½ CUP GREEN ONION, SLICED
   ½ CUP RED BELL PEPPER, DICED
   ¾ CUP FROZEN PEAS

Dressing

   ½ CUP PLAIN LOW-FAT YOGURT
   2 TABLESPOONS REDUCED-CALORIE
       MAYONNAISE
   1 TABLESPOON FRESH DILL, CHOPPED, OR
       1 TEASPOON DRIED DILL
 4–6 DASHES TABASCO SAUCE
   ½ TEASPOON LEMON JUICE
   ¼ TEASPOON SALT
   ⅛ TEASPOON BLACK PEPPER

Method

1. Combine rice, salmon, onion, red pepper, and peas.
2. Combine all ingredients for dressing: add to rice mixture and
   toss lightly. Chill.

Note: Salmon may be prepared in microwave oven. Place skin
side down on microwave roast rack. Cover with plastic wrap
and cook for 3–4 minutes on high power or until fish flakes with
fork. To cook conventionally, place fish in 8-inch skillet and add

¼ cup water. Cover and cook over medium heat for 10 minutes per inch of thickness.

*400 milligrams or more of sodium per serving.
**3 grams or more of fiber per serving.
†If fresh salmon is used, Na = 422 mg.

A Taste of California Slaw

Yield: 8 servings	Nutrient Content per Serving:			
Serving Size: ½ cup	CAL	58	PRO	4 (gm)
Exchanges:	FAT	2 (gm)	CHO	6 (gm)
Vegetable 1	Na	171 (mg)	K	214 (mg)
Fat ½	Fiber	1 (gm)	Chol	7 (mg)

Ingredients

- ½ POUND CABBAGE, SHREDDED
- 2 GREEN ONIONS, SLICED
- 1 RIB CELERY, SLICED
- 1 MEDIUM CARROT, THINLY SLICED
- 2 OUNCES PROVOLONE CHEESE, CUT INTO THIN STRIPS
- 1 CLOVE GARLIC, MINCED
- 1 SMALL JALAPEÑO PEPPER, MINCED
- ½ RED BELL PEPPER, CUT INTO THIN STRIPS
- ⅛ TEASPOON CELERY SEED

Dressing

- 1 CUP PLAIN LOW-FAT YOGURT
- 1 TEASPOON DIJON MUSTARD
- 1 TEASPOON LEMON JUICE
- ¼ TEASPOON SALT
- ⅛ TEASPOON WHITE PEPPER

Method

1. Combine first 9 ingredients in large bowl.
2. Combine all ingredients for dressing; pour over vegetables and toss. Chill several hours before serving.

Fresh Basil Tomato Mozzarella Salad* **

Yield: 2 servings†
Serving Size: 1½ cups
Exchanges:
Meat, medium-fat 2
Vegetable 2
Fat 5

Nutrient Content per Serving:

CAL	415	PRO	18 (gm)
FAT	35 (gm)	CHO	13 (gm)
Na	458 (mg)	K	458 (mg)
Fiber	3 (gm)	Chol	32 (mg)

Ingredients

1 FIRM TOMATO, CUT INTO THIN WEDGES
4 OUNCES MOZZARELLA CHEESE, CUT INTO STRIPS
¼ CUP FRESH BASIL, SHREDDED, OR 2 TEASPOONS DRIED BASIL
1 SMALL RED ONION, SLICED
¼ CUP BASIC VINAIGRETTE (PAGE 165)
2 TABLESPOONS PINE NUTS, TOASTED

Method

1. Combine all ingredients except pine nuts in serving bowl. Chill several hours. Stir in pine nuts before serving.

*400 milligrams or more of sodium per serving.
**3 grams or more of fiber per serving.
†To make 4 servings, double the recipe.

7-Layer Salad*

Yield: 8 servings
Serving Size: 1 cup
Exchanges:
Vegetable 3
Fat 3

Nutrient Content per Serving:

CAL	202	PRO	5 (gm)
FAT	15 (gm)	CHO	14 (gm)
Na	365 (mg)	K	409 (mg)
Fiber	5 (gm)	Chol	20 (mg)

Ingredients

- 1 HEAD LETTUCE, RINSED AND TORN INTO BITE-SIZE PIECES
- 3 RIBS CELERY, SLICED
- 1 BUNCH GREEN ONION, GREEN AND WHITE, SLICED
- 1 8-OUNCE CAN WATER CHESTNUTS, SLICED
- 1 CUP ZUCCHINI, SLICED
- 1 10-OUNCE PACKAGE FROZEN PEAS, DEFROSTED AND DRAINED
- 1½ CUPS REDUCED-CALORIE MAYONNAISE
- 1 TEASPOON DILL WEED
- ¼ CUP GRATED PARMESAN CHEESE

Method

1. In large bowl, layer vegetables in order as listed.
2. Cover with mayonnaise; sprinkle dill and Parmesan over mayonnaise. Cover and refrigerate overnight.
3. Toss salad before serving.

   *3 grams or more of fiber per serving.

Tuna and White Bean Salad*

Yield: 6 servings

Serving Size: ½ cup

Exchanges:

Starch/Bread	1
Meat, lean	1
Fat	1

Nutrient Content per Serving:

CAL	192	PRO	14 (gm)
FAT	10 (gm)	CHO	14 (gm)
Na	312 (mg)	K	357 (mg)
Fiber	4 (gm)	Chol	19 (mg)

Ingredients

1 6½-OUNCE CAN WATER-PACKED TUNA, DRAINED AND FLAKED

1 19-OUNCE CAN CANNELLINI OR ANY COOKED WHITE BEAN, DRAINED AND RINSED (2 CUPS)

⅓ CUP RED ONION RINGS, THINLY SLICED FRESHLY GROUND BLACK PEPPER TO TASTE

⅓ CUP BASIC VINAIGRETTE DRESSING (SEE PAGE 165)

Method

1. Combine tuna, beans, and onion rings. Mix in pepper, and vinaigrette. Chill before serving. Adjust seasonings.
2. Serve on a bed of lettuce.
3. Serve with crusty French bread, if desired.

*3 grams or more of fiber per serving.

Roasted Red and Yellow Pepper Potato Salad

Yield: 3 cups (6 servings)
Serving Size: ½ cup
Exchanges:
Starch/Bread 1
Fat 2

Nutrient Content per Serving:

CAL	167	PRO	1 (gm)
FAT	13 (gm)	CHO	13 (gm)
Na	108 (mg)	K	228 (mg)
Fiber	2 (gm)	Chol	0 (mg)

Ingredients

1 SMALL RED PEPPER
1 SMALL YELLOW PEPPER
4 MEDIUM RED POTATOES, COOKED, UNPEELED, AND SLICED
⅓ CUP SUNFLOWER OR VEGETABLE OIL
2 TABLESPOONS WHITE WINE VINEGAR
1½ TEASPOONS DIJON MUSTARD
¼ TEASPOON SALT
⅛ TEASPOON BLACK PEPPER

Method

1. Place peppers on broiling pan and broil until skin is burnt (black) on all sides. (May be done on outside grill, about 25 minutes.) Place in paper bag; let stand for 10 minutes.
2. Peel peppers and remove stems and seeds; slice into strips. Combine peppers with sliced potatoes.
3. Whisk together remaining ingredients; pour over potato-pepper mixture. Chill or serve at room temperature.

Green Bean Salad*

Yield: 4 servings	Nutrient Content per Serving:		
Serving Size: ¼ of recipe	CAL	174	PRO	2 (gm)
Exchanges:	FAT	15 (gm)	CHO	9 (gm)
Vegetable	2	Na	270 (mg)	K	328 (mg)
Fat	3	Fiber	4 (gm)	Chol	0 (mg)

Ingredients

- ¾ POUND FRESH STRING BEANS, ENDS TRIMMED
- 6 FRESH MUSHROOMS, SLICED
- 1 SMALL RED ONION, CHOPPED
- 4 TABLESPOONS SUNFLOWER OIL
- 2 TABLESPOONS BALSAMIC OR RED WINE VINEGAR
- ½ TEASPOON SALT
- ¼ TEASPOON BLACK PEPPER
- ¼ TEASPOON GARLIC POWDER

Method

1. Cook green beans in boiling water for 10 minutes, uncovered. Drain. Let chill in refrigerator.
2. Toss beans with mushrooms and onion.
3. Whisk oil into vinegar; whisk in spices; pour over string beans. Toss lightly.
4. Chill before serving. Makes an excellent side dish or first course.

*3 grams or more of fiber per serving.

Caesar Salad

Yield: 6 servings		Nutrient Content per Serving:			
Serving Size: ⅙ of salad		CAL	136	PRO	4 (gm)
Exchanges:		FAT	12 (gm)	CHO	4 (gm)
Vegetable	1	Na	122 (mg)	K	217 (mg)
Fat	2½	Fiber	1 (gm)	Chol	50 (mg)

Ingredients

   1 LARGE HEAD ROMAINE LETTUCE
  ¼ CUP OLIVE OIL
   3 CLOVES GARLIC, PEELED AND HALVED
  ½ CUP RYE OR WHOLE WHEAT CROUTONS
1½ TEASPOONS ANCHOVY PASTE
   1 EGG
   1 TEASPOON WORCESTERSHIRE SAUCE
    JUICE OF 1 SMALL LEMON
  ¼ CUP GRATED PARMESAN CHEESE
    PINCH OF FRESHLY GROUND PEPPER

Method

1. Rinse lettuce under cold running water, wrap in paper towel, and refrigerate at least 20 minutes.
2. Heat 1 teaspoon olive oil in small skillet. Add 2 of the halved garlic cloves; cook for 1 minute. Add croutons. Toss well. Cook until lightly toasted. Set aside.
3. Rub salad bowl with remaining garlic. Add anchovy paste, egg, Worcestershire sauce, and lemon juice. Beat with whisk. Slowly whisk in remaining olive oil.
4. Add lettuce leaves, Parmesan cheese, and pepper. Sprinkle with croutons. Serve immediately.

Oriental Duck Salad * **

Yield: 4 servings

Serving Size: ¼ of recipe

Exchanges:

Starch/Bread 1½

Meat, medium-fat 3

Fat 1½

Nutrient Content per Serving:

CAL	405	PRO	25 (gm)
FAT	24 (gm)	CHO	26 (gm)
Na	690 (mg)	K	615 (mg)
Fiber	6 (gm)	Chol	92 (mg)

Key Source Nutrients:
Ascorbic acid 58 (mg)

Ingredients

- 1 10- TO 12-OUNCE BONELESS DUCK BREAST
- 3 RIBS BOK CHOY, SHREDDED
- 2 OUNCES CELLOPHANE NOODLES, BOILED AND DRAINED
- 1 CUP SNOW PEAS, BLANCHED
- 4 OUNCES COOKED SHRIMP, PEELED
- 1 11-OUNCE CAN MANDARIN ORANGE SECTIONS, DRAINED
- 1 TABLESPOON SESAME SEEDS, TOASTED

Dressing

- ¼ CUP RICE VINEGAR
- ¼ CUP LOW-SODIUM SOY SAUCE
- ¼ CUP VEGETABLE OIL
- ½ TEASPOON SESAME OIL
- ⅛ TEASPOON GROUND GINGER
- ⅛ TEASPOON BLACK PEPPER

Method

1. Preheat oven to 350°F. Place small oven-proof skillet in oven to heat.
2. Score skin of duck breast; place skin side down in skillet. Cook on range over medium heat for 3–5 minutes or until skin is golden. Turn and continue cooking for 3 minutes. Place in oven; bake for 5–7 minutes or until done. Cool; remove skin and slice thin.
3. Arrange bok choy on serving platter. Place half of noodles at either end. Divide snow peas and place opposite noodles. Arrange shrimp in middle. Arrange duck slices around outer edges. Sprinkle oranges and sesame seeds over all.
4. Combine all ingredients for dressing; mix well. Pour ¼ cup dressing over salad; pass remaining dressing.

*400 milligrams or more of sodium per serving.
**3 grams or more of fiber per serving.

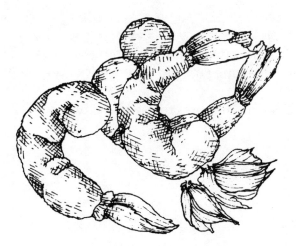

Jicama Salad

Yield: 4 ½-cup servings
Serving Size: ¼ of recipe
Exchanges:
Vegetable   2
Fat   3

Nutrient Content per Serving:

CAL	178	PRO	1 (gm)
FAT	15 (gm)	CHO	11 (gm)
Na	272 (mg)	K	253 (mg)
Fiber	2 (gm)	Chol	0 (mg)

Ingredients

8 OUNCES JICAMA, PEELED AND CUT INTO
  ½-INCH STICKS
1 SMALL CUCUMBER, THINLY SLICED
1 MEDIUM ORANGE, PEELED AND SECTIONED
⅓ CUP WHITE WINE VINEGAR
¼ CUP VEGETABLE OIL
1 TEASPOON LEMON JUICE
¼ TEASPOON CHILE POWDER
¼ TEASPOON SALT

Method

1. Combine jicama, cucumber, and orange in serving bowl.
2. Whisk together vinegar, oil, lemon juice, chile powder, and salt.
3. Pour over jicama mixture; toss well. Chill.

Basic Vinaigrette Dressing

Yield: ¾ cup
Serving Size: 1 tablespoon
Exchanges:
Fat   2

Nutrient Content per Serving:

CAL	89	PRO	0 (gm)
FAT	10 (gm)	CHO	0 (gm)
Na	89 (mg)	K	6 (mg)
Fiber	0 (gm)	Chol	0 (mg)

Ingredients

¼ CUP RED WINE VINEGAR
1 SMALL CLOVE GARLIC, MINCED
½ TEASPOON SALT
¼ TEASPOON BLACK PEPPER, FRESHLY GROUND
½ TEASPOON DRY MUSTARD
½ CUP VEGETABLE OIL

Method

1. Combine all ingredients except oil in medium bowl or food processor; blend well. Slowly add oil in a stream, mixing until thickened. Will keep 1–2 weeks refrigerated.

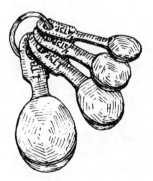

Breads, Muffins, and Biscuits

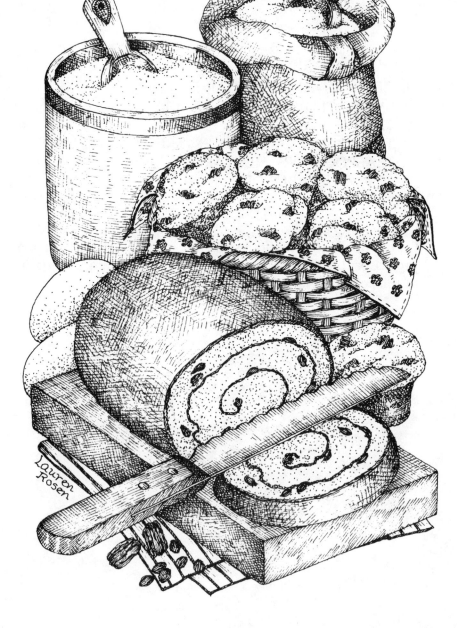

*T*here is nothing more palate-teasing than the fragrance of fresh baked bread. Our recipes taste as good as they smell! And they will prove delicious and healthy accompaniments to any meal. Try the Buttermilk Biscuits or the Quick Homemade Raisin Bread if family tastes are traditional; the Cheddar-Broccoli Corn Muffins are an unusual and substantial treat with a light supper meal. The Pizza Bread will become another easy-to-make, popular favorite.

Anadama Bread

Yield: 1 loaf (14 slices)

Serving Size: 1 slice

Exchanges:

Starch/Bread   1½

Fat   ½

Nutrient Content per Serving:

CAL	137	PRO	3 (gm)
FAT	3 (gm)	CHO	25 (gm)
Na	182 (mg)	K	92 (mg)
Fiber	1 (gm)	Chol	0 (mg)

Ingredients

2–2½ CUPS ALL-PURPOSE WHITE FLOUR
   ½ CUP YELLOW CORNMEAL
   1 PACKAGE DRY YEAST
   1 TEASPOON SALT
   1 CUP BOILING WATER
   3 TABLESPOONS MARGARINE
   ¼ CUP LIGHT MOLASSES
     NONSTICK VEGETABLE SPRAY

Method

1. Combine 1 cup flour, cornmeal, yeast, and salt.
2. In a small bowl, combine boiling water and margarine. Stir until margarine is melted; stir in molasses.
3. Stir molasses mixture into flour. Add rest of flour, a little at a time, to make a stiff dough.
4. Turn out on floured board and knead until no longer sticky, about 10 minutes.
5. Spray a large bowl with nonstick vegetable spray. Place dough in bowl, turning dough to coat it.
6. Cover; let rise in warm place 1–1½ hours, or until doubled in size.
7. Punch down, knead briefly, and shape into a round loaf. Place in 8-inch round cake tin well sprayed with nonstick vegetable spray. Cover lightly; let rise about 1 hour, or until doubled in volume.

8. Preheat oven to 350°F.
9. Bake for 45–50 minutes, or until bread sounds hollow when tapped and is deep brown in color.
10. Remove from pan and cool on rack.

Quick Homemade Raisin Bread

Yield: 18 slices
Serving Size: ½-inch slice
Exchanges:
Starch/Bread   1
Fat   ½

Nutrient Content per Serving:

CAL	93	PRO	2 (gm)
FAT	4 (gm)	CHO	14 (gm)
Na	80 (mg)	K	59 (mg)
Fiber	1 (gm)	Chol	15 (mg)

Ingredients

      NONSTICK VEGETABLE SPRAY
  ¾ CUP DARK SEEDLESS RAISINS
  1 CUP BOILING WATER
1½ CUPS ALL-PURPOSE FLOUR
  1 TEASPOON BAKING SODA
  7 PACKETS SUGAR SUBSTITUTE
  ½ TEASPOON CINNAMON
  ¼ TEASPOON SALT
  1 EGG
  1 TEASPOON VANILLA EXTRACT
  ¼ CUP VEGETABLE OIL OR MELTED MARGARINE

Method

1. Preheat oven to 350°F. Spray 9-by-5-inch loaf pan with nonstick vegetable spray. Dust lightly with flour.
2. Combine raisins and water; set aside for 30 minutes.
3. Combine flour, baking soda, sugar substitute, cinnamon, and salt in large mixing bowl. Add raisins with liquid, egg, vanilla, and oil. Mix just until dry ingredients are moistened.
4. Pour into prepared pan. Bake for 40–45 minutes or until golden brown and firm to the touch. Let stand for 5 minutes; remove to cooling rack. Serve warm or slice and toast.

Bunelos

Yield: 4 servings
Serving Size: 1 bunelo
Exchanges:
Starch/Bread   1
Fat   1

Nutrient Content per Serving:

CAL	120	PRO	3 (gm)
FAT	5 (gm)	CHO	17 (gm)
Na	33 (mg)	K	2 (mg)
Fiber	1 (gm)	Chol	0 (mg)

Ingredients

        NONSTICK VEGETABLE SPRAY
    4 (6-INCH) FLOUR TORTILLAS
    1 TABLESPOON MARGARINE, MELTED
    2 PACKETS SUGAR SUBSTITUTE
    ½ TEASPOON CINNAMON

Method

1. Preheat oven to 400°F. Spray cookie sheet with nonstick vegetable spray.
2. Brush tortillas with margarine.
3. Combine sugar substitute and cinnamon; sprinkle evenly over tortillas.
4. Place on prepared cookie sheet. Bake for 6-10 minutes or until crisp. Cut into wedges and serve warm.

Cheddar-Broccoli Corn Muffins

Yield: 1 dozen muffins (12 servings)

Serving Size: 1 muffin

Exchanges:

Starch/Bread   1½

Fat   1

Nutrient Content per Serving:

CAL	163	PRO	6 (gm)
FAT	7 (gm)	CHO	19 (gm)
Na	229 (mg)	K	97 (mg)
Fiber	1 (gm)	Chol	31 (mg)

Ingredients

NONSTICK VEGETABLE SPRAY
1½ CUPS ALL-PURPOSE FLOUR
½ CUP YELLOW CORNMEAL
1 TABLESPOON BAKING POWDER
¼ TEASPOON SALT
PINCH OF CAYENNE PEPPER
1 CUP SKIM MILK
1 EGG
¼ CUP MARGARINE, MELTED
1 CUP BROCCOLI FLORETS, BLANCHED AND CHOPPED
¾ CUP CHEDDAR CHEESE, GRATED

Method

1. Preheat oven to 425°F. Coat 12 medium muffin cups with nonstick vegetable spray or line with paper baking cups.
2. Combine flour, cornmeal, baking powder, salt, and pepper. Add milk, egg, and margarine; mix just until dry ingredients are moistened. Stir in broccoli and cheese.
3. Pour into prepared muffin cups (¾ full). Bake for 17–20 minutes or until golden brown. Remove to cooling rack. Serve warm.

Zucchini-Lemon Bread

Yield: 18 slices
Serving Size: ½-inch slice
Exchanges:
Starch/Bread   1
Fat   1

Nutrient Content per Serving:

CAL	125	PRO	3 (gm)
FAT	7 (gm)	CHO	15 (gm)
Na	179 (mg)	K	68 (mg)
Fiber	1 (gm)	Chol	31 (mg)

Ingredients

    NONSTICK VEGETABLE SPRAY
1 CUP UNSIFTED ALL-PURPOSE FLOUR
½ CUP WHOLE WHEAT FLOUR
½ CUP SUGAR
1½ TEASPOONS BAKING POWDER
1 TEASPOON SALT
½ TEASPOON BAKING SODA
½ TEASPOON GRATED LEMON PEEL
½ TEASPOON CINNAMON
1 CUP ZUCCHINI (PACKED), UNPEELED AND SHREDDED
⅓ CUP CHOPPED WALNUTS
⅓ CUP VEGETABLE OIL OR MELTED MARGARINE
½ CUP SKIM MILK
2 EGGS

Method

1. Preheat oven to 350°F. Coat 9-by-5-inch loaf pan with nonstick vegetable spray.
2. Combine flours, sugar, baking powder, salt, and baking soda in large mixing bowl. Stir in lemon peel, cinnamon, zucchini, and walnuts.
3. Add oil, milk, and eggs, mixing just until dry ingredients are moistened. Spread evenly in prepared pan. Bake for 50–60 minutes or until toothpick inserted in center comes out clean. Let stand for 5 minutes; transfer to cooling rack.

Method–Microwave

1. Line a 9-by-5-inch microwave-safe loaf dish with waxed paper. Prepare batter as directed above; pour into dish.
2. Shield ends with foil (2-inch width). Place dish on inverted saucer.
3. Cook for 8–9 minutes on medium power, rotating every 3 minutes. Remove foil. Cook for 3–5 minutes on high power or until toothpick inserted in center comes out clean. Let stand for 5 minutes; transfer to cooling rack.

Carrot-Raisin Muffins

Yield: 12 muffins
Serving Size: 1 muffin
Exchanges:
Starch/Bread   1
Fat   ½

Nutrient Content per Serving:

CAL	105	PRO	3 (gm)
FAT	4 (gm)	CHO	16 (gm)
Na	213 (mg)	K	118 (mg)
Fiber	1 (gm)	Chol	46 (mg)

Ingredients

NONSTICK VEGETABLE SPRAY
1 CUP UNSIFTED ALL-PURPOSE FLOUR
2 TABLESPOONS WHEAT GERM, TOASTED
1½ TEASPOONS BAKING POWDER
1 TEASPOON BAKING SODA
½ TEASPOON SALT
2 TEASPOONS BROWN SUGAR SUBSTITUTE
1 TEASPOON CINNAMON
⅛ TEASPOON CLOVES
⅛ TEASPOON NUTMEG
1⅓ CUPS CARROTS, SHREDDED
½ CUP DARK SEEDLESS RAISINS, SOAKED IN HOT WATER FOR 15–20 MINUTES AND DRAINED
2 EGGS
2 TABLESPOONS VEGETABLE OIL

Method

1. Preheat oven to 350°F. Spray muffin tins.
2. Combine flour, wheat germ, baking powder, baking soda, salt, brown sugar substitute, cinnamon, cloves, and nutmeg in large bowl.
3. Stir in carrots and raisins.
4. Beat eggs with oil; stir into flour–carrot mixture. Divide batter evenly among 12 tins. Bake for 30–35 minutes or until toothpick inserted in center of muffin comes out clean.

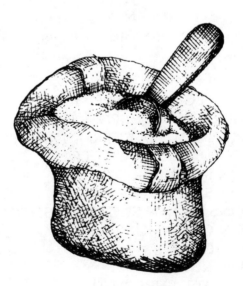

Scones

Yield: 16 scones
Serving Size: 1 scone
Exchanges:
Starch/Bread   1

Nutrient Content per Serving:

CAL	91	PRO	2 (gm)
FAT	2 (gm)	CHO	15 (gm)
Na	84 (mg)	K	48 (mg)
Fiber	1 (gm)	Chol	0 (mg)

Ingredients

   3 TABLESPOONS MARGARINE
   2 CUPS ALL-PURPOSE FLOUR
1½ TEASPOONS BAKING POWDER
 ½ TEASPOON BAKING SODA
   1 PACKET SUGAR SUBSTITUTE
 ½ CUP SKIM MILK
 ¼ CUP DARK RAISINS OR CURRANTS
 ¼ TEASPOON ORANGE PEEL
    NONSTICK VEGETABLE SPRAY

Method

1. Preheat over to 450°F.
2. In food processor or with pastry blender, mix margarine and flour until it resembles coarse crumbs. Stir in baking powder, baking soda, sugar substitute, and salt to taste.
3. Stir in milk until dry ingredients are moistened. Stir in raisins and orange peel.
4. Gather dough into a ball. Roll out on lightly floured board to ½-inch thickness. Cut into rounds using a 2½-inch cookie cutter. Place on cookie sheet well sprayed with nonstick vegetable spray.
5. Bake for 7–10 minutes or until lightly browned. Serve warm or hot with jam and margarine.

Note: Great for breakfast, snack, or afternoon tea.

Pizza Bread

Yield: 1 loaf (18 slices)
Serving Size: ½-inch slice
Exchanges:
Starch/Bread   1
Fat   ½

Nutrient Content per Serving:

CAL	110	PRO	3 (gm)
FAT	3 (gm)	CHO	18 (gm)
Na	171 (mg)	K	37 (mg)
Fiber	1 (gm)	Chol	1 (mg)

Ingredients

          3 CUPS ALL-PURPOSE FLOUR
          1 PACKAGE ACTIVE DRY YEAST
          1 CLOVE GARLIC, MINCED
          ½ TEASPOON OREGANO, CRUSHED
          ½ TEASPOON BASIL, CRUSHED
          ¼ TEASPOON GARLIC POWDER
          ⅛ TEASPOON RED PEPPER FLAKES, CRUSHED
          2 TABLESPOONS PEPPERONI, FINELY CHOPPED
          1 TABLESPOON GRATED PARMESAN CHEESE
       1¼ CUPS WATER
          2 TABLESPOONS MARGARINE
          1 TABLESPOON SUGAR
          1 TEASPOON SALT
          1 TEASPOON VEGETABLE OR OLIVE OIL

Method

1. In large mixer bowl, combine 1½ cups of the flour, yeast, garlic, oregano, basil, garlic powder, red pepper flakes, pepperoni, and cheese.
2. In small saucepan, heat water, margarine, sugar, and salt until warm (110–115°F).
3. Add to dry ingredients and beat for 3 minutes at high speed with electric mixer. Stir in enough remaining flour to make a soft dough.
4. Oil large bowl with vegetable or olive oil. Scrape dough into bowl. Cover with waxed paper, let rise in warm place for 45–60 minutes or until doubled in size.

5. Punch down. Spray a 9-by-5-inch loaf pan heavily with non-stick vegetable spray. Place dough in pan. Cover with waxed paper; let rise in warm place about 30 minutes or until doubled in size.
6. Bake in preheated 375°F over for 45–55 minutes or until bread sounds hollow when tapped. Remove from pan. Cool on rack.

Sally Lunn Bread

Yield: 8 servings
Serving Size: ⅛ of loaf
Exchanges:
Starch/Bread 3
Fat 1

Nutrient Content per Serving:

CAL	310	PRO	9 (gm)
FAT	8 (gm)	CHO	50 (gm)
Na	167 (mg)	K	140 (mg)
Fiber	2 (gm)	Chol	69 (mg)

Ingredients

    1 PACKAGE YEAST
    ¼ CUP WARM WATER (105–115°F)
    ¼ CUP MARGARINE
    1 CUP SKIM MILK
    2 EGGS, WELL BEATEN
    ¼ TEASPOON SALT
3–3½ CUPS ALL-PURPOSE FLOUR
    NONSTICK VEGETABLE SPRAY

Method

1. Dissolve yeast in water.
2. Melt margarine in milk but do not boil.
3. Stir milk into yeast, eggs, and salt.
4. Add flour in small amounts, and beat well after each addition. Make a stiff but workable batter.
5. Pour into 9-inch bundt pan, tube pan, or 2-quart baking dish well sprayed with nonstick vegetable spray. Cover and let rise in warm place until doubled (1–1½ hours).
6. Preheat oven to 375°F.

7. Bake for 30–35 minutes or until bread is golden on top and sounds hollow when rapped with knuckles. Turn out onto rack to cool or eat warm.
8. Serve warm with margarine and sugar-free jam, or cool, slice, and toast.

Note: Sally Lunn is an old quick standby for a good bread recipe when the cupboard is bare.

Challah

Yield: 1 loaf (18 slices)
Serving Size: 1/18 of loaf
Exchanges:
Starch/Bread   1½
Fat   ½

Nutrient Content per Serving:

CAL	130	PRO	3 (gm)
FAT	3 (gm)	CHO	22 (gm)
Na	95 (mg)	K	39 (mg)
Fiber	1 (gm)	Chol	61 (mg)

Ingredients

- ¼ CUP HOT WATER (105–115°F) PLUS ADDITIONAL WARM WATER
- ¼ CUP PLUS 1 TEASPOON HONEY
- 1 PACKAGE ACTIVE DRY YEAST
- 3 CUPS UNBLEACHED ALL-PURPOSE FLOUR
- ¾ TEASPOON SALT
- 1 LARGE EGG
- 2 LARGE EGG YOLKS
- 2 TABLESPOONS VEGETABLE OIL
  NONSTICK VEGETABLE SPRAY
- 1 EGG YOLK MIXED WITH 1 TABLESPOON WATER TO BRUSH ON DOUGH
- 1 TEASPOON SESAME SEEDS

Method

1. Combine hot water, 1 teaspoon honey, and yeast in small bowl to proof, about 10 minutes.
2. In large bowl, combine flour and salt.
3. Beat egg and egg yolks with vegetable oil and enough warm water to make 1 cup liquid. Stir in ¼ cup honey.
4. Stir egg mixture and yeast mixture into flour until thick and sticky.
5. Turn out onto floured board or counter; knead about 8 minutes or until dough is smooth and elastic. Place in bowl well sprayed with nonstick vegetable spray, cover, and put in warm spot to rise until doubled, about 30 minutes to 2 hours.
6. Punch dough down on floured surface and roll out into a 10-by-18-inch rectangle.
7. Roll lengthwise to form a fat sausage 18 inches long. Pinch ends closed and pinch along seam. Coil dough into itself (snail-like) and tuck end under dough. Place on cookie sheet well sprayed with nonstick vegetable spray. Cover lightly, place in warm spot, and allow to double, about 30 minutes to 1 hour.
8. Brush bread with egg mixed with water and sprinkle with sesame seeds. Bake for 35–40 minutes in preheated 375°F oven or until bread is a deep golden brown and sounds hollow when tapped on bottom.

Foccacia—Onion Flat Bread*

Yield: 6 servings
Serving Size: ⅙ loaf of bread
Exchanges:
Starch/Bread 3½
Fat 1½

Nutrient Content per Serving:

CAL	344	PRO	8 (gm)
FAT	10 (gm)	CHO	55 (gm)
Na	202 (mg)	K	133 (mg)
Fiber	4 (gm)	Chol	0 (mg)

Ingredients

> 1 PACKAGE ACTIVE DRY YEAST
> 1–1¼ CUPS WARM WATER (105–115°F)
> 3 CUPS ALL-PURPOSE FLOUR
> 1/16 TEASPOON SALT
> 4 TABLESPOONS OLIVE OIL
>   NONSTICK VEGETABLE SPRAY
> 2 MEDIUM ONIONS, THINLY SLICED
> ½ TEASPOON COARSE SALT
> ¼ TEASPOON GARLIC POWDER

Method

1. Dissolve yeast in ¼ cup warm water.
2. Put flour, pinch of salt, 2 tablespoons olive oil, and yeast into food processor fitted with steel blade.
3. With machine running slowly, pour ¾–1 cup warm water through feed tube. Add just enough water for a light dough to form.
4. Turn dough out into lightly floured board; knead for 2 minutes. Form into a ball and place in bowl well sprayed with nonstick vegetable spray. Cover and set in warm spot until dough doubles in size, rising time 1 to 1½ hours.
5. Punch down. On lightly floured board, shape into 12-by-16–inch rectangle.
6. Place on cookie sheet well sprayed with nonstick vegetable spray.
7. Cover and let rise in warm spot for 1 hour.
8. Meanwhile, prepare onion topping. Sauté onion in skillet well sprayed with nonstick vegetable spray, until soft but not brown.
9. Preheat oven to 400°F.
10. Use knuckles to poke indentations in dough. Sprinkle coarse salt and 2 tablespoons olive oil over dough.
11. Top with sautéed onion.
12. Bake for 20–25 minutes until crisp and golden.
13. Place immediately on cooling rack so bread will not become soggy.

Note: Foccacia is an Italian flat bread, wonderful served warm with margarine or at room temperature as an appetizer. May also be topped with fresh garlic, tomatoes, or sage and baked.

*3 grams or more of fiber per serving.

Buttermilk Biscuits

Yield: 18 biscuits
Serving Size: 1 biscuit
Exchanges:
Starch/Bread 1
Fat ½

Nutrient Content per Serving:

CAL	107	PRO	2 (gm)
FAT	6 (gm)	CHO	12 (gm)
Na	151 (mg)	K	31 (mg)
Fiber	1 (gm)	Chol	0 (mg)

Ingredients

NONSTICK VEGETABLE SPRAY
2 CUPS ALL-PURPOSE FLOUR
½ TEASPOON SALT
2 TEASPOONS BAKING POWDER
1 TEASPOON BAKING SODA
½ CUP VEGETABLE SHORTENING
¾ CUP LOW-FAT BUTTERMILK

Method

1. Preheat oven to 425°F. Spray cookie sheet with nonstick vegetable spray.
2. Combine flour, salt, baking powder, and baking soda. Cut in shortening until it resembles coarse crumbs.
3. Stir in buttermilk until it makes a stiff dough.
4. Roll or pat out dough on floured board to ½-inch thickness. Cut 2-inch rounds. Place biscuits 1 inch apart on prepared cookie sheet. Do not roll dough out more than twice.
5. Bake for 8–10 minutes or until puffed and golden. Serve hot or warm.

Note: These biscuits are not high, but they are light and flaky.

Meats: Beef, Pork, Veal, Lamb, Game

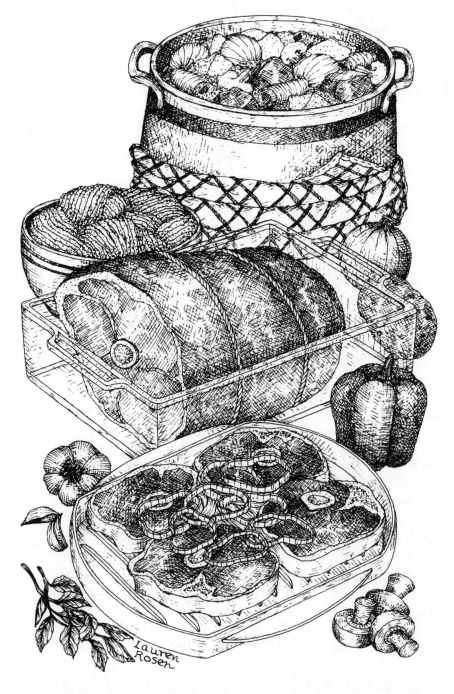

Lauren
Rosen

*M*ost of us still think of the meat course as the center of a meal: We begin by selecting the meat and plan the rest of the meal around it. The recipes in this section give you the widest possible variety in planning—everything from speedy family fare to elegant company main dishes.

Chicken Fried Steak with Pan Gravy

Yield: 4 servings
Serving Size: 1 piece with
gravy
Exchanges:
Starch/Bread   ½
Meat, lean   3

Nutrient Content per Serving:

CAL	214	PRO	21 (gm)
FAT	9 (gm)	CHO	11 (gm)
Na	323 (mg)	K	326 (mg)
Fiber	0 (gm)	Chol	52 (mg)

Ingredients

      1 POUND ROUND STEAK, POUNDED THIN
      1 EGG MIXED WITH WATER
     ½ TEASPOON SALT
 ¼–½ TEASPOON GARLIC POWDER
     ¼ TEASPOON BLACK PEPPER
     ¼ CUP FLOUR FOR DREDGING
        NONSTICK VEGETABLE SPRAY
      1 TABLESPOON VEGETABLE OIL
      1 TABLESPOON WATER

Gravy

      2 TABLESPOONS FLOUR
     ½ CUP WATER
     ½ CUP SKIM MILK

Method

1. Cut away fat from steak, remove bone, and cut into 4 pieces.
2. Beat egg with water until lemon-colored.
3. Combine salt, garlic powder, and pepper. Sprinkle seasonings on both sides of steak.
4. Dredge in flour and shake off excess; dip in egg and again in
   flour.
5. Heat large skillet, spray well with nonstick vegetable spray,
   and add vegetable oil.
6. Brown both sides of meat, turning only once. Reduce heat to
   low. Cook for 10–15 minutes until juices run clear. Add 1
   tablespoon water to skillet, cover, and cook for 5 minutes.

7. Remove steak to heated plate. Add 2 tablespoons flour to drippings; when light brown, stir in water and milk, whisking until it thickens into a gravy. Add more water if gravy is too thick.

8. Return steaks to skillet; simmer gently until ready to serve.

Fajitas* **

Yield: 4 servings
Serving Size: ¼ of recipe
Exchanges:
Starch/Bread   1
Meat, medium-
   fat   2½
Vegetable   2
Fat   ½

Nutrient Content per Serving:

CAL	345	PRO	25 (gm)
FAT	16 (gm)	CHO	25 (gm)
Na	655 (mg)	K	523 (mg)
Fiber	3 (gm)	Chol	58 (mg)

Key Source Nutrients:
Ascorbic acid   52 (mg)

Ingredients

¼ CUP LIME JUICE (2 LARGE LIMES)
1 TEASPOON SALT
½ TEASPOON GARLIC POWDER
⅛ TEASPOON CAYENNE PEPPER
¼ TEASPOON BLACK PEPPER
1 POUND FLANK STEAK, TRIMMED AND SCORED
1 MEDIUM RED ONION, THINLY SLICED
1 RED AND 1 GREEN BELL PEPPER, CUT INTO THIN STRIPS
1 TEASPOON MARGARINE
4 6–INCH FLOUR TORTILLAS, WARMED
¼ CUP CHOPPED TOMATOES
¼ CUP LETTUCE, SHREDDED
¼ CUP SALSA (SEE PAGE 384)
2 TABLESPOONS REDUCED-CALORIE SOUR CREAM

Method

1. Mix lime juice, salt, garlic powder, and cayenne and black pepper in large shallow dish. Add steak; turn to coat. Refrigerate covered, 4 hours or overnight, turning once.
2. Remove steak from marinade. Broil or grill 6 inches from heat, turning once until desired doneness (about 8–10 minutes for medium rare). Sauté onion and peppers in margarine until soft.
3. Slice steak across grain into thin strips. Divide among tortillas and top with tomatoes, lettuce, salsa, and sour cream.

*400 milligrams or more of sodium per serving.
**3 grams or more of fiber per serving.

Moussaka with Beef* **

Yield: 2 servings†   Nutrient Content per Serving:
Serving Size: ½ of recipe   CAL 484   PRO   33 (gm)
Exchanges: FAT   21 (gm) CHO   40 (gm)
Starch/Bread   3   Na   1,027 (mg) K   1,160 (mg)
Meat, medium-fat 3   Fiber   3 (gm) Chol 218 (mg)
Fat   ½

Ingredients

    ½ POUND LEAN GROUND BEEF
    ¼ CUP ONION, CHOPPED
    1 CLOVE GARLIC, MINCED
    ½ CUP TOMATO PURÉE
    ¼ CUP RED WINE
 1½ TEASPOONS PARSLEY, MINCED
    ½ TEASPOON SALT
    ⅛ TEASPOON OREGANO
    ⅛ TEASPOON BLACK PEPPER
      DASH OF CINNAMON
      NONSTICK VEGETABLE SPRAY

1½ MEDIUM POTATOES, COOKED AND PEELED
2 TABLESPOONS GRATED PARMESAN CHEESE
1 CUP PLAIN LOW-FAT YOGURT
1 EGG YOLK
1 TABLESPOON FLOUR

Method

1. Preheat oven to 350°F.
2. Sauté ground beef, onion, and garlic until beef is no longer pink; drain.
3. Stir in tomato purée, red wine, parsley, and seasonings. Simmer for 5 minutes.
4. Coat a 2- to 3-quart baking dish with nonstick vegetable spray.
5. Slice potatoes ⅛-inch thick. Arrange half of potatoes in prepared dish; top with half of meat mixture. Repeat layers. Sprinkle with half of cheese.
6. Combine yogurt, egg yolk, and flour; pour over top of casserole. Top with remaining cheese. Bake for 30 minutes or until golden brown.

Method–Microwave

1. In 2-quart microwave-safe casserole, cook ground beef, onion, and garlic on high power for about 5 minutes or until beef is no longer pink, stirring once.
2. Stir in tomato purée, wine, parsley, and seasonings. Cook on medium-high power for 5 minutes, stirring once.
3. Follow directions above for arrangement of potatoes and meat mixture. Sprinkle with paprika, if desired.
4. Cover with waxed paper. Cook on medium-high power for 13–15 minutes, rotating dish once halfway through cooking time. Let stand for 10 minutes, covered, before serving.

*400 milligrams or more of sodium per serving.
**3 grams or more of fiber per serving.
†To make 4 servings, double the recipe.

Broiled Liver and Onions* **

Yield: 4 servings
Serving Size: ¼ of recipe
Exchanges:
Meat, lean   2½
Vegetable   1

Nutrient Content per Serving:

CAL	171	PRO	21 (gm)
FAT	5 (gm)	CHO	9 (gm)
Na	338 (mg)	K	322 (mg)
Fiber	3 (gm)	Chol	324 (mg)

Key Source Nutrients:
Vitamin A   30,012 (IU)
Riboflavin   3.5 (mg)
Vitamin B$_{12}$ 60 (mcg)

Ingredients

NONSTICK VEGETABLE SPRAY
1 TEASPOON MARGARINE
2 CUPS ONIONS, THINLY SLICED
1 POUND BEEF OR CALF'S LIVER, CUT
1–1½ INCHES THICK
½ TEASPOON SALT
⅛ TEASPOON PEPPER
CHOPPED PARSLEY FOR GARNISH

Method

1. Preheat broiler. Heat skillet; spray well with nonstick vegetable spray and add margarine.
2. Separate onions into rings and sauté until golden brown.
3. Rinse liver and pat dry. Season with salt and pepper. Broil for 5 minutes for rare and 7 minutes for medium, per side.
4. Place liver on warm platter. Top with onions and chopped parsley.

*3 grams or more of fiber per serving.
**This recipe is an excellent source of iron but is also high in cholesterol. Its use should be limited.

Flank Steak with Bean Sprouts and Snow Peas

Yield: 4 servings
Serving Size: ¼ of recipe
Exchanges:
Meat, medium-fat 3
Vegetable 1

Nutrient Content per Serving:

CAL	251	PRO	23 (gm)
FAT	14 (gm)	CHO	8 (gm)
Na	356 (mg)	K	475 (mg)
Fiber	2 (gm)	Chol	58 (mg)

Ingredients

- 1 TABLESPOON LOW-SODIUM SOY SAUCE
- 1 TABLESPOON DRY SHERRY
- 1 TEASPOON VEGETABLE OIL
- 1 TEASPOON CORNSTARCH
- ½ TEASPOON SUGAR
- ¼ TEASPOON BLACK PEPPER
- 1 POUND FLANK STEAK, CUT INTO THIN STRIPS ACROSS GRAIN
  NONSTICK VEGETABLE SPRAY
- 1 CLOVE GARLIC, CHOPPED
- 1 TEASPOON FRESH GINGER, MINCED
- ¼ TEASPOON SALT
- 2 OUNCES (ABOUT ½ CUP) BEAN SPROUTS
- 2 OUNCES (ABOUT ½ CUP) SNOW PEAS
- 1 TABLESPOON CHINESE TREE EAR MUSHROOMS, SOAKED IN HOT WATER FOR 30 MINUTES AND DRAINED
- 1 TABLESPOON CORNSTARCH
- 3 TABLESPOONS WATER
- 2 SMALL GREEN ONIONS, SLICED

Method

1. Combine first 6 ingredients in shallow bowl. Add steak slices; toss well. Let stand at room temperature for 30 minutes.
2. Heat a large skillet or wok and coat with nonstick vegetable spray. Add steak mixture, garlic, and ginger. Stir-fry for 2 minutes or until steak is still pink; set aside.

3. Respray skillet. Add salt, bean sprouts, snow peas, and mushrooms. Stir-fry about 1 minute. Cover and cook for 1 minute.
4. Uncover; add beef mixture and cornstarch dissolved in water. Stir-fry until slightly thickened. Add green onions and heat thoroughly.

Method–Microwave

1. In a 1½-quart microwave-safe casserole (do not spray casserole) cook meat mixture, garlic, and ginger uncovered on high power for 4–5 minutes or until meat is still pink, stirring once. Set aside.
2. Cook salt, bean sprouts, snow peas, and mushrooms in same casserole on high power for 2 minutes.
3. Add beef mixture and cornstarch dissolved in water. Cook for 1–2 minutes on high power or until slightly thickened, stirring once. Stir in green onions.

Note: Serve over hot cooked rice, if desired.

Broiled Flank Steak with Mustard Butter*

Yield: 5 servings

Serving Size: ⅕ of recipe

Exchanges:

		Nutrient Content per Serving:			
		CAL	248	PRO	21 (gm)
		FAT	17 (gm)	CHO	1 (gm)
Meat, lean	3	Na	424 (mg)	K	348 (mg)
Fat	2	Fiber	0 (gm)	Chol	58 (mg)

Ingredients

    2 TABLESPOONS PREPARED MUSTARD
    1 TEASPOON ONION POWDER
    ½ TEASPOON SALT
    ¼ TEASPOON BLACK PEPPER
    1¼ POUND FLANK STEAK, TRIMMED AND SCORED

Mustard Butter

> 2 TABLESPOONS MARGARINE, SOFTENED
> 1 TABLESPOON FRESH PARSLEY, CHOPPED, OR 1
>   TEASPOON DRIED PARSLEY
> 1 TEASPOON LEMON JUICE
> 1 TEASPOON PREPARED MUSTARD

Method

1. Combine first 4 ingredients. Rub mixture on both sides of flank steak. Marinate at room temperature for at least 1 hour.
2. Preheat broiler. Broil steak for 8–10 minutes (medium).
3. In small bowl, combine all ingredients for mustard butter. Blend until smooth.
4. Slice cooked steak, spread butter over slices, and serve.

*400 milligrams or more of sodium per serving.

Texas Beef Brisket

Yield: 8 servings	Nutrient Content per Serving:			
Serving Size: ⅛ of recipe	CAL	250	PRO	29 (gm)
Exchanges:	FAT	12 (gm)	CHO	5 (gm)
Meat, lean	4	Na 398 (mg)	K	386 (mg)
Vegetable	1	Fiber 1 (gm)	Chol	88 (mg)

Ingredients

> 2 MEDIUM ONIONS, FINELY CHOPPED
> 2 GARLIC CLOVES, FINELY CHOPPED
> 2 TABLESPOONS PREPARED MUSTARD
> 1¼ TEASPOONS BROWN SUGAR SUBSTITUTE
> 1 TABLESPOON WORCESTERSHIRE SAUCE
> 1 TEASPOON CHILE POWDER
> ¼ CUP LOW-SODIUM SOY SAUCE
> ¼ CUP RED WINE
> 1 TABLESPOON LIGHT MOLASSES
> 3½-POUND CENTER-CUT BEEF BRISKET

Method

1. Preheat oven to 325°F.
2. Center a 24-inch length of 18-inch wide heavy-duty foil in a 13-by-9-inch baking pan.
3. Combine all marinade ingredients.
4. Place brisket on center of foil.
5. Pour sauce over meat. Bring ends of foil together evenly; fold over and continue folding down to top of meat. Fold sides up to make a neatly sealed package.
6. Bake 3–3½ hours or until meat is tender.
7. Remove from oven. Put meat on heated serving platter; trim excess fat and slice.
8. Skim excess fat from sauce. Serve sauce with meat.

New England Beef Boil* **

Yield: 10 servings
Serving Size: ¹/₁₀ of cooked corned beef and vegetables
Exchanges:
Starch/Bread   1
Meat, medium-fat 3
Fat   2

Nutrient Content per Serving:

CAL	391	PRO	25 (gm)
FAT	25 (gm)	CHO	15 (gm)
Na	1,590 (mg)	K	522 (mg)
Fiber	4 (gm)	Chol	126 (mg)

Key Source Nutrients:
Vitamin A   4,166 (IU)

Ingredients

    4-POUND CORNED BEEF BRISKET, RINSED
    6 WHITE BOILING ONIONS, PEELED
    4 MEDIUM TURNIPS, PEELED
    6 RED BOILING POTATOES, SCRUBBED
    6 SMALL CARROTS (6–8 OUNCES), PEELED AND CUT INTO 1-INCH PIECES
    1 POUND WHITE CABBAGE, CUT INTO WEDGES

Mustard Sauce (optional)

⅓ CUP PREPARED MUSTARD
1 TABLESPOON PREPARED HORSERADISH

Method

1. Place corned beef in 6½-quart Dutch oven; cover with cold water. Bring to a boil; reduce heat and simmer for 2½–3 hours or until almost tender. Turn beef once and skim foam if necessary.
2. Add onions and turnips; cook for 30 minutes.
3. Add potatoes, carrots, and cabbage. Cook for 20 minutes or until meat and vegetables are tender.
4. Trim fat from beef; slice. Combine mustard and horseradish and serve with beef and vegetables, if desired.

*400 milligrams or more of sodium per serving.
**3 grams or more of fiber per serving.

English Muffin Pizza Melt*

Yield: 6 servings
Serving Size: ½ muffin plus ⅙ topping
Exchanges:
Starch/Bread 1
Meat, medium-fat 2

Nutrient Content per Serving:

CAL	244	PRO	17 (gm)
FAT	12 (gm)	CHO	17 (gm)
Na	497 (mg)	K	488 (mg)
Fiber	1 (gm)	Chol	50 (mg)

Ingredients

- 1 POUND LEAN GROUND BEEF
- ¼ CUP ONION, CHOPPED
  NONSTICK VEGETABLE SPRAY
- 1 8-OUNCE CAN PIZZA SAUCE
- 1 TEASPOON DRIED PARSLEY FLAKES
- ½ TEASPOON BASIL
- ¼ TEASPOON GARLIC POWDER
- 2 TABLESPOONS MOZZARELLA CHEESE, SHREDDED
- 3 WHOLE WHEAT OR PLAIN ENGLISH MUFFINS, SPLIT

Method

1. Preheat oven to 350°F.
2. Cook beef and onion in skillet sprayed with nonstick vegetable spray. Cook until meat is no longer pink. Drain and pat dry with paper towels to reduce fat. Stir in pizza sauce and seasonings. Top each muffin with ⅙ cup beef mixture. May pretoast muffins before adding meat and cheese.
3. Top each muffin with 1 teaspoon cheese. Place in oven and bake for 10–15 minutes or until heated thoroughly and cheese is melted.

Method–Microwave

1. Place beef and onion in colander set into 2-quart microwave-safe saucepan. Cook for 5–7 minutes on high power or until meat is no longer pink; stir once. Drain fat from saucepan.
2. Add pizza sauce and seasonings; stir well. Cook for 2 minutes on high power.
3. Spread mixture on English muffins; top with cheese. Cook for 1–2 minutes on high power until cheese melts and beef is heated thoroughly.

*400 milligrams or more of sodium per serving.

Sloppy Joe Pitas*

Yield: 4 servings
Serving Size: ½ large pita plus ½ cup filling
Exchanges:
Starch/Bread 1
Meat, lean 3
Vegetable ½
Fat 1

Nutrient Content per Serving:

CAL	302	PRO	24 (gm)
FAT	15 (gm)	CHO	17 (gm)
Na	839 (mg)	K	515 (mg)
Fiber	2 (gm)	Chol	71 (mg)

Ingredients

      NONSTICK VEGETABLE SPRAY
  1 POUND LEAN GROUND BEEF
  ¼ CUP ONION, CHOPPED
  ¼ CUP GREEN PEPPER, CHOPPED
  1 8-OUNCE CAN TOMATO SAUCE
  ½ TEASPOON GARLIC POWDER
  ½ TEASPOON ONION POWDER
  ½ TEASPOON SALT
  ⅛–¼ TEASPOON BLACK PEPPER
  2 LARGE PITAS

Method

1. Spray large skillet with nonstick vegetable spray. Cook ground beef, onion, and green pepper until meat is no longer pink. Drain and pat dry. Stir in tomato sauce and seasonings. Cook for 5–10 minutes or until heated thoroughly. Stir several times.
2. Cut large pitas in half and stuff with ½ cup meat mixture. May heat pitas in 350°F oven to crisp before stuffing, about 5 minutes.

Method–Microwave

1. Cook ground beef, onion, and green pepper in colander set into 1½-quart microwave-safe casserole for 7 minutes on high power; stir once. Drain fat from casserole.
2. Put ground beef mixture into casserole. Stir in tomato sauce and seasonings. Cook for 3–5 minutes on high power or until heated thoroughly; stir once.
3. Stuff into pitas.

*400 milligrams or more of sodium per serving.

Moo Shu Pork* **

Yield: 4 dinner, 8 appetizer, or 4 lunchbox entrées

Serving Size: 2 filled pancakes

Exchanges:

Starch/Bread	2½
Meat, lean	2
Vegetable	1
Fat	1

Nutrient Content per Serving:

CAL	374	PRO	21 (gm)
FAT	14 (gm)	CHO	42 (gm)
Na	457 (mg)	K	480 (mg)
Fiber	5 (gm)	Chol	171 (mg)

Key Source Nutrients:
Vitamin A   6,175 (IU)

Ingredients

- ½ POUND BONELESS PORK LOIN, CUT INTO MATCHSTICK SHREDS
- 1 CARROT, SHREDDED
- 2 TEASPOONS LOW-SODIUM SOY SAUCE
- 1 TEASPOON DRY SHERRY
- 1 CLOVE GARLIC, CHOPPED
- 1 PACKET SUGAR SUBSTITUTE
- 2 TEASPOONS CORNSTARCH
  NONSTICK VEGETABLE SPRAY
- ¼ CUP CLOUD EAR MUSHROOMS, SOAKED, DRAINED, AND SHREDDED
- ½ CUP BAMBOO SHOOTS, SHREDDED
- 2 EGGS
- ½ CUP CHICKEN BROTH†
- 2 GREEN ONIONS, THINLY SLICED ON AN ANGLE
- 1 CUP CHINESE CABBAGE, SHREDDED
- 1 TEASPOON SESAME OIL
- 8 MANDARIN PANCAKES
  HOISIN OR PLUM SAUCE

Method

1. Combine pork, carrot, soy sauce, sherry, garlic, sugar substitute, and cornstarch. Marinate for 20 minutes at room temperature.
2. Heat wok or large skillet; spray well with nonstick vegetable

spray. Add pork mixture and cook, stirring for 2 minutes or until pork turns a grayish color.

3. Add cloud ears and bamboo shoots. Cook, stirring for 1 minute. Remove from wok.
4. Wipe out wok. Spray again. Scramble eggs to hard stage. Add chicken broth and cook for 1 minute, stirring to blend. Add green onions and cabbage. Stir in pork mixture and sesame oil. Cook for 1 minute. Pour into serving dish.
5. Heat pancakes for 5 minutes in a steamer.
6. To serve, place one pancake flat on dish. Spread 1 teaspoon hoisin or plum sauce on pancake. Spoon generous amount of filling on pancake. Roll up to enclose filling, folding one end over. Eat from opposite end with fingers.

Method–Microwave

1. Cook pork mixture in a 2-quart microwave-safe casserole for 3–4 minutes on high poer, stirring once, or until pork turns a grayish color.
2. Stir in cloud ears, bamboo shoots, chicken broth, green onions, cabbage, and sesame oil. Cook for 4–5 minutes or until meat is tender. Stir once. Set aside. Keep warm.
3. Scramble eggs in 2–cup glass measure on high power until well done, about 1½–2 minutes; stir once. Stir eggs into pork mixture.
4. Heat mixture for 3–4 more minutes or until heated thoroughly.
5. Wrap pancakes in plastic wrap and heat for 20–25 seconds on high power.

Notes: Beef or chicken may be used in place of pork. Partially frozen meat slices are better. One-half cup plain mushrooms may be used in place of cloud ears. (Cloud ears are Chinese mushrooms found in Oriental food markets or in the Oriental section of the grocery store.) Mandarin pancakes are also found in Oriental food markets or the Oriental section of the grocery store.

*400 milligrams or more of sodium per serving.
**3 grams or more of fiber per serving.
†For reduced salt and fat, use homemade chicken broth.

Russian Pork Chops

Yield: 2 servings*
Serving Size: 1 chop
Exchanges:
Starch/Bread   1
Meat, lean   4
Fat   ½

Nutrient Content per Serving:

CAL	330	PRO	31 (gm)
FAT	17 (gm)	CHO	14 (gm)
Na	253 (mg)	K	594 (mg)
Fiber	1 (gm)	Chol	92 (mg)

Ingredients

NONSTICK VEGETABLE SPRAY
¼ POUND POTATOES, PEELED AND SLICED
2 CENTER-CUT PORK CHOPS, WELL TRIMMED
⅛ TEASPOON SALT
⅛ TEASPOON GARLIC POWDER
⅛ TEASPOON ONION POWDER
⅛ TEASPOON BLACK PEPPER
1½ TABLESPOONS WATER
2 OUNCES (½ CUP) MUSHROOMS, SLICED
¼ CUP REDUCED-CALORIE SOUR CREAM
1½ TEASPOONS FRESH PARSLEY, MINCED, OR
½ TEASPOON DRIED PARSLEY

Method

1. Heat skillet over medium heat. Spray with nonstick vegetable spray. Add potatoes; brown lightly and set aside.
2. Season pork chops with salt, garlic powder, onion powder, and black pepper. Respray skillet. Cook chops for 1 minute on each side; drain fat.
3. Add water, cover, and cook for 10 minutes. Add sliced potatoes and mushrooms; cook for 10 minutes more. Stir in sour cream; heat thoroughly, but do not boil. Sprinkle with parsley.

*To make 4 servings, double the recipe.

B.B.Q. Pork*

Yield: 4 servings
Serving Size: 4 ounces pork
plus sauce, without bun
Exchanges:
Meat, lean   4
Vegetable   1
Fat   1

Nutrient Content per Serving:

CAL	293	PRO	32 (gm)
FAT	16 (gm)	CHO	4 (gm)
Na	451 (mg)	K	642 (mg)
Fiber	1 (gm)	Chol	102 (mg)

Ingredients

B.B.Q. Sauce

    1 8-OUNCE CAN TOMATO SAUCE
    1 TEASPOON PREPARED YELLOW MUSTARD
    1 TEASPOON MINCED DRIED ONION FLAKES
    1 TEASPOON WORCESTERSHIRE SAUCE
    ¼ TEASPOON BROWN SUGAR SUBSTITUTE
    ¼ TEASPOON GARLIC POWDER
  4-6 DASHES TABASCO SAUCE OR TO TASTE
    1 POUND COOKED BONELESS PORK, THINLY
      SLICED

Method

1. Combine all B.B.Q. sauce ingredients in 10-inch skillet. Bring to boil; then reduce heat to simmer. Add pork slices and stir to coat. Cover and heat for 5 minutes, or until heated thoroughly.
2. Serve on buns for sandwiches or as an entrée.

   *400 milligrams or more of sodium per serving.

Scandinavian Pork with Prunes

Yield: 4 servings
Serving Size: 5 ounces pork
plus 1 tablespoon reduced
glaze and 1¼ prunes (¼ of
recipe)
Exchanges:
Meat, lean   4
Fruit   ½

Nutrient Content per Serving:
CAL	259	PRO	26 (gm)
FAT	13 (gm)	CHO	8 (gm)
Na	254 (mg)	K	450 (mg)
Fiber	1 (gm)	Chol	85 (mg)

Ingredients

  6 PITTED PRUNES
  ½ CUP BEEF BROTH
  ¼ TEASPOON BLACK PEPPER
  ¼ TEASPOON GROUND GINGER
  1¼ POUNDS BONELESS ROLLED PORK ROAST

Glaze

  ¼ CUP DRY SHERRY
  4 TEASPOONS KETCHUP
  ¾ TEASPOON LOW-SODIUM SOY SAUCE
  ¾ TEASPOON HONEY

Method

1. Preheat oven to 375°F.
2. Heat broth to boiling; soak prunes for 30 minutes. Drain prunes, reserving broth. Mix prunes with pepper and ginger.
3. Make 6 slits in roast, about 1½ inches deep. Place a prune in each slit.
4. Place in shallow roasting pan.
5. Combine all ingredients for glaze. Pour over roast.
6. Bake for 50 minutes or until thermometer reads 160°F, basting occasionally. Allow roast to stand covered with foil for 10 minutes.
7. Spoon fat from drippings; add broth. Pour into a 1-quart saucepan and cook over high heat until reduced to ¼ cup. Serve with roast.

Method–Microwave

1. Place roast with prunes fat side down on microwave-safe roast rack. Brush some of glaze onto roast. Cover with waxed paper. Cook for 10–12 minutes per pound on medium-high power or until thermometer reads 160°F. Turn roast and baste with remaining glaze halfway through cooking.
2. Spoon fat from drippings; add broth. Cook in 2-cup glass measure on high power for 10–12 minutes or until reduced to ¼ cup.
3. Allow roast to stand covered with foil while preparing sauce as directed above.

Veal Française

Yield: 4 servings
Serving Size: 1 slice
Exchanges:
Meat, lean   4
Vegetable   1

Nutrient Content per Serving:

CAL	242	PRO	39 (gm)
FAT	8 (gm)	CHO	1 (gm)
Na	345 (mg)	K	603 (mg)
Fiber	0 (gm)	Chol	112 (mg)

Ingredients

1 POUND (4 SLICES) VEAL SCALLOPINI
½ CUP TOMATO, COARSELY CHOPPED
½ CUP FRESH MUSHROOMS, SLICED
1 CLOVE GARLIC, CHOPPED
1 TABLESPOON FRESH PARSLEY, CHOPPED
½ TEASPOON SALT
¼ TEASPOON BLACK PEPPER
¼ CUP DRY WHITE WINE
1 TABLESPOON LEMON JUICE

Method

1. Preheat over to 350°F.
2. Rinse and pat dry veal. Place 2 scallopini side by side on a long sheet of aluminum foil. Reserve other scallopini.
3. Combine tomato, mushrooms, garlic, parsley, salt, and pepper. Top veal on foil with half of tomato mixture. Top with remaining scallopini and finish with tomato mixture.
4. Combine wine and lemon juice; pour over veal. Wrap veal in neat package with foil. Place on cookie sheet and bake for 20 minutes. Serve each scallopini with some of the sauce and vegetable mixture.

Method–Microwave

1. Place scallopini stacks in 2–quart microwave-safe baking dish. Cover with plastic wrap. Cook for 8–10 minutes on medium power. Let stand covered for 5 minutes before serving.

Crustless Veal Pizza*

Yield: 4 servings
Serving Size: ¼ pie
Exchanges:
Meat, medium-
  fat   2½
Vegetable   1

Nutrient Content per Serving:

CAL	212	PRO	22 (gm)
FAT	13 (gm)	CHO	5 (gm)
Na	505 (mg)	K	522 (mg)
Fiber	1 (gm)	Chol	47 (mg)

Ingredients

    NONSTICK VEGETABLE SPRAY
½ POUND GROUND VEAL
2 TABLESPOONS ONION, CHOPPED
½ TEASPOON OREGANO
¼ TEASPOON GARLIC POWDER
⅛ TEASPOON BLACK PEPPER
1 TEASPOON DRIED PARSLEY FLAKES
1 8-OUNCE CAN TOMATO SAUCE
4 OUNCES MOZZARELLA CHEESE, SLICED

Method

1. Preheat oven to 350°F.
2. Cook veal and onion in a small skillet sprayed with nonstick vegetable spray until brown, about 5 minutes. Drain.
3. Stir in seasonings and tomato sauce. Simmer for 5 minutes, or until sauce thickens.
4. Pat into 8–inch pie plate. Top with cheese.
5. Bake 10–15 minutes, or until cheese is melted and bubbly.

Method–Microwave

1. Put veal and onion in plastic colander set into 2-quart micro-wave-safe casserole. Cook for 2–2½ minutes on high power, stirring once.
2. Remove fat from pan. Put veal mixture into pan along with tomato sauce and seasonings. Cook for 4–5 minutes on me-dium-high power, or until slightly thickened.

3. Pat into 8-inch microwave-safe casserole or pie plate. Top with cheese. Cook for 2–3 minutes on high power, or until cheese melts.

*400 milligrams or more of sodium per serving.

Veal Patties

Yield: 4 servings
Serving Size: 1 patty
Exchanges:
Meat, lean 4
Fat 1

Nutrient Content per Serving:

CAL	255	PRO	29 (gm)
FAT	16 (gm)	CHO	2 (gm)
Na	224 (mg)	K	609 (mg)
Fiber	1 (gm)	Chol	61 (mg)

Ingredients

    1 POUND GROUND VEAL
    ½ SMALL ONION, CHOPPED
    2 TABLESPOONS GREEN PEPPER, CHOPPED
    2 TABLESPOONS BREAD CRUMBS (DRY)
    2 TEASPOONS WORCESTERSHIRE SAUCE
    ¼ TEASPOON GARLIC POWDER
    ¼ TEASPOON ONION POWDER
    ¼ TEASPOON SALT
    ⅛ TEASPOON BLACK PEPPER

Method

1. Preheat broiler.
2. Combine all ingredients and form into 4 patties.
3. Broil for 3–4 minutes per side.

Veal Roast

Yield: 4 servings
Serving Size: ¼ of recipe
Exchanges:
Starch/Bread   1
Meat, lean   4

Nutrient Content per Serving:
CAL 316   PRO   43 (gm)
FAT   8 (gm)   CHO   15 (gm)
Na   166 (mg)   K   84 (mg)
Fiber 2 (gm)   Chol 119 (mg)

Key Source Nutrients:
Vitamin A   3,926 (IU)

Ingredients

   1 CARROT, PEELED AND COARSELY CHOPPED
   ½ LARGE ONION, PEELED AND COARSELY
     CHOPPED
   3 SMALL RED POTATOES, PEELED AND
     QUARTERED
   ¼ CUP DRY WHITE WINE
   ½ CUP WATER
   1½ POUNDS VEAL BREAST, DEBONED AND ROLLED
   ¼ TEASPOON ROSEMARY
   ¼ TEASPOON THYME
   ¼ TEASPOON GARLIC POWDER
   ¼ TEASPOON ONION POWDER
   ⅛ TEASPOON SALT
   ⅛ TEASPOON BLACK PEPPER

Method

1. Preheat oven to 325°F.
2. Combine carrot, onion, and potatoes in bottom of shallow roasting pan. Add wine and water. Put veal in pan and surround with vegetables. Rub seasonings on both sides of roast. Cover with foil. Roast for 2–3 hours or until tender. If necessary, add additional water to pan.
3. Remove roast to heated platter. Separate fat from pan juices by skimming off with a spoon. Serve natural juice with cooked vegetables along with roast.

Veal Stew*

Yield: 4 servings**
Serving Size: ¼ recipe
without rice or noodles
added
Exchanges:
Meat, lean   3
Vegetable   2

Nutrient Content per Serving:

CAL	208	PRO	28 (gm)
FAT	5 (gm)	CHO	12 (gm)
Na	656 (mg)	K	704 (mg)
Fiber	2 (gm)	Chol	75 (mg)

Ingredients

    NONSTICK VEGETABLE SPRAY
1 POUND VEAL SHOULDER OR STEW MEAT, CUT
    INTO 1-INCH CUBES
¾ CUP ONION, CHOPPED
1 LEEK, SLICED, WHITE PART ONLY
¼ CUP CARROT, SLICED
1 CLOVE GARLIC, CRUSHED
2 OUNCES (½ CUP) FRESH MUSHROOMS, SLICED
¼ TEASPOON ROSEMARY
¼ TEASPOON SALT
⅛ TEASPOON BLACK PEPPER
1 CUP CHICKEN BROTH†
½ CUP DRY WHITE WINE

Sauce

1 TABLESPOON CORNSTARCH
1 TABLESPOON WATER
1 TABLESPOON DIJON MUSTARD
¼ CUP EVAPORATED SKIM MILK

Method

1. Preheat oven to 325°F.
2. Spray 4-quart Dutch oven with nonstick vegetable spray.
   Brown veal on both sides. Stir in onion, leek, carrot, garlic,
   mushrooms, rosemary, salt, and pepper. Cook for 5 minutes.
   Remove from heat.

3. Stir in chicken broth and wine. Cover.
4. Bake for 1–1½ hours or until veal is tender.
5. Strain liquid into saucepan. Combine all ingredients for sauce and whisk into cooking liquid. Whisk over medium heat until sauce is thickened. Do not boil. Stir sauce back into veal.
6. Serve over rice or noodles, if desired.

*400 milligrams or more of sodium per serving.
**To make 8 servings, double the recipe.
†For reduced salt and fat, use homemade chicken broth.

Veal Medallions with Blueberry Sauce*

Yield: 4 servings
Serving Size: ¼ of recipe
Exchanges:
Starch/Bread   ½
Meat, medium-fat 4
Fat   ½

Nutrient Content per Serving:

CAL	366	PRO	32 (gm)
FAT	23 (gm)	CHO	11 (gm)
Na	488 (mg)	K	664 (mg)
Fiber	1 (gm)	Chol	62 (mg)

Ingredients

  1 POUND VEAL MEDALLIONS OR CUTLETS, POUNDED THIN
  ⅓ CUP ALL-PURPOSE FLOUR
  ½ TEASPOON PAPRIKA
  ¼ TEASPOON SALT
  ⅛ TEASPOON WHITE PEPPER
    NONSTICK VEGETABLE SPRAY
  2 TABLESPOONS OLIVE OIL
  1 CLOVE GARLIC, MINCED
  6 OUNCES CANNED CHICKEN BROTH**
  3 OUNCES DRY WHITE WINE
  ⅓ CUP BLUEBERRIES, FRESH OR FROZEN, RINSED AND DRAINED

Method

1. Rinse veal and pat dry. Dredge in flour mixed with paprika, salt, and pepper.
2. Spray hot skillet with nonstick vegetable spray and add olive oil. Sauté veal until golden brown on both sides and veal tests done. Place on warm platter.
3. Add garlic, broth, and wine to skillet. Bring to boil and scrape up loose bits. Reduce sauce to ½ cup. Bring to simmer; add blueberries and heat thoroughly. Pour sauce over veal.

*400 milligrams or more of sodium per serving.
**For reduced salt and fat, use homemade chicken broth.

Stuffed Peppers with Ground Lamb* **

Yield: 4 servings
Serving Size: 1 pepper
Exchanges:
Starch/Bread   ½
Meat, medium-fat 1
Vegetable   3

Nutrient Content per Serving:
CAL   189   PRO   14 (gm)
FAT   5 (gm)   CHO   23 (gm)
Na   514 (mg)   K   682 (mg)
Fiber   5 (gm)   Chol   37 (mg)

Key Source Nutrients:
Ascorbic acid   227 (mg)

Ingredients

4 MEDIUM-SIZE GREEN PEPPERS
½ POUND GROUND LAMB
¼ CUP ONION, CHOPPED
1 CUP COOKED RICE
1 8-OUNCE CAN TOMATO SAUCE
¼ TEASPOON GARLIC POWDER
¼ TEASPOON SALT
¼ TEASPOON NUTMEG
⅛ TEASPOON BLACK PEPPER
  PINCH OF DRIED MINT, CRUSHED

Method

1. Preheat oven to 350°F.
2. Cut thin slice from stem end of each pepper. Remove all seeds and membranes.
3. Cook peppers in boiling water for 5 minutes. Drain and set aside.
4. In 10-inch skillet, cook ground lamb and onion until lamb is brown and onion is tender; drain off fat.
5. Stir in rice, ½ cup tomato sauce, garlic powder, salt, nutmeg, pepper, and mint. Heat thoroughly.
6. Divide mixture evenly among peppers. Stand peppers upright in 8-inch baking dish.

7. Top with rest of tomato sauce.
8. Cover with foil and bake for 40–45 minutes. Uncover and bake for 10–15 minutes.

Method–Microwave

1. Place cleaned peppers upside-down in round 8-inch micro-wave-safe casserole. Cover with plastic wrap and cook on high power for 3–5 minutes.
2. Drain peppers on paper towel and discard liquid.
3. Place ground lamb and onion in plastic colander set into a 2-quart microwave-safe saucepan.
4. Cook for 2½ minutes on high power (lamb may still be a bit pink).
5. Drain fat from saucepan.
6. Crumble lamb mixture into saucepan with rice, ½ cup to-mato sauce, garlic powder, salt, nutmeg, pepper, and mint.
7. Cook for 2 minutes on high power or until heated thor-oughly.
8. Divide mixture among peppers. Stand upright in 8-inch microwave-safe dish. Top with remaining tomato sauce.
9. Cover with waxed paper. Cook on medium-high power for 8–10 minutes, rotating dish once.
10. Let stand for 5 minutes before serving.

*400 milligrams or more of sodium per serving.
**3 grams or more of fiber per serving.

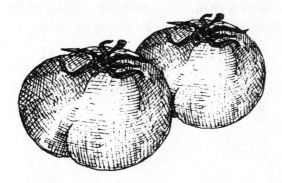

Souvlakia—Lamb Shish-Kabobs

Yield: 4 servings
Serving Size: ¼ pound
marinated lamb, without
rice

Exchanges:

Meat, lean   4
Fat   1

Nutrient Content per Serving:

CAL	271	PRO	27 (gm)
FAT	17 (gm)	CHO	1 (gm)
Na	345 (mg)	K	284 (mg)
Fiber	0 (gm)	Chol	86 (mg)

Ingredients

    2 TABLESPOONS VEGETABLE OIL
    2 TABLESPOONS LEMON JUICE
    2 TABLESPOONS WHITE WINE VINEGAR
    1 CLOVE GARLIC, SLICED
    1 BAY LEAF, HALVED
    1 TEASPOON OREGANO
    ½ TEASPOON SALT
    ⅛ TEASPOON BLACK PEPPER
    1 POUND BONELESS LAMB, CUBED

Method

1. Combine all ingredients except lamb. Place lamb in shallow dish and cover with marinade. Cover and marinate in refrigerator for at least 2 hours, turning meat over.
2. Preheat broiler.
3. Put meat through oiled skewers, if desired, or on broiling pan. Broil 6 inches from heat, turning often and basting with marinade. Broil until meat is brown and crispy, about 10–15 minutes.
4. Serve with rice.

Note: Beef may be substituted for lamb in this recipe.

Grilled Venison Steak

Yield: 4 servings
Serving Size: 1 steak
Exchanges:
Meat, lean   3½

Nutrient Content per Serving:

CAL	187	PRO	31 (gm)
FAT	5 (gm)	CHO	1 (gm)
Na	305 (mg)	K	375 (mg)
Fiber	0 (gm)	Chol	23 (mg)

Ingredients

    4 VENISON STEAKS (4 OUNCES EACH), TRIMMED
    2 CLOVES GARLIC, SPLIT
    ¼ TEASPOON ONION POWDER
    ¼ TEASPOON SALT
    ¼ TEASPOON BLACK PEPPER
    4 STRIPS BACON
    2 TEASPOONS DRY WHITE WINE (OPTIONAL)

Method

1. Preheat broiler or prepare grill.
2. Rub each steak on both sides with garlic.
3. Combine onion powder, salt, and pepper; rub on both sides of steaks.
4. Place 1 strip of bacon on each steak. Roll up and secure with a bamboo skewer.
5. Grill for 3–5 minutes per side over moderately hot fire or broiler. Steaks should be well done.
6. Transfer to a warm platter, remove skewers, and sprinkle with wine.

Venison Roast*

Yield: 8 servings
Serving Size: ⅛ of recipe
Exchanges:
Starch/Bread 1
Meat, lean 3

Nutrient Content per Serving:

CAL	235	PRO	28 (gm)
FAT	4 (gm)	CHO	20 (gm)
Na	137 (mg)	K	681 (mg)
Fiber	3 (gm)	Chol	18 (mg)

Key Source Nutrients:
Vitamin A   7,001 (IU)

Ingredients

- 1 CLOVE GARLIC, SPLIT
- ½ TEASPOON ROSEMARY
- 2 POUNDS VENISON ROAST
- 5 STRIPS BACON
- 2 BAKING POTATOES (10–12 OUNCES EACH), UNPEELED AND CUT INTO EIGHTHS
- 2 CARROTS, PEELED AND CUT INTO ½-INCH PIECES
- 1 MEDIUM ONION, CUT INTO EIGHTHS
- ¼ CUP DRY RED WINE
- ¼ CUP WATER

Method

1. Preheat oven to 350°F.
2. Rub garlic and rosemary over roast. Insert garlic in roast. Place in shallow roasting pan. Cover with bacon strips and tie with string. Add potatoes, carrots, and onion to pan. Pour wine and water into pan.
3. Insert meat thermometer into roast and cook until thermometer reaches 170°F, about 1½ hours. Baste often; if needed, add more water during cooking. Allow roast to stand covered about 10 minutes before carving. Remove string and bacon before carving. Serve with vegetables and natural pan juices.

*3 grams or more of fiber per serving.

Venison Chile* **

Yield: 4 servings†
Serving Size: ¼ recipe
Exchanges:
Starch/Bread 1
Meat, lean 2½
Vegetable 2

Nutrient Content per Serving:

CAL	257	PRO	33 (gm)
FAT	3 (gm)	CHO	25 (gm)
Na	688 (mg)	K	858 (mg)
Fiber	6 (gm)	Chol	15 (mg)

Ingredients

1 POUND VENISON, CUBED
2 CLOVES GARLIC
1 15-OUNCE CAN KIDNEY BEANS, RINSED AND DRAINED
1 MEDIUM ONION, CHOPPED
1 8-OUNCE CAN TOMATO SAUCE
16 OUNCES WATER
2 TEASPOONS CHILE POWDER
½ TEASPOON SALT
¼ TEASPOON CUMIN

Method

1. Trim fat from venison. Grind venison with garlic in food processor or meat grinder. Remove any bits of fat not processed.
2. Combine venison, beans, onion, tomato sauce, water, chile powder, salt, and cumin in large pot.
3. Cover; cook over moderate heat, stirring occasionally, for 2–2½ hours or until tender. Adjust seasonings.

*400 milligrams or more of sodium per serving.
**3 grams or more of fiber per serving.
†To make 8 servings, double recipe.

Poultry

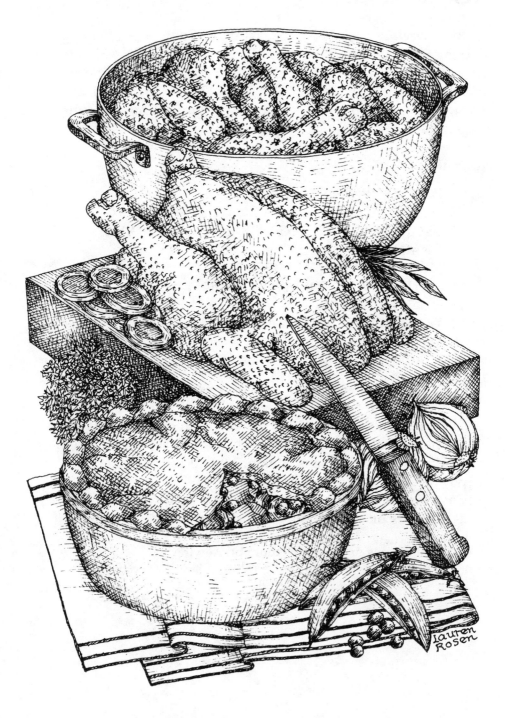

Lauren Rosen

*N*owadays, there *is* a chicken in nearly every pot— or under every broiler or stir-fried in every wok. It's hard to think of a more versatile main dish than poultry, and it's generally economical and low in fat as well.

Tandoori Chicken*

Yield: 4 servings
Serving Size: ¼ chicken
Exchanges:
Meat, medium-fat 3

Nutrient Content per Serving:

CAL	231	PRO	26 (gm)
FAT	13 (gm)	CHO	2 (gm)
Na	621 (mg)	K	259 (mg)
Fiber	0 (gm)	Chol	81 (mg)

Ingredients

    1 2-POUND CHICKEN, CUT UP
    1 TEASPOON SALT
    ¼ CUP LEMON JUICE

Marinade

    1 CLOVE GARLIC, CHOPPED
    2 TEASPOONS GINGER ROOT, CHOPPED
    2 TEASPOONS PAPRIKA
    ½ TEASPOON GROUND CUMIN
    ¼ TEASPOON CARDAMOM
    ¼ TEASPOON RED PEPPER FLAKES, CRUSHED
    ¼ CUP PLAIN LOW-FAT YOGURT

Method

1. Prick chicken with a fork. Make diagonal slashes ½ inch deep, 1 inch apart in chicken. Place in 2-quart baking dish. Rub with salt and lemon juice. Cover; marinate for 30 minutes.
2. Combine all ingredients for marinade. Pour over chicken. Marinate for 4 hours at room temperature or overnight in refrigerator.
3. Preheat oven to 500°F.
4. Bring chicken to room temperature. Bake for 30–35 minutes or until chicken is cooked thoroughly. Serve with rice.**

*400 milligrams or more of sodium per serving.
**Rice not included in nutritional analysis.

New England Chicken Croquettes*

Yield: 8 croquettes (4 servings)

Serving Size: 2 croquettes

Exchanges:

Starch/Bread	1
Meat, lean	3
Fat	1

Nutrient Content per Serving:

CAL	305	PRO	24 (gm)
FAT	14 (gm)	CHO	20 (gm)
Na	589 (mg)	K	316 (mg)
Fiber	1 (gm)	Chol	188 (mg)

Ingredients

        2 TABLESPOONS MARGARINE
        2 TABLESPOONS FLOUR
        1 CUP SKIM MILK
        1 TEASPOON WORCESTERSHIRE SAUCE
    ½ TEASPOON CHERVIL
    ½ TEASPOON SALT
    ⅛ TEASPOON WHITE PEPPER
        2 CUPS COOKED CHICKEN, FINELY CHOPPED
    ⅔ CUP BREAD CRUMBS
        2 EGGS, LIGHTLY BEATEN
        NONSTICK VEGETABLE SPRAY

Method

1. Preheat oven to 375°F.
2. Melt margarine over low heat; stir in flour until smooth. Add milk gradually, whisk until smooth; add Worcestershire sauce, chervil, salt, pepper, and chicken. Cool.
3. When cold, form into 8 balls, using ⅓ cup of mixture per ball.
4. Roll in bread crumbs, egg, and again in bread crumbs.
5. Place on cookie sheet well sprayed with nonstick vegetable spray. Bake for 25–30 minutes until a light golden brown. Serve with cranberry sauce, if desired.

*400 milligrams or more of sodium per serving.

Chicken Nuggets with B.B.Q. Dipping Sauce

Yield: 12 nuggets (4 servings)

Serving Size: 3 nuggets with 1 teaspoon sauce

Exchanges:

Starch/Bread   1
Meat, lean   3

Nutrient Content per Serving:

CAL	225	PRO	30 (gm)
FAT	5 (gm)	CHO	12 (gm)
Na	358 (mg)	K	302 (mg)
Fiber	0 (gm)	Chol	140 (mg)

Ingredients

    12 CHICKEN NUGGETS (MAY FIND READY MADE
       AT GROCERY OR CUBE 2 WHOLE BONELESS
       BREASTS, ABOUT 1 POUND)
    ½ TEASPOON SALT
       PEPPER TO TASTE
     1 EGG, BEATEN
    ½ CUP DRY BREAD CRUMBS

B.B.Q. Sauce (Yield: ⅓ cup)

     2 TABLESPOONS PREPARED MUSTARD
     2 TABLESPOONS KETCHUP
     1 TEASPOON WORCESTERSHIRE SAUCE
    ½ TEASPOON DRIED MINCED ONION FLAKES
    ½ TEASPOON BROWN SUGAR SUBSTITUTE

Method

1. Preheat oven to 350°F.
2. Sprinkle nuggets with salt and pepper.
3. Dip nuggets in egg, then bread crumbs. Place on cookie sheet.
4. Bake for 20–25 minutes or until lightly golden brown and juices run clear.
5. For sauce, combine mustard, ketchup, Worcestershire sauce, onion, and brown sugar substitute. Mix well. Serve with nuggets, about ¼ of the sauce per serving.

Note: Instead of B.B.Q. sauce, try low-salt teriyaki, sweet and sour, or hot mustard sauce.

Spinach-Stuffed Chicken Breasts

Yield: 4 servings*
Serving Size: ½ breast plus
stuffing (with skin)
Exchanges:
Meat, medium-fat 3
Vegetable   2

Nutrient Content per Serving:
CAL 257   PRO   34 (gm)
FAT   11 (gm)   CHO   4 (gm)
Na   336 (mg)   K   420 (mg)
Fiber 1 (gm)   Chol   90 (mg)

Key Source Nutrients:
Vitamin A   4,545 (IU)

Serving Size: ½ breast plus
stuffing (without skin)
Exchanges:
Meat, lean   3
Vegetable   2

Nutrient Content per Serving:
CAL 218   PRO   33 (gm)
FAT   8 (gm)   CHO   4 (gm)
Na   335 (mg)   K   415 (mg)
Fiber 1 (gm)   Chol   85 (mg)

Key Source Nutrients:
Vitamin A   4,476 (IU)

Ingredients

- ½ 10-OUNCE PACKAGE FROZEN CHOPPED
  SPINACH, DEFROSTED AND DRAINED
- 2 OUNCES (¼ CUP) LOW-FAT RICOTTA CHEESE
- 2 OUNCES LOW-FAT MOZZARELLA CHEESE,
  FINELY DICED OR SHREDDED
- ¼ TEASPOON TARRAGON
- ¼ TEASPOON SALT
- ⅛ TEASPOON BLACK PEPPER
- 2 WHOLE CHICKEN BREASTS, DEBONED (LEAVE
  SKIN INTACT)
- ½ TEASPOON MARGARINE, MELTED

Method

1. Preheat oven to 350°F.
2. Combine spinach, cheeses, and seasonings.

3. Lift up skin of each chicken breast and divide mixture evenly among them. Be careful not to tear skins. Smooth skin over stuffing; tuck underneath to form a neat package.
4. Brush with melted margarine. Place in 2-quart baking dish.
5. Bake uncovered for 45–50 minutes.

Method–Microwave

1. Follow directions above for preparation of chicken breasts.
2. Place on microwave roast rack skin side up; brush with 2 teaspoons of a commercial browning sauce mixed with 1 teaspoon water in place of margarine.
3. Cover with waxed paper for the first half of cooking time. Cook for 6–7 minutes per pound on medium-high power, rotating dish halfway through cooking time.

*To make 8 servings, double the recipe.

Chicken Marengo* **

Yield: 4 servings
Serving Size: ¼ chicken
(with skin)
Exchanges:
Meat, medium-
   fat   4½
Vegetable   3

Nutrient Content per Serving:
CAL 421   PRO   44 (gm)
FAT   21 (gm) CHO   16 (gm)
Na   711 (mg) K   1,068 (mg)
Fiber 5 (gm) Chol   127 (mg)

Serving Size: ¼ chicken
(without skin)
Exchanges:
Meat, lean   4
Vegetable   3

Nutrient Content per Serving:
CAL 279   PRO   35 (gm)
FAT   9 (gm) CHO   16 (gm)
Na   689 (mg) K   1,003 (mg)
Fiber 5 (gm) Chol   95 (mg)

Ingredients

    NONSTICK VEGETABLE SPRAY
1 2½-POUND FRYING CHICKEN, CUT INTO
  EIGHTHS
½ POUND FRESH MUSHROOMS, SLICED
2 ONIONS, PEELED AND QUARTERED
1 28-OUNCE CAN PLUM TOMATOES, SLIGHTLY
  CRUSHED, WITH JUICE
½ CUP DRY WHITE WINE
½ TEASPOON GARLIC POWDER
½ TEASPOON SALT
⅛ TEASPOON BLACK PEPPER

Method

1. Preheat oven to 350°F.
2. Spray large oven-proof skillet with nonstick vegetable spray. Sauté chicken until brown on all sides, about 15 minutes. Add mushrooms, onions, tomatoes with juice, wine, and seasonings. Stir into chicken. Cover with foil and bake for 1–1½ hours or until tender.

*400 milligrams or more of sodium per serving.
**3 grams or more of fiber per serving.

California-Style Chicken*

Yield: 4 servings
Serving Size: ¼ chicken
(with skin)
Exchanges:
Meat, medium-fat 5
Vegetable 1

Nutrient Content per Serving:
CAL 388   PRO   41 (gm)
FAT   22 (gm)   CHO   5 (gm)
Na   424 (mg)   K   518 (mg)
Fiber   2 (gm)   Chol 127 (mg)

Serving Size: ¼ chicken
(without skin)
Exchanges:
Meat, lean   4
Vegetable   1

Nutrient Content per Serving:
CAL 247   PRO   32 (gm)
FAT   10 (gm)   CHO   5 (gm)
Na   402 (mg)   K   454 (mg)
Fiber   2 (gm)   Chol   95 (mg)

Ingredients

    2 TEASPOONS OLIVE OIL
    1 BROILER-FRYER CHICKEN, CUT UP (ABOUT 2½–3
      POUNDS)
    2 TEASPOONS BASIL
    1 TEASPOON OREGANO
    ½ TEASPOON SALT
    ¼ TEASPOON BLACK PEPPER
   40 CLOVES GARLIC, UNPEELED
    4 RIBS CELERY, CUT INTO 1-INCH PIECES
    1 CUP ONION, CHOPPED
    ¼ CUP PARSLEY, CHOPPED
    ½ CUP DRY WHITE WINE
    2 TABLESPOONS LEMON JUICE

Method

1. Preheat oven to 375°F.
2. Place oil in 2-quart baking dish. Coat chicken with oil.
3. Combine seasonings and sprinkle over chicken.
4. Sprinkle garlic, celery, onion, and parsley over chicken.
5. Pour wine and lemon juice over chicken.
6. Cover with foil and bake for 40 minutes. Uncover and bake for an additional 30 minutes. Squeeze garlic out of skin and spread on toasted French bread, if desired.

Method–Microwave

1. Place oil in 2-quart microwave-safe baking dish.
2. Follow instructions above for preparing chicken.
3. Cover with waxed paper. Cook on medium-high power for 24–26 minutes, rotating dish halfway through cooking time. Let stand for 10 minutes before serving.

*400 milligrams or more of sodium per serving.

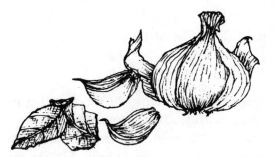

Southern Chicken Hash

Yield: 4 servings
Serving Size: 1 cup

Nutrient Content per Serving:

CAL	254	PRO	28 (gm)
FAT	11 (gm)	CHO	11 (gm)
Na	378 (mg)	K	438 (mg)
Fiber	2 (gm)	Chol	79 (mg)

Exchanges:
Starch/Bread   ½
Meat, lean   3½
Vegetable   1

Ingredients

   ½ CUP ONION, CHOPPED
   ¼ CUP GREEN PEPPER, CHOPPED
   1 TABLESPOON VEGETABLE OIL
      NONSTICK VEGETABLE SPRAY
 2½ CUPS COOKED CHICKEN, COARSELY CHOPPED
   1 CUP RED POTATOES, COOKED, PEELED, AND
      DICED
   1 TEASPOON WORCESTERSHIRE SAUCE
   ½ TEASPOON SALT
   ½ TEASPOON PAPRIKA
   ⅛ TEASPOON MACE
      PINCH OF CAYENNE PEPPER
   ¼ CUP EVAPORATED SKIM MILK

Method

1. Sauté onion and green pepper with oil for about 5 minutes in skillet well sprayed with nonstick vegetable spray.
2. Stir in chicken, potatoes, Worcestershire sauce, salt, paprika, mace, cayenne pepper, and evaporated milk. Flatten out thin. Cover pan and cook for 5 minutes until hash is heated thoroughly. Uncover and cook on low; allow hash to brown. Flip over; hash will break apart. Pat down, brown, and serve.

Method–Microwave

1. Sauté onion and green pepper in oil in 1½-quart microwave-safe casserole for 5 minutes on high power. Stir once.
2. Stir in chicken, potatoes, Worcestershire sauce, salt, paprika, mace, cayenne pepper, and evaporated milk. Cover and cook for 5–6 minutes or until hash is heated thoroughly on high power. Stir once and serve.

Chicken Pot Pie* **

Yield: 4 servings
Serving Size: 1 cup
Exchanges:
Starch/Bread   2
Meat, medium-
   fat   4½
Vegetable   2

Nutrient Content per Serving:

CAL	552	PRO	41 (gm)
FAT	25 (gm)	CHO	39 (gm)
Na	791 (mg)	K	645 (mg)
Fiber	5 (gm)	Chol	163 (mg)

Ingredients

    NONSTICK VEGETABLE SPRAY
 2 TABLESPOONS FLOUR
 1 CUP CANNED CHICKEN BROTH†
 1 TEASPOON DRIED PARSLEY FLAKES
½ TEASPOON TARRAGON
¼ TEASPOON GARLIC POWDER
⅛ TEASPOON BLACK PEPPER
 3 CUPS COOKED CHICKEN, CUBED
 1 10-OUNCE PACKAGE FROZEN MIXED
   VEGETABLES
 1 8-OUNCE CAN TINY WHOLE ONIONS, DRAINED
4–6 FRESH MUSHROOMS, SLICED
 1 9-INCH READY-MADE OR HOMEMADE PIE
   CRUST
 1 EGG YOLK MIXED WITH 1 TABLESPOON WATER

Method

1. Preheat oven to 425°F. Spray 1½-quart casserole with non-stick vegetable spray.
2. Whisk flour into chicken broth in 1½-quart saucepan. Whisk in seasonings. Cook over medium heat, stirring constantly until sauce thickens.
3. Combine chicken, vegetables, onions, and mushrooms. Stir in sauce. Pour into prepared casserole.
4. Top with pie crust; mold crust to sides of casserole. Brush with egg yolk mixture, cut steam vents, and bake for 20–25 minutes or until crust is golden brown.

*400 milligrams or more of sodium per serving.
**3 grams or more of fiber per serving.
†For reduced salt and fat, use homemade chicken broth.

Stuffed Baked Chicken

Yield: 4 servings
Serving Size: ¼ chicken
(with skin)
Exchanges:
Meat, medium-fat 5
Vegetable   1

Nutrient Content per Serving:

CAL	398	PRO	41 (gm)
FAT	23 (gm)	CHO	5 (gm)
Na	299 (mg)	K	538 (mg)
Fiber	2 (gm)	Chol	127 (mg)

Serving Size: ¼ chicken
(without skin)
Exchanges:
Meat, lean   4
Vegetable   1

Nutrient Content per Serving:

CAL	256	PRO	32 (gm)
FAT	11 (gm)	CHO	5 (gm)
Na	277 (mg)	K	474 (mg)
Fiber	2 (gm)	Chol	95 (mg)

Ingredients

NONSTICK VEGETABLE SPRAY
2 RIBS CELERY, CHOPPED
1 LARGE ONION, CHOPPED
1 CLOVE GARLIC, CHOPPED
1 CUP CLOUD EARS OR FRESH WHITE
MUSHROOMS, CHOPPED, SOAKED, AND
DRAINED
2 TEASPOONS MARGARINE
¼ TEASPOON GARLIC POWDER
¼ TEASPOON SALT
⅛ TEASPOON BLACK PEPPER
1 WHOLE FRYER CHICKEN (2½ POUNDS)
1 TEASPOON VEGETABLE OIL

Method

1. Preheat oven to 400°F. Spray shallow roasting pan with non-stick vegetable spray.
2. Sauté celery, onion, garlic, and mushrooms in margarine until soft, but not brown. Stir in seasonings.
3. Rinse and pat dry chicken. Stuff cavity with celery mixture. Rub with vegetable oil. Place in roasting pan. Bake for 1 hour at 400°F. Reduce heat to 350°F and bake for 1½ hours until skin is brown and crisp and juices run clear.

Method–Microwave

1. Cook celery, onion, garlic, and mushrooms in margarine in 1½-quart microwave saucepan for 4–5 minutes or until soft on high power; stir once. Stir in seasonings.
2. Stuff cavity. Rub chicken with vegetable oil. Tie legs and wings with string. Place chicken breast side down on microwave roast rack. Cover with waxed paper.
3. Cook for 6–7 minutes per pound on medium-high power. Halfway through cooking time, place chicken breast side up. Allow chicken to stand for 10 minutes before carving.

Chicken and Cheese Puff*

Yield: 6 servings
Serving Size: 1½ cups
Exchanges:
Starch/Bread   1
Meat, medium-fat 3

Nutrient Content per Serving:
CAL 317   PRO   26 (gm)
FAT   17 (gm)   CHO 16 (gm)
Na   424 (mg)   K   359 (mg)
Fiber   1 (gm)   Chol 204 (mg)

Ingredients

    2 CUPS COOKED CHICKEN, CUBED
    1 TABLESPOON PIMIENTO, CHOPPED
    ½ TEASPOON DRY MUSTARD
    2 TEASPOONS WORCESTERSHIRE SAUCE
    ⅛ TEASPOON WHITE PEPPER
    ¼ CUP REDUCED-CALORIE MAYONNAISE
    3 EGGS, SLIGHTLY BEATEN
    1¾ CUPS SKIM MILK
       NONSTICK VEGETABLE SPRAY
    6 SLICES WHOLE WHEAT BREAD, CUT INTO
       CUBES AND CRUSTS REMOVED
    1 CUP MEDIUM-SHARP CHEDDAR CHEESE,
       SHREDDED

Method

1. Combine chicken, pimiento, mustard, Worcestershire sauce, pepper, and mayonnaise; set aside.
2. In separate bowl, beat eggs with milk.
3. Spray 8-by-8 inch baking dish with nonstick vegetable spray. Place half of bread cubes on bottom of dish. Top with all of chicken mixture and cheese. Sprinkle remaining bread cubes over cheese. Pour egg mixture over casserole. Cover and refrigerate overnight.
4. Allow casserole to come to room temperature. Preheat oven to 325°F. Bake for 1 hour or until firm and set. Serve immediately.

*400 milligrams or more of sodium per serving.

Peachy Chicken*

Yield: 2 servings**

Serving Size: ½ recipe

Exchanges:

Meat, lean	4
Fruit	1
Fat	½

Nutrient Content per Serving:

CAL	311	PRO	28 (gm)
FAT	15 (gm)	CHO	16 (gm)
Na	462 (mg)	K	394 (mg)
Fiber	2 (gm)	Chol	72 (mg)

Ingredients

    1 MEDIUM PEACH, SLICED ¼ INCH THICK
    1 WHOLE CHICKEN BREAST, DEBONED, SKINNED,
      AND CUT IN HALF
    2 TABLESPOONS ALL-PURPOSE FLOUR
    ¼ TEASPOON SALT
    ⅛ TEASPOON WHITE PEPPER
      NONSTICK VEGETABLE SPRAY
    2 TABLESPOONS MARGARINE
    ¼ TEASPOON CURRY POWDER
    ¼ TEASPOON GROUND GINGER
    ¼ CUP RED ONION, SLICED
    2 TABLESPOONS BRANDY

Method

1. Reserve sliced peach.
2. Lightly flatten chicken breast. Season flour with salt and pepper and dredge chicken in flour. Spray hot 10-inch skillet very well with nonstick vegetable spray. Melt margarine in skillet, add chicken breast, and sauté until done, about 5 minutes. Remove to a warm platter.
3. Stir curry and ginger into skillet. Add onion and stir until tender and crisp, about 1–2 minutes.
4. Add brandy; flame.
5. Add peach; cook until heated thoroughly. Remove from heat and pour over chicken.

Method–Microwave

1. Melt 2 teaspoons margarine in 1½-quart microwave casserole. Add chicken dredged in flour. Cook for 3–5 minutes on high power, turning once, or until opaque. Remove to warm platter.
2. Stir curry and ginger into margarine. Add onion and cook for 1½–2 minutes.
3. Add brandy; heat for 45 seconds; remove brandy; flame.
4. Stir in peaches, cook for 45 seconds to 1 minute or until heated thoroughly. Pour over chicken.

   *400 milligrams or more of sodium per serving.
   **To make 4 servings, double the recipe.

Hunan Chicken

Yield: 4 servings*
Serving Size: ¼ of recipe,
rice not included
Exchanges:
Meat, lean   2½
Vegetable   1

Nutrient Content per Serving:

CAL	158		PRO	20 (gm)
FAT	6 (gm)		CHO	6 (gm)
Na	331 (mg)		K	301 (gm)
Fiber	2 (gm)		Chol	48 (mg)

Ingredients

   1½ TEASPOONS VEGETABLE OIL
   ½ POUND BONELESS CHICKEN BREAST, SKINNED AND CUT INTO CUBES
   2 FRESH MUSHROOMS, SLICED
   1 GREEN ONION, SLICED ON ANGLE
   ¼ RED PEPPER, SEEDED, CORED, AND CUT INTO STRIPS
   1 CLOVE GARLIC, CHOPPED
   ½ CUP BOK CHOY, SLICED
   1 OUNCE BEAN SPROUTS

  1 OUNCE SNOW PEAS, STRINGS REMOVED
  1 TABLESPOON SOY SAUCE
  ⅛ TEASPOON GARLIC POWDER
    PINCH OF CRUSHED RED PEPPER FLAKES
1½ TEASPOONS CORNSTARCH
  1 TABLESPOON WATER
  2 TABLESPOONS UNSALTED CASHEWS

Method

1. Heat oil in large frying pan or wok. Stir-fry chicken until opaque, about 10 minutes. Set aside; keep warm.
2. In same pan, cook mushrooms, green onion, red pepper, garlic, and bok choy. Stir constantly for about 5 minutes. Add bean sprouts and snow peas. Cook for 2 minutes.
3. Stir in chicken, soy sauce, garlic powder, and crushed red pepper. Cook for 2 minutes or until chicken is heated thoroughly. Stir in cornstarch mixed with water. Stir until thickened. Stir in cashews.
4. Serve over hot rice or cold as a salad.

Method–Microwave

1. Combine chicken with vegetable oil in 2-quart microwave-safe casserole. Cover with plastic wrap, and cook for 3–4 minutes (5–6 minutes for 8 servings) on high power. Stir once. Chicken should be opaque. Set aside.
2. In same casserole, cook mushrooms, green onion, red pepper, garlic, and bok choy. Cover and cook for 2–3 minutes (3–4 minutes for 8 servings) on high power; stir once.
3. Add chicken, bean sprouts, snow peas, soy sauce, garlic powder, and crushed red pepper. Cook for 2 minutes on high power.
4. Stir in cornstarch mixed with water. Cook for 2–3 minutes on high power or until slightly thickened. Stir in cashews.

*To make 8 servings, double the recipe.

Chicken Veronique

Yield: 2 servings*
Serving Size: ½ recipe
Exchanges:
Meat, lean   3
Fruit   1

Nutrient Content per Serving:
CAL 213   PRO   30 (gm)
FAT   3 (gm)   CHO   15 (gm)
Na   241 (mg)   K   446 (mg)
Fiber 1 (gm)   Chol 74 (mg)

Ingredients

   1 SHALLOT, MINCED
   1 WHOLE CHICKEN BREAST, SKINNED AND
     DEBONED
  ⅛ TEASPOON SALT
     PINCH OF WHITE PEPPER
  ¼ CUP DRY WHITE WINE
   2 TABLESPOONS WATER
  ¼ CUP EVAPORATED SKIM MILK
  1½ TEASPOONS CORNSTARCH
  ½ CUP SEEDLESS GREEN GRAPES

Method

1. Place shallot in bottom of 10-inch skillet. Add chicken; season
   with salt and pepper. Pour wine and water over chicken.
   Bring to a boil; cover. Reduce heat; simmer for 10 minutes or
   until chicken is cooked thoroughly.
2. Remove chicken and keep warm. Strain poaching liquid into
   1-quart saucepan and cook over high heat until reduced to
   ⅓ cup.
3. Stir in milk mixed with cornstarch. Whisk until thickened over
   medium heat; stir in grapes. Serve over chicken.

Method–Microwave

1. Place shallot in bottom of shallow microwave-safe casserole. Add chicken; season with salt and pepper. Pour wine and water over chicken. Cover with plastic wrap; cook for 6–7 minutes (8–10 minutes for 4 servings) on high power; rotate dish halfway through cooking.
2. Remove chicken to heated plate and keep warm. Strain liquid into a 1-quart microwave-safe saucepan. Cook on high power for 4–5 minutes (8–10 minutes for 4 servings) or until reduced to ⅓ cup (⅔ cup for 4 servings).
3. Whisk in milk mixed with cornstarch. Cook on medium-high power for 1½–2½ minutes (2½–3½ minutes for 4 servings) or until thickened. Whisk once halfway through cooking.
4. Stir in grapes; pour over chicken.

*To make 4 servings, double the recipe.

Turkey in White Wine and Marsala

Yield: 4 3-ounce servings	Nutrient Content per Serving:	
Serving Size: 1 slice	CAL 181	PRO 30 (gm)
Exchanges:	FAT 1 (gm)	CHO 8 (gm)
Starch/Bread ½	Na 246 (mg)	K 342 (mg)
Meat, lean 3	Fiber 0 (gm)	Chol 77 (mg)

Ingredients

    1 POUND TURKEY BREAST, SLICED
    3 TABLESPOONS ALL-PURPOSE FLOUR
   ¼ TEASPOON WHITE PEPPER
      NONSTICK VEGETABLE SPRAY
   ¼ CUP DRY WHITE WINE
   ¼ CUP SWEET MARSALA WINE
   ½ CUP CANNED CHICKEN BROTH
    1 CLOVE GARLIC, MINCED
   ¼ TEASPOON BROWN SUGAR SUBSTITUTE
    1 TEASPOON CORNSTARCH
    2 TABLESPOONS WATER
   ½ TEASPOON LEMON ZEST

Method

1. Rinse turkey slices and pat dry. Mix flour with pepper. Dredge turkey in flour and shake off excess.
2. Heat skillet and spray well with nonstick vegetable spray. Cook cutlets in single layer over medium-high heat, about 2 minutes. Turn over and cook for an additional 2 minutes, or until light tan in color. Remove turkey to a warm platter.
3. Add wine, Marsala, chicken broth, garlic, and brown sugar to skillet. Stir, scraping up bits from pan. Bring to boil and reduce sauce to ½ cup.
4. Stir in cornstarch mixed with water. Bring to boil. Stir in lemon zest.
5. Return turkey to skillet, coat with sauce, and heat thoroughly, about 5 minutes.

Croque Madame*

Yield: 6 sandwiches or 12 appetizers

Serving Size: 1 sandwich

Exchanges:

Starch/Bread 1

Meat, medium-fat 2

Fat ½

Nutrient Content per Serving:

CAL	254	PRO	18 (gm)
FAT	12 (gm)	CHO	16 (gm)
Na	419 (mg)	K	158 (mg)
Fiber	1 (gm)	Chol	85 (mg)

Ingredients

1 LONG LOAF FRENCH OR ITALIAN BREAD
2 TABLESPOONS MARGARINE, MELTED
2 TABLESPOONS DIJON MUSTARD
6 THIN TURKEY SLICES, COOKED
1 TABLESPOON WONDRA FLOUR
1 LARGE EGG, SLIGHTLY BEATEN
¼ CUP LIGHT BEER
½ TEASPOON BRANDY EXTRACT
¼ TEASPOON SALT
⅛ TEASPOON CAYENNE PEPPER
1 CUP SWISS CHEESE, SHREDDED

Method

1. Preheat oven to 450°F.
2. Cut off top and bottom crusts of bread. Cut lengthwise into 2¾-inch slices.
3. Brush both slices of bread with margarine-mustard combination. Top half of bread with turkey slices.
4. Combine Wondra flour, egg, beer, brandy extract, salt, cayenne, and Swiss cheese. Brush onto turkey.
5. Top with remaining bread slice, mustard side up. Bake for 15 minutes or until brown and crisp. Slice and serve.

*400 milligrams or more of sodium per serving.

Turkey Creole* **

Yield: 2 servings†

Serving Size: ½ 2-serving recipe

Exchanges:

Meat, lean   2½

Vegetable   3

Nutrient Content per Serving:

CAL	222	PRO	38 (gm)
FAT	2 (gm)	CHO	14 (gm)
Na	828 (mg)	K	851 (mg)
Fiber	3 (gm)	Chol	96 (mg)

Key Source Nutrients:
Ascorbic acid   73 (mg)

Ingredients

- ½ BAY LEAF
- ¼ TEASPOON OREGANO
- ¼ TEASPOON SALT
- ¼ TEASPOON BASIL
- ⅛ TEASPOON BLACK PEPPER
- ⅛ TEASPOON PAPRIKA
- ⅛ TEASPOON CAYENNE PEPPER
- ⅛ TEASPOON THYME
- ⅛ TEASPOON GARLIC POWDER
  NONSTICK VEGETABLE SPRAY
- ½ POUND TURKEY CUTLETS
- ½ GREEN PEPPER, CHOPPED
- ¼ CUP FRESH MUSHROOMS, SLICED
- ¼ CUP CELERY, CHOPPED
- ¼ CUP ONION, CHOPPED
- ½ CLOVE GARLIC, CHOPPED
- 1 8-OUNCE CAN STEWED TOMATOES, UNDRAINED
- ½ CUP CHICKEN BROTH‡
- 2 DROPS TABASCO SAUCE
- 1½ TEASPOONS CORNSTARCH
- 1½ TEASPOONS WATER

Method

1. Combine seasonings. Set aside.
2. Spray large frying pan with nonstick vegetable spray. Heat pan.
3. Sear turkey cutlets quickly on both sides. Set aside.
4. Sauté green pepper, mushrooms, celery, onion, and garlic, about 5 minutes.
5. Add seasonings, tomatoes with juice, chicken broth, Tabasco sauce, and cornstarch mixed with water. Bring to a boil. Simmer for 20–30 minutes.
6. Add cutlets; spoon sauce over them and simmer for another 4–6 minutes.
7. Remove bay leaf before serving. Serve over hot cooked rice.

Method–Microwave

1. Place turkey cutlets in 8-inch round microwave-safe casserole (may need to cook in batches); cover with waxed paper. Cook for 2½–3 minutes per batch on high power. Set aside.
2. In same casserole, cook green peppers, mushrooms, celery, onion, and garlic for 3–4 minutes uncovered on high power, stirring once.
3. Stir in seasonings, tomatoes with juice, chicken broth, Tabasco sauce, and cornstarch mixed with water. Bring to a boil for 3–5 minutes uncovered on high power. Continue to cook for 6–8 minutes on medium power or until bubbly and thickened, stirring once.
4. Bury turkey in sauce. Cover with waxed paper and cook for 3–4 minutes on medium-high power or until heated thoroughly.

*400 milligrams or more of sodium per serving.
**3 grams or more of fiber per serving.
†To make 4 servings, double the recipe.
‡For reduced salt and fat, use homemade chicken broth.

Hawaiian Turkey Burgers*

Yield: 4 servings
Serving Size: 1 patty plus
sauce
Exchanges:
Meat, medium-
   fat   2½
Fruit   1

Nutrient Content per Serving:

CAL	227	PRO	16 (gm)
FAT	12 (gm)	CHO	17 (gm)
Na	763 (mg)	K	387 (mg)
Fiber	2 (gm)	Chol	47 (mg)

Ingredients

   1 POUND GROUND TURKEY
   1 TABLESPOON BREAD CRUMBS
   1 TEASPOON PREPARED MUSTARD
  ¼ TEASPOON GARLIC POWDER
  ¼ TEASPOON ONION POWDER
  ⅛ TEASPOON SALT
  ⅛ TEASPOON BLACK PEPPER

Sauce

   1 16-OUNCE CAN MIXED FRUITS PACKED IN
     LIGHT SYRUP OR PINEAPPLE CHUNKS IN OWN
     JUICE, DRAINED AND RESERVED
   1 TABLESPOON VINEGAR
   2 TEASPOONS SOY SAUCE
   1 TEASPOON CORNSTARCH
   1 TABLESPOON WATER
   1 SMALL GREEN PEPPER, CUT INTO CHUNKS AND
     BLANCHED

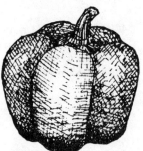

Method

1. Preheat broiler.
2. Mix turkey with bread crumbs and seasonings. Shape into 4 patties.
3. Broil for 3–4 minutes per side.
4. In 2-quart saucepan, combine reserved juice, vinegar, soy sauce, and cornstarch mixed with water.
5. Bring to a boil; reduce heat and simmer, whisking until thickened.
6. Stir in green pepper and fruit.
7. Pour over "burgers."

Method–Microwave (sauce only)

1. In 2-quart microwave-safe saucepan, combine juice, vinegar, soy sauce, and cornstarch mixed with water. Cook for 3–5 minutes on medium-high power; stir once.
2. Stir in green pepper and fruit.

*400 milligrams or more of sodium per serving.

Braised Quail

Yield: 4 servings
Serving Size: 1 quail plus
sauce
Exchanges:
Meat, lean   3
Fat   2

Nutrient Content per Serving:

CAL	266	PRO	22 (gm)
FAT	19 (gm)	CHO	1 (gm)
Na	258 (mg)	K	262 (mg)
Fiber	0 (gm)	Chol	14 (mg)

Ingredients

NONSTICK VEGETABLE SPRAY
2 TABLESPOONS MARGARINE
1/3 CUP ONION, CHOPPED
1 LARGE CLOVE GARLIC, CHOPPED
1/2 BAY LEAF
4 QUAIL (3 OUNCES EACH), SEMI-BONELESS OR
   WITH BONE, TRUSSED AND CLEANED
3/4 CUP DRY WHITE WINE
3/4 CUP WATER
1/4 TEASPOON SALT
1/8 TEASPOON BLACK PEPPER

Method

1. Spray large skillet with nonstick vegetable spray and melt margarine. Sauté onion, garlic, and bay leaf for 5 minutes.
2. Add quail and brown on all sides.
3. Add wine, water, and seasonings. Cover and simmer slowly for 30 minutes or until tender.
4. Remove quail to individual serving plates and spoon sauce over each quail.

Fish and Seafood

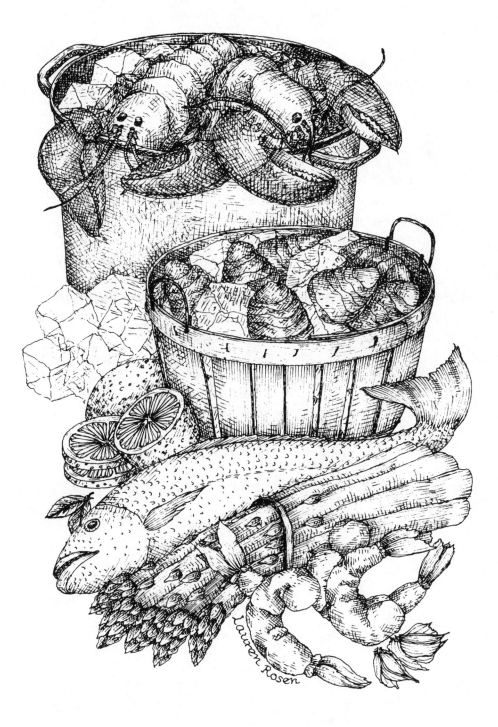

Lauren Rosen

*E*ven if you don't eat much fish—perhaps fresh fish isn't readily available in your region of the country— do try some of these recipes. Many can be made quite easily using canned or frozen alternatives. Sole, crab, lobster, shrimp, and oysters are widely available in frozen or canned form. Unless otherwise noted, they are acceptable for use in the recipes in this section (although when using nonfresh products, you should check the label for sodium content).

Fillet of Sole Italiano*

Yield: 2 servings**
Serving Size: 3½ ounces
plus sauce
Exchanges:
Meat, lean   2
Vegetable   2½

Nutrient Content per Serving:

CAL	167	PRO	32 (gm)
FAT	1 (gm)	CHO	6 (gm)
Na	1,046 (mg)	K	913 (mg)
Fiber	0 (gm)	Chol	47 (mg)

Ingredients

1 CUP TOMATO JUICE
1 TABLESPOON DEHYDRATED ONION FLAKES
½ TEASPOON CHICKEN BOUILLON GRANULES
¼ TEASPOON GARLIC POWDER
¼ TEASPOON OREGANO
¼ TEASPOON BLACK PEPPER
2 FRESH MUSHROOMS, SLICED
½ POUND FILLET OF SOLE

Method

1. Preheat oven to 350°F.
2. Combine all ingredients except fish in 2-quart saucepan.
3. Bring to a boil; cook for 8–10 minutes until slightly thickened.
4. Place fillets in 2-quart baking dish.
5. Pour sauce over fillets; cover with foil.
6. Bake for 20 minutes or until fish flakes with a fork.

Method–Microwave

1. Combine all ingredients except fish in 2-quart microwave-safe casserole.
2. Cook for 8–10 minutes on high power until mixture comes to a boil, stirring once.
3. Bury fish in sauce; cover with waxed paper.
4. Cook for 4–5 minutes on high power or until fish flakes with a fork. Let stand covered for 5 minutes before serving.

*400 milligrams or more of sodium per serving.
**To make 4 servings, double the recipe.

Shrimp and Asparagus in Fettucini with Mustard Cream Sauce*

Yield: 4 servings
Serving Size: 1 cup
Exchanges:
Starch/Bread 2
Meat, lean 1
Fat 2
Vegetable 1

Nutrient Content per Serving:
CAL 306   PRO   16 (gm)
FAT   14 (gm)   CHO 28 (gm)
Na   756 (mg)   K   295 (mg)
Fiber   1 (gm)   Chol 103 (mg)

Ingredients

    4 OUNCES FETTUCINI NOODLES
    8 OUNCES SHRIMP, PEELED AND DEVEINED
    4 OUNCES ASPARAGUS, CUT INTO 1-INCH PIECES
    1 CLOVE GARLIC, MINCED
    2 TABLESPOONS OLIVE OIL
    2 TABLESPOONS MARGARINE
    2 TABLESPOONS FLOUR
    1 CUP SKIM MILK
    ¼ TEASPOON SALT
    ⅛ TEASPOON BLACK PEPPER
    1 TABLESPOON DIJON MUSTARD

Method

1. Cook fettucini in 6 cups boiling water until *al dente*. Drain.
2. Sauté shrimp and asparagus and garlic in oil just until shrimp is cooked thoroughly.
3. Melt margarine in 1-quart saucepan over medium heat. Add flour; cook until bubbly. Gradually stir in milk, cooking and stirring until thickened. Add salt and pepper; remove from heat and stir in mustard.
4. In a large bowl, combine fettucini, shrimp mixture, and sauce; toss to coat. Serve immediately.

*400 milligrams or more of sodium per serving.

Fillet of Sole Etoufee*

Yield: 4 servings

Serving Size: 1 sandwich

Exchanges:

Starch/Bread	1
Meat, lean	3

Nutrient Content per Serving:

CAL	267	PRO	37 (gm)
FAT	5 (gm)	CHO	17 (gm)
Na	625 (mg)	K	826 (mg)
Fiber	2 (gm)	Chol	116 (mg)

Ingredients

1 POUND FILLET OF SOLE, DEBONED (4 SLICES)

Stuffing

1 RIB CELERY, CHOPPED
1 SMALL ONION, CHOPPED
4 FRESH MUSHROOMS, SLICED
1 TEASPOON MARGARINE
1½ CUPS UNSEASONED BREAD CUBES FOR STUFFING
½ CUP CHICKEN BROTH**
1 EGG, LIGHTLY BEATEN
PEPPER, TO TASTE

Method

1. Preheat oven to 350°F.
2. Sauté celery, mushrooms, and onion in margarine, about 5 minutes.
3. In bowl, combine bread cubes, chicken broth, egg, and pepper. Stir in celery mixture.
4. Place 2 slices fish on cookie sheet side by side. Top with stuffing (about 2–3 tablespoons each). Top with remaining fish.
5. Bake covered with foil for 15–20 minutes or until fish flakes with a fork.
6. Divide the two filled "sandwiches" into four servings.

Method–Microwave

1. Combine margarine, celery, onion, and mushrooms in 2-quart microwave-safe saucepan. Cook for 4–5 minutes on high power; stir once.
2. In bowl, combine bread cubes, chicken broth, egg, and pepper. Stir in celery mixture.
3. Place 2 slices fish on microwave roast rack. Top with stuffing and remaining fish.
4. Cover with plastic wrap; cook for 4–5 minutes or until fish flakes with a fork. Let stand covered for 5 minutes before serving.
5. Divide the two fillet "sandwiches" into four servings.

Note: You can also roll fillets with stuffing inside and use a toothpick to hold together.

*400 milligrams or more of sodium per serving.
**For reduced salt and fat, use homemade chicken broth.

Swordfish with Red Pepper Sauce

Yield: 4 servings with 1 cup sauce

Serving size: ¼ fish plus ¼ cup sauce

Exchanges:

Meat, lean	3
Vegetable	1
Fat	1½

Nutrient Content per Serving:

CAL	253	PRO	23 (gm)
FAT	16 (gm)	CHO	3 (gm)
Na	145 (mg)	K	91 (mg)
Fiber	1 (gm)	Chol	44 (mg)

Ingredients

1 CUP WATER
1 TABLESPOON LEMON JUICE
1 POUND SWORDFISH STEAK

Red Pepper Sauce

    1 7-OUNCE JAR ROASTED RED PEPPERS, DRAINED
      AND RINSED
    2 TABLESPOONS EVAPORATED SKIM MILK
    ½ CUP DRY WHITE WINE
    2 TABLESPOONS LEMON JUICE
  1½ TEASPOONS SHALLOT, MINCED
    2 TEASPOONS FRESH GINGER, CHOPPED,
      (½-INCH PIECES)
    4 TABLESPOONS MARGARINE, SOFTENED

Method

1. Fill 8- to 10-inch skillet with water and lemon juice. Bring to a boil. Add fish, cover, reduce heat to simmer, and cook for 10 minutes per inch of thickness. Remove to a warm plate.
2. Purée peppers with milk in food processor or blender.
3. In 1-quart saucepan, combine wine, lemon juice, shallot, and ginger. Cook over high heat until sauce is reduced to 1 tablespoon, about 5 minutes.
4. Stir in pepper purée. Add margarine 1 tablespoon at a time, whisking over low heat until just melted. Serve with fish.

Method–Microwave

1. In 1-quart microwave-safe saucepan, combine wine, lemon juice, shallot, and ginger. Cook uncovered for 8–9 minutes on high power or until sauce is reduced to 1 tablespoon.
2. Stir in pepper purée. Cook for 2 minutes on medium power. Add margarine 1 tablespoon at a time, whisking until just melted. Keep sauce warm while preparing fish.
3. Place swordfish on microwave roast rack (without water and lemon juice). Cover with plastic wrap. Cook for 5–6 minutes on high power, or until fish is opaque and flakes easily with a fork. Do not overcook. Let stand covered for 2–3 minutes. Serve fish with sauce.

Baked Orange Roughy with Tomatoes and Herbs*

Yield: 2 servings**
Serving Size: ½ of recipe
Exchanges:

		Nutrient Content per Serving:		
		CAL	144	PRO	26 (gm)
		FAT	2 (gm)	CHO	5 (gm)
Meat, lean	2	Na	510 (mg)	K	672 (mg)
Vegetable	1	Fiber	1 (gm)	Chol	37 (mg)

Ingredients

- ¼ CUP ONION, CHOPPED
- 1 CLOVE GARLIC, MINCED
- ½ TEASPOON MARGARINE
- ½ LARGE TOMATO, SEEDED AND CHOPPED
- ¼ TEASPOON SALT
- ⅛ TEASPOON OREGANO
- ⅛ TEASPOON THYME
  - PINCH OF BLACK PEPPER
- ½ POUND ORANGE ROUGHY FISH FILLETS, DEFROSTED IF FROZEN
- ¼ CUP DRY WHITE WINE
- 1½ TEASPOONS TOMATO PASTE

Method

1. Preheat oven to 350°F.
2. In oven-proof skillet over medium heat, sauté onion and garlic in margarine until soft, about 5 minutes. Stir in tomato and seasonings. Cover and simmer for 5 minutes.
3. Place fish in skillet; cover with sauce. Pour wine over fish. Cover and bake for 15–20 minutes or until fish just flakes with fork.
4. Remove fish to heated platter. Reduce sauce on top of range to ⅓ cup (⅔ cup for 4 servings). Stir in tomato paste and pour over fish. Serve with lemon wedges, if desired.

Method–Microwave

1. In 2-quart microwave-safe saucepan, cook onion and garlic in margarine for 4–5 minutes on high power, stirring once.
2. Stir in tomato and seasonings. Cook for 3 minutes on medium power, stirring once.
3. Place fish in 8-inch microwave-safe dish; pour sauce and wine over fish. Cover with plastic wrap; cook for 5–6 minutes on high power or just until fish flakes with a fork.
4. Remove fish to heated platter. Reduce sauce in dish to ⅓ cup (⅔ cup for 4 servings), about 5–6 minutes (6–8 minutes for 4 servings) on high power.
5. Stir in tomato paste; cook for 1 more minute at high power. Pour over fish. Serve with lemon wedges, if desired.

   *400 milligrams or more of sodium per serving.
   **To make 4 servings, double the recipe.

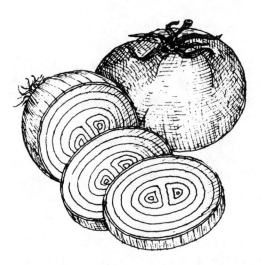

Broiled Maine Lobster Tail

Yield: 2 servings*		Nutrient Content per Serving:	
Serving Size: 1 tail		CAL 174	PRO 24 (gm)
Exchanges:		FAT 6 (gm)	CHO 3 (gm)
Meat, lean	3	Na 317 (mg)	K 252 (mg)
		Fiber 0 (gm)	Chol 108 (mg)

Ingredients

- 2 LOBSTER TAILS (ABOUT 1 POUND)
- 1 TEASPOON MARGARINE, MELTED
- 1 TEASPOON LEMON JUICE
- 2 TEASPOONS SHALLOT OR FRESH GARLIC, CHOPPED
- 1 TEASPOON OLIVE OIL
- 1 TEASPOON FINES HERBES OR ½ TEASPOON THYME AND ½ TEASPOON TARRAGON
- 1 TABLESPOON FRESH PARSLEY, CHOPPED
- ¼–½ TEASPOON GARLIC POWDER
- 1 TEASPOON LEMON JUICE
- 1 TABLESPOON BREAD CRUMBS

Method

1. Preheat broiler.
2. Split tails halfway up middle so as not to curl while broiling. Place shell side up on broiler pan. Broil for 7–8 minutes. Turn over and brush with melted margarine and 1 teaspoon lemon juice. Broil for 7–8 minutes.
3. To prepare topping, sauté shallot in olive oil until soft. Stir in fines herbes, parsley, garlic powder, lemon juice, and bread crumbs. Cook until crumbs are lightly browned.
4. Place topping on lobster tails; broil for 30 seconds. May serve with lemon wedges, if desired.

Note: Monk fish may be used in place of lobster. Monk fish is known as poor man's lobster tail. Broil monk fish for 8–10 minutes total.

*To make 4 servings, double the recipe.

Crabcakes

Yield: 4 servings*	Nutrient Content per Serving:			
Serving Size: 1 crabcake	CAL	109	PRO	11 (gm)
Exchanges:	FAT	5 (gm)	CHO	4 (gm)
Meat, lean 2	Na	202 (mg)	K	88 (mg)
	Fiber	0 (gm)	Chol	117 (mg)

Ingredients

> NONSTICK VEGETABLE SPRAY
> ½ POUND LUMP CRAB MEAT, FLAKED
> 1 TABLESPOON DIJON MUSTARD
> 1 TABLESPOON MARGARINE, MELTED
> 1 EGG
> 1½ TEASPOONS LEMON JUICE
> ½ TEASPOON WORCESTERSHIRE SAUCE
> PINCH OF CAYENNE PEPPER
> ⅛ TEASPOON SALT
> 2 DASHES TABASCO SAUCE
> ½ CUP SOFT BREAD CRUMBS

Method

1. Preheat oven to 400°F. Spray cookie sheet with nonstick vegetable spray.
2. Combine crab meat, mustard, margarine, egg, lemon juice, Worcestershire sauce, and seasonings. Add 2–4 tablespoons bread crumbs to bind.
3. Shape into 4 cakes (use about ½ cup mixture each). Roll in remaining bread crumbs; place on prepared cookie sheet.
4. Bake for 20–25 minutes or until lightly browned, turning crabcakes over halfway through cooking time. Serve with lemon wedges, if desired.

*To make 8 servings, double the recipe.

Quenelles of Sole with Shrimp Sauce*

Yield: 6 servings	Nutrient Content per Serving:
Serving Size: 4 or 5	CAL 262 PRO 25 (gm)
quenelles and ¼ cup sauce	FAT 10 (gm) CHO 16 (gm)
Exchanges:	Na 769 (mg) K 506 (mg)
Starch/Bread 1	Fiber 1 (gm) Chol 132 (mg)
Meat, lean 3½	

Ingredients

- ½ CUP WATER PLUS 2 QUARTS
- 2 TABLESPOONS MARGARINE
- ⅛ TEASPOON SALT PLUS ½ TEASPOON SALT
- ½ CUP ALL-PURPOSE FLOUR
- 2 EGGS
- ¾ POUND FILLETS OF SOLE
- ¼ TEASPOON WHITE PEPPER
- ¼ TEASPOON NUTMEG
- 1 EGG WHITE
- ¼ CUP EVAPORATED SKIM MILK, CHILLED

Method

1. Combine ½ cup water, margarine, and ⅛ teaspoon salt in 1-quart saucepan; bring to a boil. Remove from heat and stir in flour. Beat vigorously with a wooden spoon until mixture forms a ball. Allow to cool slightly.
2. Beat in eggs one at a time. Chill until cold.
3. Cut fillets into pieces; place in food processor fitted with steel blade.
4. Add remaining salt, pepper, and nutmeg; process until smooth.
5. Add egg white slowly through feed tube while processing to blend.
6. Add chilled flour mixture and mix with several on/off pulses just until blended.
7. Pour milk through feed tube while processing to blend. Chill until ready to poach.
8. Heat 2 quarts water to a slow simmer.

9. Shape rounded teaspoonfuls of the mixture and drop into water. Cook for 12–15 minutes; drain. Serve with shrimp sauce (recipe below).

Method–Microwave

1. Prepare quenelle mixture as directed above.
2. Fill 2-quart microwave-safe casserole halfway with hot water. Bring to a simmer, about 5–7 minutes on high power.
3. Cook quenelles in batches, about 8 at a time, for 5–7 minutes on high power.

Shrimp Sauce

    2 TABLESPOONS MARGARINE
    2 TABLESPOONS FLOUR
    1 CUP SKIM MILK
    ½ TEASPOON SALT
    ¼ TEASPOON GROUND WHITE PEPPER
    ⅛ TEASPOON NUTMEG
    ¼ CUP EVAPORATED SKIM MILK
    1 TEASPOON TOMATO PASTE
    2 TABLESPOONS DRY SHERRY (OPTIONAL)
    ½ CUP COOKED SHRIMP, CHOPPED

Method

1. Heat margarine in 1-quart saucepan over medium heat. Blend in flour and cook until bubbly. Whisk in milk, salt, pepper, and nutmeg. Cook over medium heat until thickened, whisking often.
2. Stir in evaporated milk, tomato paste, sherry, and shrimp. Simmer for 5 minutes or until heated thoroughly. Serve with quenelles.

Method–Microwave

1. In 2-quart microwave-safe saucepan, heat milk with margarine for 2 minutes on high power.

2. Whisk in flour and seasonings. Cook for 1½–3 minutes or until thickened on medium-high power, stirring once.
3. Stir in evaporated milk, tomato paste, sherry, and shrimp. Cook for 3–5 minutes or until heated thoroughly on medium-high power, stirring once.

*400 milligrams or more of sodium per serving.

Oyster Stir Fry* **

Yield: 4 servings
Serving Size: ¼ of recipe
Exchanges:
Meat, lean   1
Vegetable   3

Nutrient Content per Serving:

CAL	140	PRO	12 (gm)
FAT	4 (gm)	CHO	16 (gm)
Na	419 (mg)	K	400 (mg)
Fiber	4 (gm)	Chol	60 (mg)

Key Source Nutrients:
Ascorbic acid   65 (mg)

Ingredients

    1 PINT SHUCKED OYSTERS, DRAINED AND
      PATTED DRY
 1½ TABLESPOONS LOW-SODIUM SOY SAUCE
    2 TEASPOONS CORNSTARCH
    1 TABLESPOON DRY SHERRY
    1 TEASPOON FRESH GINGER, CHOPPED
    1 GREEN ONION, SLICED
  ½ TEASPOON SESAME OIL
      NONSTICK VEGETABLE SPRAY
    1 TABLESPOON VEGETABLE OIL
    1 SMALL RED BELL PEPPER, CUBED

Lemon Sauce

>   2 TEASPOONS CORNSTARCH
>   3 TABLESPOONS LEMON JUICE
>   ¼ CUP CHICKEN BROTH†
>   1 TABLESPOON LEMON PEEL, GRATED
>   ¼ TEASPOON RED PEPPER FLAKES, CRUSHED
>   1 TABLESPOON HONEY
>   4–5 RIBS BOK CHOY

Method

1. Combine oysters with soy sauce, cornstarch, sherry, ginger, green onion, and sesame oil.
2. Spray large skillet with nonstick vegetable spray. Heat vegetable oil over medium-high heat. Add oyster mixture and stir-fry for 3 minutes or until oysters are just cooked and edges curl.
3. Set oysters aside; add red pepper to skillet. Stir-fry for 1 minute. Add to oysters.
4. Combine cornstarch, lemon juice, and chicken broth, whisking over medium heat until thickened.
5. Stir in lemon peel, red pepper flakes, and honey; cool.
6. To serve, line a serving bowl with bok choy. Pour oyster mixture into bowl; top with lemon sauce. Serve at room temperature.

*400 milligrams or more of sodium per serving.
**3 grams or more of fiber per serving.
†For reduced salt and fat, use homemade chicken broth.

Catfish aux Epinards

Yield: 4 servings
Serving Size: ¼ of recipe
Exchanges:

Meat, lean	3
Vegetable	2
Fat	½

Nutrient Content per Serving:

CAL	240	PRO	25 (gm)
FAT	10 (gm)	CHO	12 (gm)
Na	392 (mg)	K	652 (mg)
Fiber	1 (gm)	Chol	85 (mg)

Key Source Nutrients:
Vitamin A   4,810 (IU)

Ingredients

- 1 CUP SKIM MILK
- 2 TABLESPOONS MARGARINE PLUS 1 TEASPOON, MELTED
- 2 TABLESPOONS FLOUR
- ¼ TEASPOON SALT
- ⅛ TEASPOON BLACK PEPPER
  PINCH OF NUTMEG
- 1 10-OUNCE PACKAGE FROZEN CHOPPED SPINACH, DEFROSTED AND DRAINED
- 1 POUND CATFISH OR SOLE FILLETS, DIVIDED INTO 4 PIECES
  NONSTICK VEGETABLE SPRAY
- ¼ CUP CORNFLAKE CRUMBS

Method

1. Preheat oven to 375°F.
2. Heat milk and 2 tablespoons margarine in 1-quart saucepan.
3. Whisk in flour, salt, pepper, and nutmeg. Continue to whisk until sauce is thickened.
4. Stir in spinach and heat for 5 minutes.
5. Spread a heaping tablespoon of spinach down middle of each fillet. Roll up lengthwise.

6. Spray 8-inch square baking dish with nonstick vegetable spray. Place fish fillets seam side down in dish.
7. Combine cornflake crumbs and 1 teaspoon melted margarine; sprinkle over fillets.
8. Bake for 25–30 minutes or until fish flakes easily with a fork. Serve with remaining heated spinach.

Method–Microwave

1. Heat milk and margarine in 2-quart microwave-safe saucepan on high power.
2. Whisk flour and seasonings into milk mixture. Cook for 1½–2½ minutes on medium-high power or until sauce coats back of spoon; whisk once.
3. Stir in spinach. Cook for 3 minutes on high power.
4. Spray 8-inch round microwave-safe casserole with nonstick vegetable spray.
5. Follow method above for preparing fish; place seam side down in prepared dish.
6. Cover with waxed paper, cook 4–5 minutes on high power or until fish flakes easily with fork. Let stand covered for 5 minutes. Serve with remaining heated spinach.

Red Snapper Provençale

		Nutrient Content per Serving:		
Yield: 4 servings				
Serving Size: ¼ of recipe		CAL 173	PRO	24 (gm)
Exchanges:		FAT 5 (gm)	CHO	8 (gm)
Meat, lean	2	Na 284 (mg)	K	696 (mg)
Vegetable	2	Fiber 2 (gm)	Chol	52 (mg)

Ingredients

- 1 MEDIUM ONION, FINELY CHOPPED
- 2 CLOVES GARLIC, MINCED
- 1 TABLESPOON OLIVE OIL
- 1 ZUCCHINI, JULIENNED
- 2 MEDIUM TOMATOES, SEEDED AND DICED
- 2 TABLESPOONS PARSLEY, CHOPPED
- 2 TABLESPOONS TOMATO PASTE
- ½ TEASPOON BASIL
- ½ TEASPOON OREGANO
- ¼ TEASPOON SALT
- ⅛ TEASPOON BLACK PEPPER
- ⅛ TEASPOON THYME
- 1 POUND RED SNAPPER FILLETS

Method

1. Preheat oven to 350°F.
2. Sauté onion and garlic in oil for 5 minutes or until soft.
3. Stir in zucchini, tomatoes, parsley, tomato paste, and seasonings. Simmer for 10–15 minutes.
4. Rinse and pat dry fillets. Pour half of sauce on bottom of 8-inch square baking dish. Top with fillets and remaining sauce.
5. Cover with foil and bake for 20–25 minutes or until fish flakes with fork.

Method–Microwave

1. In 1-quart microwave-safe casserole, cook onion and garlic in oil for 2–3 minutes on high power, stirring once.
2. Stir in zucchini, tomatoes, parsley, tomato paste, and seasonings.

3. Cook for 6–7 minutes or until thickened on medium power, stirring once.
4. Pour half of sauce in bottom of 8-inch microwave-safe baking dish. Top with fillets and remaining sauce.
5. Cover with plastic wrap. Cook for 4–5 minutes on high power or until fish flakes easily with a fork. Let stand covered for 5 minutes before serving.

Broiled Scallops*

Yield: 2 servings
Serving Size: ½ of recipe
Exchanges:

		Nutrient Content per Serving:		
		CAL	243	PRO	26 (gm)
		FAT	6 (gm)	CHO	19 (gm)
Starch/Bread	1	Na	491 (mg)	K	511 (mg)
Meat, lean	3	Fiber	1 (gm)	Chol	51 (mg)

Ingredients

        NONSTICK VEGETABLE SPRAY
    8 OUNCES SEA SCALLOPS
    ¼ CUP DRY BREAD CRUMBS
    1 TABLESPOON FRESH LEMON JUICE
    2 TEASPOONS MARGARINE, MELTED

Method

1. Preheat broiler. Spray broiler pan with nonstick vegetable spray.
2. Coat scallops lightly in bread crumbs; place on prepared pan.
3. Combine lemon juice and margarine; sprinkle over scallops.
4. Broil for 3–5 minutes or until cooked thoroughly. Serve immediately with lemon wedges, if desired.

*400 milligrams or more of sodium per serving.

Poached Scallops
with Cran-Horseradish Sauce

		Nutrient Content per Serving:		
Yield: 4 servings				
Serving Size: ¼ of recipe		CAL	78	PRO	11 (gm)
Exchanges:		FAT	1 (gm)	CHO	8 (gm)
Meat, lean	1	Na	140 (mg)	K	350 (mg)
Fruit	½	Fiber	2 (gm)	Chol	23 (mg)

Ingredients

Cran-Horseradish Sauce

- ¼ CUP WATER
- ½ CUP WHOLE FRESH OR FROZEN CRANBERRIES
- 3 PACKETS SUGAR SUBSTITUTE (NOT ASPARTAME) OR 2 TABLESPOONS SUGAR
- 2 TABLESPOONS RAISINS
- 2 TABLESPOONS CELERY, CHOPPED
- 1–2 TABLESPOONS PREPARED HORSERADISH

Poaching liquid

- ½ CUP WATER
- ¼ CUP DRY WHITE WINE
- 1 RIB CELERY, COARSELY CHOPPED
- 1 SMALL CARROT, COARSELY CHOPPED
- 2 TABLESPOONS ONION, CHOPPED
- 2 SPRIGS PARSLEY
- 1 LEMON SLICE
- ½ BAY LEAF
- 4 WHOLE BLACK PEPPERCORNS
- 8 OUNCES SEA SCALLOPS

Method

1. Combine water and cranberries in 1-quart saucepan. Bring to a boil; stir in sugar substitute. Reduce heat to simmer and cook for 3–5 minutes or until thickened.
2. Remove from heat; stir in raisins and celery. Cool for 15 minutes before adding horseradish.
3. Combine all ingredients for poaching liquid except scallops in 2-quart saucepan.
4. Bring to a boil. Add scallops, cover, and simmer. Cook for 5 minutes. Remove scallops with slotted spoon to serving bowl. Serve with cran-horseradish sauce.

Method–Microwave

1. Combine cranberries and water in 2-quart microwave-safe saucepan. Cover and cook for 3–4 minutes on high power or until boiling. Stir in sugar; cover and cook for 4–5 minutes on medium-high power or until mixture is thick. Stir in celery and raisins. Allow to cool for 15 minutes before adding horseradish.
2. Combine all ingredients for poaching liquid in 2-quart microwave-safe casserole. Cover and cook for 5–6 minutes or until boiling on high power.
3. Add scallops. Cover and cook for 3–4 minutes on high power until scallops are opaque and firm; let stand covered for 3 minutes.
4. Remove scallops with slotted spoon; serve with cran-horseradish sauce.

Shrimp with Curry Sauce

Yield: 4 servings
Serving Size: ¼ pound
shrimp plus 4½ tablespoons
sauce
Exchanges:
Starch/Bread   ½
Meat, lean   3

Nutrient Content per Serving:

CAL	197	PRO	24 (gm)
FAT	7 (gm)	CHO	9 (gm)
Na	391 (mg)	K	379 (mg)
Fiber	1 (gm)	Chol	173 (mg)

Ingredients

    2 TABLESPOONS MARGARINE
    ¼ CUP ONION, CHOPPED
    1 SMALL CLOVE GARLIC, MINCED
    1 CUP SKIM MILK
    2 TABLESPOONS FLOUR
    ½ TEASPOON SALT
 ¼–½ TEASPOON CURRY POWDER
    ⅛ TEASPOON BLACK PEPPER
    3 CUPS WATER
    1 POUND MEDIUM RAW SHRIMP, PEELED AND
      DEVEINED

Method

1. Melt margarine in small saucepan. Sauté onion and garlic until soft, about 5 minutes. Stir in milk, flour, salt, curry powder, and pepper. Whisk and cook until sauce is thickened, about 5 minutes.
2. Bring water to a boil; drop in shrimp and return to a boil. Reduce heat; simmer for 5 minutes or until shrimp turn pink and are just cooked through (do not overcook).
3. Stir shrimp into sauce; heat for 4 minutes or until heated thoroughly.

Method–Microwave

1. Place shrimp in 2-quart microwave-safe casserole with thick part of shrimp toward outside of casserole (omit water). Cover with plastic wrap; cook for 2½–3 minutes on high power or until shrimp turn pink and are just cooked through, stirring once. Keep shrimp covered while preparing sauce.
2. Combine margarine, onion, and garlic in 1½-quart microwave-safe casserole. Cook for 2–3 minutes on high power or until softened.
3. Heat milk in 1- or 2-cup measure for 2 minutes at high power. Whisk flour and milk into onion mixture; stir in seasonings.
4. Cook at medium-high power for 2–3 minutes or until sauce reaches desired thickness, stirring once. Stir drained shrimp into sauce.

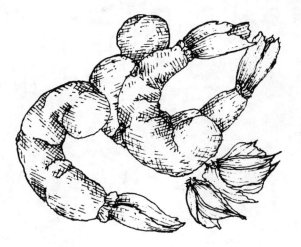

Combination Dishes

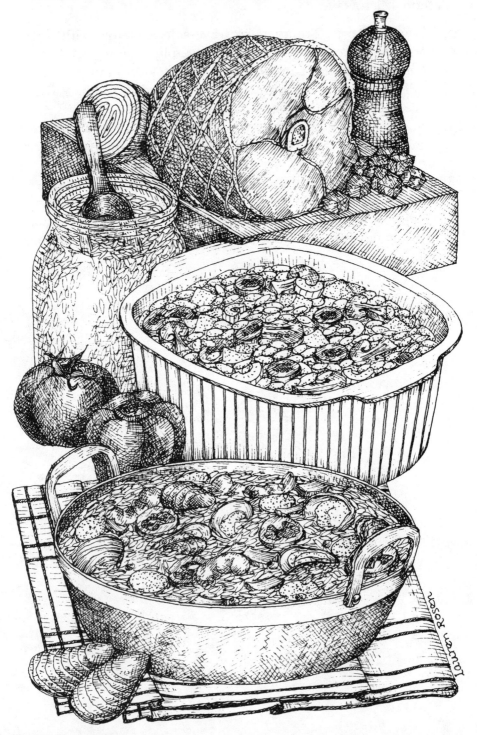

*A*s its name suggests, Jambalaya is a jumbled mix of good edibles—shrimp, ham, and chicken. Each combination dish provides its own special array of flavors, textures, and colors. Paella combines mussels, clams, shrimp, and chicken, while the Hearty Lentil Stew is a one-pot meal chock full of potatoes, mushrooms, celery, carrots, and more than half a dozen different herbs and spices. Try the Tuna Noodle Bake, with its crunchy water chestnuts, or the Nasi Gorenj if your food budget is tight. Chicken Cannelloni with Red and White Sauce is an elegant disguise for leftover chicken.

Jambalaya*

Yield: 8 servings
Serving Size: 1¼ cups
Exchanges:

Starch/Bread	1½
Meat, lean	1½
Vegetable	2½

Nutrient Content per Serving:

CAL	266	PRO	21 (gm)
FAT	4.2 (gm)	CHO	35 (gm)
Na	1,052 (mg)	K	563 (mg)
Fiber	2 (gm)	Chol	59 (mg)

Ingredients

2 MEDIUM ONIONS, CHOPPED
1 SMALL GREEN BELL PEPPER, CHOPPED
2 RIBS CELERY, CHOPPED
2 CLOVES GARLIC, MINCED
1 TABLESPOON MARGARINE
1 16-OUNCE CAN DICED TOMATOES IN PURÉE,
  UNDRAINED
2 CUPS CHICKEN BROTH**
2 TABLESPOONS TOMATO PASTE
1 TEASPOON SALT
½ TEASPOON THYME
¼ TEASPOON BLACK PEPPER
¼ TEASPOON CAYENNE PEPPER
1 BAY LEAF
8 DROPS TABASCO SAUCE
1½ CUPS RAW CONVERTED RICE
¼ POUND (1 CUP) COOKED HAM, CUBED
1 WHOLE CHICKEN BREAST (1 CUP), SKINNED,
  DEBONED, AND CUBED
6 OUNCES MEDIUM SHRIMP, PEELED

Method

1. Sauté onions, green pepper, celery, and garlic in margarine in 4-quart Dutch oven over medium heat until softened.
2. Add tomatoes, chicken broth, tomato paste, and seasonings; simmer for 10 minutes.
3. Add rice; cover and simmer for 10 minutes. Add ham, chicken, and shrimp. Continue cooking covered for 10–15 minutes or until rice absorbs liquid. Remove bay leaf before serving.

Method–Microwave

1. In a 4-quart microwave-safe casserole, cook onions, green pepper, celery, and garlic in 1 tablespoon margarine for 4 minutes on high power, stirring once.
2. Add tomatoes, chicken broth, tomato paste, and seasonings. Cook on medium-high power for 10 minutes. Stir in rice; cook for 10 minutes.
3. Stir in ham, chicken, and shrimp; continue cooking for 15–20 minutes on medium power, stirring once, until all liquid is absorbed.

*400 milligrams or more of sodium per serving.
**For reduced salt and fat, use homemade chicken broth.

Paella* **

Yield: 4 servings†
Serving Size: ¼ of recipe
(without skin)
Exchanges:

Starch/Bread	3½
Meat, lean	4
Vegetable	3
Fat	1

Nutrient Content per Serving:

CAL	627	PRO	42 (gm)
FAT	20 (gm)	CHO	67 (gm)
Na	617 (mg)	K	778 (mg)
Fiber	4 (gm)	Chol	117 (mg)

Key Source Nutrients:
Ascorbic acid   48 (mg)

Serving Size: ¼ of recipe
(with skin)
Exchanges:

Starch/Bread	4½
Meat, medium-fat	5

Nutrient Content per Serving:

CAL	740	PRO	49 (gm)
FAT	30 (gm)	CHO	67 (gm)
Na	635 (mg)	K	830 (mg)
Fiber	4 (gm)	Chol	143 (mg)

Key Source Nutrients:
Ascorbic acid   48 (mg)

Ingredients

1½–2 POUNDS CHICKEN, CUT UP
   2 TABLESPOONS OLIVE OIL
   ¼ MEDIUM RED PEPPER, CUT INTO STRIPS
   ¼ MEDIUM GREEN PEPPER, CUT INTO STRIPS
   ½ CUP ONION, COARSELY CHOPPED
   1 CLOVE GARLIC, CHOPPED
   4 OUNCES MILD ITALIAN SAUSAGE OR LEAN
      CHORIZO
1½ CUPS RAW RICE
   1 15½- OR 16-OUNCE CAN WHOLE TOMATOES,
      COARSELY CHOPPED AND UNDRAINED
   ½ TEASPOON SALT
   ⅛ TEASPOON GROUND SAFFRON
   3 CUPS BOILING WATER
   4 CLAMS, SCRUBBED
   4 MUSSELS, SCRUBBED
   8 MEDIUM SHRIMP, IN SHELL
   ½ CUP FROZEN PEAS, DEFROSTED

Method

1. Preheat oven to 400°F.
2. Rinse chicken and pat dry. Heat paella pan or large oven-proof skillet. Add olive oil.
3. Sauté chicken over medium heat for 10–15 minutes or until browned on both sides. Drain on paper towel and set aside.
4. In same pan sauté red and green peppers, onion, and garlic for 5 minutes, stirring often; set aside.
5. Cook sausage for 10–15 minutes or until browned; drain, slice, and set aside.
6. In same pan, combine rice, vegetable mixture, tomatoes, salt, saffron, and water; bring to a boil, stirring constantly. Remove from heat.
7. Add chicken and sausage to rice. Cover and bake for 30 minutes.
8. Add clams, mussels, shrimp, and peas; arrange around chicken. Bake for 10 minutes, or until mussels and clams open. (Discard any that do not open.)
9. Serve out of pan with a good crusty bread and a salad.

   *400 milligrams or more of sodium per serving.
   **3 grams or more of fiber per serving.
   †To make 8 servings, double the recipe.

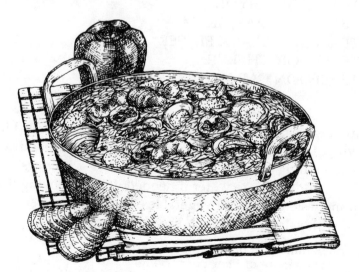

Hearty Lentil Stew* **

Yield: 6 servings
Serving Size: ¹⁄₆ of recipe
Exchanges:
Starch/Bread 2
Vegetable 2

Nutrient Content per Serving:

CAL	212	PRO	14 (gm)
FAT	1 (gm)	CHO	40 (gm)
Na	423 (mg)	K	846 (mg)
Fiber	9 (gm)	Chol	0 (mg)

Ingredients

        NONSTICK VEGETABLE SPRAY
    1 BAKING POTATO, PEELED AND CUBED
    2 MEDIUM ONIONS, PEELED AND CHOPPED
    ¼ POUND FRESH MUSHROOMS, SLICED
    1 CLOVE GARLIC, CHOPPED
    1 MEDIUM CARROT, PEELED AND SLICED
    2 RIBS CELERY, CHOPPED
  1½ CUPS LENTILS, WASHED AND DRAINED
    1 16-OUNCE CAN TOMATOES WITH JUICE,
        SLIGHTLY CRUSHED
    2 CUPS BEEF BROTH†
    1 CUP WATER
    ½ CUP DRY RED WINE
    1 BAY LEAF, HALVED
    1 TABLESPOON WORCESTERSHIRE SAUCE
    ½ TEASPOON THYME
    ½ TEASPOON MARJORAM
    ¼ TEASPOON BLACK PEPPER
    ¼ TEASPOON CHERVIL
    ¼ TEASPOON CARAWAY SEED

Method

1. Spray large casserole with nonstick vegetable spray. Lightly brown potato, onions, mushrooms, garlic, carrot, and celery.
2. Add remaining ingredients. Simmer for 1–1½ hours, partly covered, adding more water if needed during cooking. Check for doneness; cook until vegetables and lentils are soft.
3. Serve with salad and French bread, if desired.

   *400 milligrams or more of sodium per serving.
   **3 grams or more of fiber per serving.
   †For reduced salt and fat, use homemade beef broth.

Tuna Noodle Bake* **

Yield: 2 servings†
Serving Size: ½ of recipe
Exchanges:
Starch/Bread   2
Meat, lean   1½

Nutrient Content per Serving:
CAL 237   PRO   15 (gm)
FAT   7 (gm)   CHO   31 (gm)
Na   648 (mg)   K   307 (mg)
Fiber   4 (gm)   Chol   20 (mg)

Ingredients

NONSTICK VEGETABLE SPRAY
2 OUNCES MOSTACCIOLI (PREFERABLY WHOLE WHEAT OR SPINACH)
2 OUNCES WATER-PACKED TUNA, DRAINED AND FLAKED
¼ CUP FRESH MUSHROOMS, SLICED
¼ CUP WATER CHESTNUTS, SLICED, RINSED, AND DRAINED
¼ TEASPOON SALT
½ TEASPOON GARLIC POWDER
¼ TEASPOON WHITE PEPPER

White Sauce

1 TABLESPOON MARGARINE
1 TABLESPOON FLOUR
½ CUP SKIM MILK
PINCH OF NUTMEG

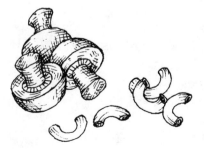

Method
1. Preheat oven to 350°F. Spray 1½-quart casserole with non-stick vegetable spray.
2. Cook mostaccioli; drain.
3. Prepare white sauce. Melt margarine in 1-quart saucepan. Whisk in flour, slowly whisk in milk, and add nutmeg. Cook over medium heat until sauce is thickened, 5–7 minutes.
4. Combine mostaccioli, tuna, mushrooms, water chestnuts, salt, pepper, garlic powder, and white sauce. Pour into prepared casserole. Bake for 15–20 minutes or until heated thoroughly.

Method–Microwave
1. Cook mostaccioli using stove-top method; drain.
2. Prepare white sauce. Melt margarine in 2-cup glass measure. Whisk in flour. Heat milk 1 minute on high power in 1-cup glass measure, whisk slowly into flour, and add nutmeg. Cook for 3–5 minutes on medium-high power; whisk once. Cook until thickened.
3. Combine mostaccioli, tuna, mushrooms, water chestnuts, salt, pepper, garlic powder, and white sauce. Pour into un-greased microwave-safe 1½-quart casserole. Cook for 5 minutes on high power or until heated thoroughly.

*400 milligrams or more of sodium per serving.
**3 grams or more of fiber per serving.
†To make 6 servings, triple the recipe.

Chicken Cannelloni with Red and White Sauce*

Yield: 5 servings
Serving Size: 2 crêpes and sauce

Exchanges:
Starch/Bread   1½
Meat, lean   3
Vegetable   1
Fat   1

Nutrient Content per Serving:

CAL	363	PRO	26 (gm)
FAT	15 (gm)	CHO	28 (gm)
Na	954 (mg)	K	610 (mg)
Fiber	2 (gm)	Chol	152 (mg)

Key Source Nutrients:
Vitamin A   4,426 (IU)

Ingredients

Crêpes

¾ CUP WATER
¾ CUP FLOUR
⅛ TEASPOON SALT
2 EGGS
   NONSTICK VEGETABLE SPRAY

Filling

1 CHICKEN BREAST (1 CUP), COOKED, DEBONED,
   AND CUBED
1 10-OUNCE BOX FROZEN CHOPPED SPINACH,
   DEFROSTED AND SQUEEZED DRY

White Sauce

4 TABLESPOONS MARGARINE
4 TABLESPOONS FLOUR
1 CUP CHICKEN BROTH**
⅓ CUP SKIM MILK
¼ CUP DRY WHITE WINE
⅛ TEASPOON WHITE PEPPER
   PINCH OF NUTMEG

Red Sauce

1 8-OUNCE CAN TOMATO SAUCE
¼–½ TEASPOON GARLIC POWDER
¼–½ TEASPOON OREGANO
¼–½ TEASPOON BASIL
¼ CUP GRATED PARMESAN CHEESE

Method

1. Combine first 4 ingredients in food processor or blender until smooth.
2. Heat 5- or 6-inch skillet or crêpe pan until moderately hot. Spray with nonstick vegetable spray.

3. Pour 1 ounce (2 tablespoons) of batter into pan; tilt quickly to cover pan with thinnest possible layer.
4. Cook until bottom is lightly browned and edges lift easily. Turn and cook on other side for a few minutes. Remove each crêpe to sheet of waxed paper and repeat process until all batter is used.
5. To make filling, place chicken and spinach in food processor fitted with steel blade, or use a sharp knife; chop until well blended. Add enough white sauce to make a spreadable mixture (about ¼ cup).
6. For white sauce, melt margarine in 1-quart saucepan over medium-high heat. Whisk in flour and cook until blended.
7. Gradually add chicken broth and milk. Cook, whisking until smooth and thickened.
8. Remove from heat; stir in wine, pepper, and nutmeg. Taste for seasonings.
9. For red sauce, combine tomato sauce and seasonings.
10. Preheat oven to 350°F. Spray 2-quart shallow baking dish with nonstick vegetable spray.
11. Place 1½ tablespoons filling in center of each crêpe; roll up. Place seam side down in baking dish.
12. Top with remaining white sauce.
13. Pour red sauce in a strip over white sauce. Sprinkle Parmesan cheese over all.
14. Bake for 30 minutes or until cheese is brown and bubbly.

Method–Microwave

1. To cook chicken breast, place on microwave-safe roast rack, cover with plastic wrap, and cook for 3 minutes on high power.
2. To defrost spinach, remove wrapper and place box on microwave-safe plate. Defrost for 5 minutes on defrost cycle. Squeeze dry.
3. To prepare white sauce, heat milk and margarine for 2–3 minutes on high power in 2-quart microwave-safe saucepan.
4. Whisk flour, chicken broth, wine, and seasonings into milk. Cook 1½–2½ minutes on medium-high power or until sauce coats back of spoon; stir once.

5. Follow filling and preparation directions given above, except do not spray 2-quart microwave-safe baking dish.
6. Cover and cook for 20–25 minutes on medium power or until cheese is melted and cannelloni is heated thoroughly. Let stand for 10 minutes, covered, before serving.

*400 milligrams or more of sodium per serving.
**For reduced salt and fat, use homemade chicken broth.

Nasi Goreng*

Yield: 2 servings**
Serving Size: ½ of recipe
Exchanges:
Starch/Bread   2½
Meat, medium-fat 2
Fat   ½

Nutrient Content per Serving:

CAL	381	PRO	23 (gm)
FAT	16 (gm)	CHO	37 (gm)
Na	334 (mg)	K	543 (mg)
Fiber	3 (gm)	Chol	71 (mg)

Ingredients

      NONSTICK VEGETABLE SPRAY
  ½ POUND LEAN GROUND BEEF
  ½ MEDIUM ONION, THINLY SLICED
  ½ SMALL GREEN PEPPER, CORED, SEEDED, AND
      CUT INTO ½-INCH DICES
  ½ TOMATO, SEEDED AND DICED
  ½ MEDIUM TART APPLE, PEELED, CORED AND
      DICED
  1 TEASPOON CURRY POWDER OR TO TASTE
  ¼ TEASPOON SALT
  ¼ TEASPOON CRUSHED RED PEPPER FLAKES
  1 CUP COOKED WHITE RICE

Method

1. Spray large skillet with nonstick vegetable spray; brown ground beef. Drain fat.
2. Add onion, green pepper, tomato, and apple. Continue cooking until vegetables are tender-crisp.
3. Stir in curry powder, salt, and crushed red pepper flakes. Cook for 5 minutes.
4. Stir in rice and cook for 5 minutes.

Method–Microwave

1. Place beef in plastic colander set into 2-quart microwave-safe casserole dish. Cook for 2½ minutes on high power. Drain fat from casserole.
2. Stir in meat, onion, green pepper, tomato, and apple. Cover and cook for 3–5 minutes on high power.
3. Stir in curry, salt, and red pepper flakes. Cover and cook for 2½ minutes on high power.
4. Stir in rice; heat for 2½–5 minutes, depending on temperature of rice. Cook, covered, on high power; stir once.

Note: Nasi goreng is a quick and easy rice and beef dish from Indonesia. May serve hot or at room temperature. Serve with chutney, banana slices, raisins, peanuts or shredded coconut, and Indian bread.

*3 grams or more of fiber per serving.
**To make 4 servings, double the recipe.

Bobotie—South African Beef Casserole*

Yield: 6 servings
Serving Size: ⅙ of recipe
Exchanges:
Meat, medium-fat 4
Fruit   1

Nutrient Content per Serving:

CAL	371	PRO	30 (gm)
FAT	20 (gm)	CHO	18 (gm)
Na	502 (mg)	K	529 (mg)
Fiber	2 (gm)	Chol	97 (mg)

Ingredients

        NONSTICK VEGETABLE SPRAY
     2 MEDIUM ONIONS, FINELY CHOPPED
     2 CLOVES GARLIC, CHOPPED
     1 POUND LEAN GROUND BEEF
     1 POUND GROUND LAMB
     1 SLICE WHITE BREAD
     1 CUP SKIM MILK
     2 PACKETS SUGAR SUBSTITUTE
     1 TEASPOON SALT
   2-3 TEASPOONS CURRY POWDER
    ½ TEASPOON TURMERIC
    ½ TEASPOON BLACK PEPPER
     2 TABLESPOONS LEMON JUICE
     3 TABLESPOONS PLUM OR ANY TYPE CHUTNEY
    ¼ CUP RAISINS
    ¼ CUP SLICED ALMONDS, BLANCHED
        PEEL OF 1 LEMON, COARSELY CHOPPED
     2 BAY LEAVES, BROKEN INTO 4 PIECES
     1 EGG

Method

1. Preheat oven to 350°F.
2. Spray 10-inch oven-proof skillet with nonstick vegetable spray. Brown onions, garlic, beef, and lamb.
3. Soak bread in milk, squeeze dry, and reserve milk.
4. Crumble bread into meat. Add remaining ingredients except for reserved milk, egg, and bay leaves.
5. Tuck bay leaves around mixture. Bake for 1 hour.
6. Remove bay leaves. Beat egg with milk. Pour on top of meat mixture. Bake for 20–30 minutes or until top is golden brown.

Note: Bobotie comes from the Malays who were enslaved by 17th-century Dutch settlers. It can be served with rice and additional chutney. May use all beef or all lamb.

*400 milligrams or more of sodium per serving.

Whole Wheat Roulade with Filling*

Yield: 6 servings
Serving Size: ⅙ of recipe
(with ham filling)
Exchanges:
Starch/Bread   1
Meat, medium-
  fat   1½
Fat   1

Nutrient Content per Serving:
CAL 224   PRO   15 (gm)
FAT   14 (gm)   CHO   11 (gm)
Na   557 (mg)   K   239 (mg)
Fiber   1 (gm)   Chol 165 (mg)

Serving Size: ⅙ of recipe
(with mushroom filling)
Exchanges:
Starch/Bread   1
Meat, medium-fat   1
Fat   1

Nutrient Content per Serving:
CAL 197   PRO   10 (gm)
FAT   13 (gm)   CHO   12 (gm)
Na   307 (mg)   K   223 (mg)
Fiber   1 (gm)   Chol 155 (mg)

Ingredients

Roulade

    NONSTICK VEGETABLE SPRAY
 1 CUP SKIM MILK
 3 EGG YOLKS
½ CUP WHOLE WHEAT FLOUR
 5 EGG WHITES, BEATEN STIFF

Filling

 1 CUP HAM, CHOPPED (SUBSTITUTE 1 CUP
   MUSHROOMS, CHOPPED, IF DESIRED)
½ CUP MEDIUM-SHARP CHEDDAR CHEESE,
   SHREDDED
 2 GREEN ONIONS, SLICED
 1 TABLESPOON PREPARED MUSTARD

Sauce

   1 TABLESPOON DIJON OR PREPARED MUSTARD
   ½ CUP REDUCED-CALORIE MAYONNAISE
   1 TEASPOON DRIED CHIVES OR 1 TABLESPOON
   FRESH CHIVES

Method

1. Preheat oven to 400°F. Spray a 15½-by-10½ jelly-roll pan with nonstick vegetable spray. Line with waxed paper and spray with nonstick vegetable spray.
2. Cook milk and egg yolks until thickened. Do not boil; stir constantly.
3. Cook for 15 minutes. Stir in flour. Fold in beaten egg whites. Pour into prepared pan.
4. Bake for 20 minutes. Invert pan on towel and carefully remove waxed paper. Allow to cool while preparing filling and sauce.
5. For filling, combine ham, cheese, and onions. For sauce, combine mustard, mayonnaise, and chives.
6. Spread roulade with mustard; leave 1-inch border all around. Spread filling over mustard and leave 1-inch border all around. Roll up jelly-roll style, lifting with towel as rolling. Place seam side down on serving platter. Slice off ends. Slice remaining roll. Serve with sauce. Serve at room temperature, or heat at 350°F for 10–15 minutes before slicing.

Note: A roulade is a flat soufflé, perfect for lunch box, breakfast, or buffet.

   *400 milligrams or more of sodium per serving when prepared with ham filling.

Vegetarian Dishes

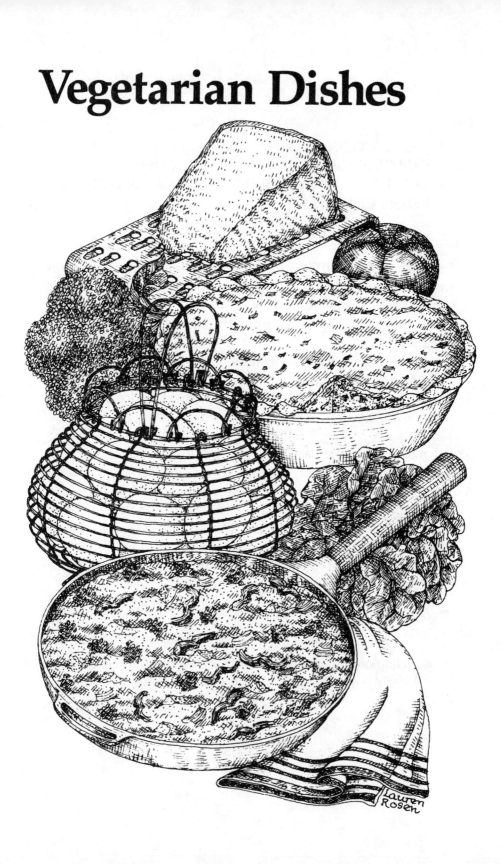

Lauren
Rosen

*M*any dishes you enjoy right now are vegetarian, although you may not think of them as such—spaghetti with tomato sauce, pancakes and maple syrup, a cheese soufflé. If you're trying to increase your intake of no-meat dishes, try doing so at meals *other than* dinner—the time when people customarily expect a meat course and may feel deprived if they don't get it. Instead, introduce vegetarian dishes at breakfast, brunch, lunch, or supper. Once their appeal has been established, try them as a dinner main course.

American-Style Toad in the Hole

Yield: 1 serving
Serving Size: 1 toad
Exchanges:
Starch/Bread   1
Meat, medium-fat 1
Fat   1

Nutrient Content per Serving:

CAL	181	PRO	9 (gm)
FAT	10 (gm)	CHO	14 (gm)
Na	261 (mg)	K	143 (mg)
Fiber	2 (gm)	Chol	274 (mg)

Ingredients

> 1 SLICE WHOLE WHEAT BREAD
> 1 TEASPOON MARGARINE
>   NONSTICK VEGETABLE SPRAY
> 1 EGG
>   PEPPER TO TASTE

Method

1. Spread half of margarine on one side of bread and cut out a 2-inch square.
2. Preheat skillet and spray well with nonstick vegetable spray. Place bread and cube buttered side down in skillet. Brown. Spread remaining margarine on bread and turn over. Brown slightly; drop egg in middle of square. Sprinkle with pepper. Cook over moderate heat for 3–5 minutes; flip over and cook for 1 minute. Serve egg yolk side up. Serve extra square of bread for dunking.
3. For more servings, use 1 slice of bread and 1 egg per serving.

Baked Polenta with Mushroom Sauce

Yield: 12 3-inch squares
Serving Size: 3-inch square
Exchanges:
Starch/Bread   1
Fat   ½

Nutrient Content per Serving:

CAL	89	PRO	4 (gm)
FAT	3 (gm)	CHO	12 (gm)
Na	213 (mg)	K	123 (mg)
Fiber	1 (gm)	Chol	3 (mg)

Ingredients

> 2 CUPS SKIM MILK
> 2 CUPS WATER
> 1 TABLESPOON MARGARINE
> ½ TEASPOON SALT
> 1 CUP STONE-GROUND YELLOW CORNMEAL
> ¼ CUP ASIAGO OR MOZZARELLA CHEESE, GRATED
> 2 TABLESPOONS GRATED PARMESAN CHEESE
> ⅛ TEASPOON WHITE PEPPER
> NONSTICK VEGETABLE SPRAY

Mushroom Sauce

> 2 SHALLOTS, SLICED, OR 1 CLOVE GARLIC, SLICED
> 1 TABLESPOON OLIVE OIL
> 1 CUP PLAIN MUSHROOMS
> 1 CUP BEEF BROTH*

Method

1. Heat milk, water, margarine, and salt to boiling. Reduce to medium heat and whisk in cornmeal. Continue stirring and cooking until mixture pulls away from sides of pan, about 10 minutes. Stir in cheeses and pepper.
2. Pour onto large cookie sheet well sprayed with nonstick vegetable spray. Let cool to room temperature.
3. Preheat oven to 350°F.
4. Bake for 15–20 minutes or until edges are brown and bubbly.
5. Meanwhile, prepare sauce. Sauté shallots in olive oil until soft. Stir in mushrooms and cook for 5 minutes. Add beef broth and simmer for 5 minutes. Add salt and pepper to taste, if desired.

Note: In place of mushroom sauce, you can use a small can of tomato sauce and combine with chopped, sauteéd onion and garlic. Top with shredded mozzarella and bake at 350°F for 15–20 minutes or until cheese is melted.

*For reduced salt and fat, use homemade beef broth.

Nutty Rice Loaf*

Yield: 6 servings
Serving Size: 1 slice
Exchanges:
Starch/Bread 1
Meat, medium-fat 1
Vegetable 1
Fat ½

Nutrient Content per Serving:

CAL	247	PRO	13 (gm)
FAT	13 (gm)	CHO	20 (gm)
Na	154 (mg)	K	269 (mg)
Fiber	4 (gm)	Chol	157 (mg)

Ingredients

     NONSTICK VEGETABLE SPRAY
1½ CUPS COOKED BROWN RICE
  1 CUP ZUCCHINI, SHREDDED
 ¼ CUP ONION, CHOPPED
 ½ CUP WHEAT GERM
 ¼ CUP WALNUTS, CHOPPED
  1 CUP MEDIUM-SHARP CHEDDAR CHEESE,
     SHREDDED
  3 EGGS, LIGHTLY BEATEN
 ½ TEASPOON THYME
 ½ TEASPOON MARJORAM
 ¼ TEASPOON BLACK PEPPER

Method

1. Preheat oven to 350°F. Spray a 9-by-5-inch loaf pan with non-stick vegetable spray.
2. Combine all ingredients. Pack into loaf pan.
3. Bake for 40–45 minutes or until brown on edges and firm to touch.
4. Cut into slices. Serve hot or at room temperature.

Method–Microwave

1. Combine all ingredients. Pack into microwave loaf pan or glass loaf pan. Cover with waxed paper. Cook for 8 minutes on high power. Rotate dish once during cooking.

Note: Good for lunch, side dish, or meatless entrée. Serve with fresh fruit and a salad.

*3 grams or more of fiber per serving.

Cheese Tortellini with Creamy Spinach*

Yield: 4 servings
Serving Size: 1 cup
Exchanges:
Starch/Bread 2
Vegetable 2

Nutrient Content per Serving:
CAL 244   PRO 12 (gm)
FAT 3 (gm)   CHO 43 (gm)
Na 448 (mg)   K 309 (mg)
Fiber 2 (gm)   Chol 5 (mg)

Key Source Nutrients:
Vitamin A 4,449 (IU)

Ingredients

1 7-OUNCE BOX CHEESE TORTELLINI
1 10-OUNCE PACKAGE FROZEN, CHOPPED SPINACH, DEFROSTED AND DRAINED
1 CUP SKIM MILK
1 TEASPOON BASIL
½ TEASPOON OREGANO
½ TEASPOON SALT
¼ TEASPOON BLACK PEPPER
¼ TEASPOON GARLIC POWDER
¼ TEASPOON GRATED PARMESAN CHEESE

Method

1. Prepare tortellini according to directions on package. Drain and keep warm.
2. Combine all ingredients for sauce except Parmesan cheese. Boil 3–5 minutes. Stir in cheese and remove from heat. Pour over tortellini. Serve hot.

*400 milligrams or more of sodium per serving.

Ricotta Cheese Dumplings*

Yield: 4 servings (about 8
dumplings)
Serving Size: 2 dumplings
Exchanges:
Starch/Bread   2½
Meat, medium-fat 2
Fat   1

Nutrient Content per Serving:

CAL	389	PRO	21 (gm)
FAT	18 (gm)	CHO	35 (gm)
Na	620 (mg)	K	236 (mg)
Fiber	1 (gm)	Chol	170 (mg)

Ingredients

    15 OUNCES PART-SKIM RICOTTA CHEESE
    ¾ CUP ALL-PURPOSE FLOUR
    2 WHOLE EGGS
    2 EGG WHITES
    ½ TEASPOON SALT
    ¼ TEASPOON BASIL
    ¼ TEASPOON GARLIC POWDER
    ¼ TEASPOON OREGANO
    2 TABLESPOONS MARGARINE, MELTED
    ½ CUP BREAD CRUMBS

Method

1. Mix ricotta cheese, flour, whole eggs, egg whites, salt, and seasonings until smooth.
2. Wet hands and form mixture into balls. Drop them into a pot of boiling water and cook for 20 minutes. Drain.
3. Melt margarine in skillet large enough to hold the dumplings. Brown bread crumbs in margarine.
4. Put dumplings into skillet and shake to cover.
5. Serve warm with light sour cream or cinnamon**, if desired.

Note: May be used as a light lunch with a salad, side dish, or dessert. These dumplings are of Hungarian origin.

*400 milligrams or more of sodium per serving.
**Sour cream and cinnamon not included in nutritional analysis.

Vegetable Frittata

Yield: 4 main-dish servings
Serving Size: ¼ pie
Exchanges:
Meat, medium-fat 1
Vegetable   1½

Nutrient Content per Serving:

CAL	107	PRO	8 (gm)
FAT	5 (gm)	CHO	8 (gm)
Na	174 (mg)	K	282 (mg)
Fiber	2 (gm)	Chol	141 (mg)

Key Source Nutrients:
Riboflavin 62 (mg)

Ingredients

- 1 TEASPOON MARGARINE
- 1 SMALL ONION, THINLY SLICED
- 1 SMALL RED PEPPER, SLICED INTO THIN STRIPS
- 1 RED POTATO, COOKED, SLICED, AND UNPEELED
- 1 CUP BROCCOLI FLORETS
- ¼ TEASPOON SALT
- ⅛ TEASPOON BLACK PEPPER
- ¼ CUP SWISS CHEESE, SHREDDED
- 3 WHOLE EGGS, LIGHTLY BEATEN
- 3 EGG WHITES, LIGHTLY BEATEN
- PINCH OF PAPRIKA

Method

1. Preheat oven to 450°F.
2. Melt margarine in 8-inch pie plate or quiche pan in oven. Arrange onion slices on bottom and cook in hot oven for 5 minutes.
3. Remove pan from oven; arrange red pepper, potato, and broccoli on top of onion. Add salt and pepper. Top with cheese and pour whole eggs and egg whites over vegetables. Sprinkle with paprika. Bake for 10–15 minutes or until eggs are set in middle. Serve immediately.

Method–Microwave

1. Melt margarine in glass or microwave-safe 9-inch pie plate. Add onion and red pepper. Cook for 2 minutes on high power.
2. Arrange potato and broccoli on onion mixture. Top with cheese and pour whole eggs and egg whites over vegetables. Sprinkle with paprika.
3. Cover with waxed paper. Cook for 6–8 minutes on medium-high power. Rotate dish ¼ turn every 2 minutes. Cook for 2 minutes on high power or until set. Serve immediately.

Baked Apple Pancake

Yield: 6 servings
Serving Size: ⅙ pancake
Exchanges:
Starch/Bread   1
Meat, lean   ½
Fat   ½

Nutrient Content per Serving:

CAL	139	PRO	6 (gm)
FAT	5 (gm)	CHO	19 (gm)
Na	120 (mg)	K	196 (mg)
Fiber	2 (gm)	Chol	46 (mg)

Ingredients

    NONSTICK VEGETABLE SPRAY
1 CUP SKIM MILK
¾ CUP UNSIFTED ALL-PURPOSE FLOUR
2 EGG WHITES
1 WHOLE EGG
½ TEASPOON BAKING POWDER
3 PACKETS SUGAR SUBSTITUTE (NOT ASPARTAME)
2 TABLESPOONS MARGARINE, MELTED
2 TEASPOONS VANILLA
1 TEASPOON GRATED LEMON PEEL
1 TART LARGE APPLE, CUT INTO ¼-INCH SLICES
2 TEASPOONS LEMON JUICE
½ TEASPOON CINNAMON
¼ TEASPOON BROWN SUGAR SUBSTITUTE

Method

1. Preheat oven to 400°F. Coat a 10-inch oven-proof skillet with nonstick vegetable spray.
2. Combine milk, flour, egg whites, whole egg, baking powder, sugar substitute, margarine, vanilla, and lemon peel in blender or food processor; blend until smooth.
3. Pour into prepared skillet; bake for 20–25 minutes or until puffed and browned.
4. Meanwhile, spray a small skillet with nonstick vegetable spray. Combine apple with lemon juice, cinnamon, and brown sugar substitute.
5. Sauté over medium heat until softened, about 7–10 minutes. Pour over pancake. Cut into 6 servings and serve immediately with lemon wedges, if desired.

Method–Microwave

1. Prepare pancake using instructions above. Meanwhile, combine apple, lemon juice, cinnamon, and brown sugar substitute in 8-inch microwave-safe pie plate. Cover with plastic wrap.
2. Cook on high power for 2 minutes or until apples are softened. Mix well; let stand covered for 2–3 minutes. Pour over pancake. Cut into 6 servings and serve immediately with lemon wedges, if desired.

Hot Brown Rice with Chiles* **

Yield: 2 servings as main course, 4 servings as side dish.
Serving Size: 1 cup
Exchanges:
Starch/Bread 3
Meat, medium-fat 1

Nutrient Content per Serving:

CAL	307	PRO	13 (gm)
FAT	7 (gm)	CHO	48 (gm)
Na	424 (mg)	K	382 (mg)
Fiber	4 (gm)	Chol	20 (mg)

Ingredients

> NONSTICK VEGETABLE SPRAY
> 1½ CUPS COOKED BROWN RICE (½ CUP RAW)
> 1 CUP PLAIN LOW-FAT YOGURT
> ¼ TEASPOON SALT
> ⅛ TEASPOON BLACK PEPPER
> 2 OUNCES (½ CAN) GREEN CHILES, CHOPPED
> AND DRAINED
> ¼ CUP MONTEREY JACK CHEESE, SHREDDED

Method

1. Preheat oven to 350°F. Spray 1½-quart casserole with nonstick vegetable spray.
2. Combine rice with yogurt, salt, and pepper. Place half of mixture in bottom of casserole.
3. Top with half of chiles and half of cheese. Repeat layers, ending with cheese on top.
4. Bake uncovered for 25–30 minutes or until top is lightly browned.

Method–Microwave
1. Combine rice with yogurt, salt, and pepper. Place half in 1½-quart microwave-safe casserole.
2. Top with half of chiles and half of cheese. Repeat layers, ending with cheese on top.
3. Cook uncovered for 6½–7 minutes on high power, or until heated thoroughly. Rotate dish once during cooking time.

*400 milligrams or more of sodium per serving.
**3 grams or more of fiber per serving.

Cheese Soufflé

Yield: 6 servings
Serving Size: ⅙ of recipe
Exchanges:
Starch/Bread ½
Meat, lean 2
Fat 1½

Nutrient Content per Serving:
CAL 222   PRO 12 (gm)
FAT 15 (gm)   CHO 10 (gm)
Na 210 (mg)   K 205 (mg)
Fiber 0 (gm) Chol 67 (mg)

Ingredients

NONSTICK VEGETABLE SPRAY
¼ CUP UNSALTED MARGARINE
¼ CUP ALL-PURPOSE FLOUR
1 CUP EVAPORATED SKIM MILK
1 CUP MEDIUM-SHARP CHEDDAR CHEESE, SHREDDED
¼ TEASPOON BASIL OR OREGANO, CRUSHED
DASH OF CAYENNE PEPPER
2 EGG YOLKS
5 EGG WHITES, BEATEN STIFF BUT NOT DRY

Method

1. Preheat oven to 400°F. Spray 2-quart soufflé dish with non-stick vegetable spray.
2. Melt margarine over low heat; add flour, stirring until smooth. Cook for 1 minute, stirring constantly. Gradually add evaporated milk; cook over medium heat, stirring constantly, until mixture is thickened and bubbly.
3. Add cheese and seasonings; stir until cheese melts. Gradually stir one-fourth of hot mixture into egg yolks; add to remaining hot ingredients. Fold beaten whites into egg mixture.
4. Pour into prepared soufflé dish. Bake for 30 minutes or until puffed and golden. Serve immediately.

Method–Microwave

1. In 1½-quart microwave-safe saucepan, melt margarine. Stir in flour until smooth. Gradually whisk in evaporated milk. Cook for 3–6 minutes on high power, stirring every 1½ minutes. Cook until thickened. Stir in cheese until melted and add seasonings.
2. Gradually stir one-fourth of hot mixture into egg yolks; add to remaining hot ingredients. Fold in beaten egg whites.
3. Pour into ungreased 2-quart microwave-safe soufflé or casserole dish. Cook for 25–35 minutes or until top is dry, on medium-low power. Rotate dish ¼ turn every 7 minutes.

Baked Farfel*

Yield: 4 servings**
Serving Size: ¼ of recipe
Exchanges:
Starch/Bread 2½
Fat 1

Nutrient Content per Serving:

CAL	232	PRO	7 (gm)
FAT	8 (gm)	CHO	34 (gm)
Na	166 (mg)	K	214 (mg)
Fiber	3 (gm)	Chol	40 (mg)

Ingredients

     NONSTICK VEGETABLE SPRAY
6 OUNCES TOASTED FARFEL
1 MEDIUM ONION, SLICED (ABOUT 1 CUP)
2 TABLESPOONS MARGARINE
½ CUP FRESH MUSHROOMS, SLICED
1½ TEASPOONS WORCESTERSHIRE SAUCE
¼ TEASPOON GARLIC POWDER
⅛ TEASPOON SALT
     PINCH OF BLACK PEPPER

Method

1. Preheat oven to 350°F. Spray a 1½- or 2-quart casserole with nonstick vegetable spray.
2. Cook toasted farfel in boiling water for 10 minutes. Drain well.
3. Sauté onion in margarine until golden brown. Stir in mushrooms, Worcestershire sauce, garlic powder, salt, and pepper. Cook for 5 minutes.
4. Combine farfel with mushroom mixture and pour into prepared casserole. Bake for 30–45 minutes.

Method–Microwave

1. Cook farfel as directed above.
2. Cook onion in margarine in covered 2-quart casserole dish for 3–5 minutes on high power. Stir once.
3. Uncover; cook for 8–10 minutes on high power until lightly browned. Stir in mushrooms, Worcestershire sauce, garlic powder, salt, and pepper. Cook for 2 minutes on high power. Stir in farfel. Cook for 8–10 minutes on high power, rotating dish once during cooking time.

Note: Farfel is a Jewish egg-and-flour noodle that is used in soup or as a side dish. Serve as a meatless main dish or as an accompaniment to meat or chicken.

    *3 grams or more of fiber per serving.
    **To make 8 servings, double the recipe.

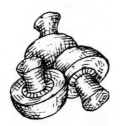

Vegetable Stir-Fry with Tofu Sauce*

Yield: 4 servings
Serving Size: ¼ of recipe
Exchanges:
Meat, medium-
  fat   ½
Vegetable   1

Nutrient Content per Serving:

CAL	58	PRO	6 (gm)
FAT	2 (gm)	CHO	6 (gm)
Na	314 (mg)	K	293 (mg)
Fiber	3 (gm)	Chol	0 (mg)

Key Source Nutrients:
Ascorbic acid   46 (mg)

Ingredients

- 1 GREEN ONION, CHOPPED
- 1 CLOVE GARLIC, CHOPPED
- 1 TEASPOON FRESH GINGER, CHOPPED
  PINCH OF CRUSHED RED PEPPER FLAKES OR TO
  TASTE
- 1 CUP BROCCOLI FLORETS
- 1 CUP ZUCCHINI, SLICED
- ½ CUP FRESH MUSHROOMS, SLICED
- ½ CUP RED PEPPER STRIPS

Sauce

- 6 OUNCES TOFU, DRAINED
- ⅓ CUP WATER
- 2 TABLESPOONS LOW-SODIUM SOY SAUCE
- 1 TABLESPOON RICE VINEGAR
- 1 PACKET SUGAR SUBSTITUTE
  NONSTICK VEGETABLE SPRAY

Method

1. Purée tofu with water, soy sauce, rice vinegar, and sugar substitute. Set aside.
2. Heat wok or large skillet; spray well with nonstick vegetable spray. Stir-fry onion, garlic, ginger, and crushed red pepper for 15 seconds.
3. Stir in broccoli and zucchini; stir and cook for 4 minutes. Stir in mushrooms and red peppers; cover and cook for 3–4 minutes. Set aside until ready to serve.
4. Just before serving, stir tofu sauce into vegetables. Cook until heated thoroughly, about 5 minutes.

Method–Microwave

1. Combine onion, garlic, ginger, and crushed red pepper in 2-quart microwave-safe casserole. Cook for 15–20 seconds on high power.
2. Add broccoli and zucchini. Cook for 3–4 minutes on high power; stir once.
3. Stir in mushrooms and peppers; cover with plastic wrap. Cook for 2–3 minutes on high power.
4. Just before serving, stir tofu sauce (prepared according to conventional method) into vegetables. Heat for 3–4 minutes on high power or until heated thoroughly.

*3 grams or more of fiber per serving.

Crustless Zucchini Quiche* **

Yield: 4 servings
Serving Size: ¼ pie
Exchanges:
Meat, medium-fat 1
Vegetable 2
Fat ½

Nutrient Content per Serving:
CAL 142 PRO 10 (gm)
FAT 8 (gm) CHO 7 (gm)
Na 427 (mg) K 342 (mg)
Fiber 3 (gm) Chol 152 (mg)

Ingredients

½ CUP ONION, CHOPPED
1 TEASPOON MARGARINE
2 CUPS ZUCCHINI, SLICED ¼-INCH THICK
2 EGGS
½ CUP EVAPORATED SKIM MILK
½ TEASPOON SALT
⅛ TEASPOON GROUND WHITE PEPPER
PINCH OF NUTMEG
½ CUP MONTEREY JACK CHEESE, SHREDDED
PINCH OF PAPRIKA

Method

1. Preheat oven to 350°F.
2. Sauté onion in margarine for 2–3 minutes; add zucchini and sauté for 5 more minutes.
3. Beat eggs with milk and seasonings.
4. Place zucchini mixture in 8-inch glass pie plate.
5. Pour egg mixture over zucchini mixture and top with cheese.
6. Bake for 45–50 minutes or until edges are brown and eggs are set in center.

Method–Microwave

1. Melt margarine in 8-inch glass pie plate, about 30 seconds on high power.
2. Cook onion in margarine for 2 minutes on high power.
3. Add zucchini; continue cooking on high power for 2 minutes.

4. Combine eggs, milk, and seasonings; pour over zucchini. Top with cheese. Sprinkle with paprika, if desired.
5. Cover with waxed paper; cook on medium-high power for 10 minutes, rotating dish halfway through cooking. Cook 1½ minutes on high power. Let stand for 5 minutes.

   *400 milligrams or more of sodium per serving.
   **3 grams or more of fiber per serving.

Whole Wheat Blueberry Rice Pancakes

Yield: 12 pancakes
Serving Size: 2 4-inch
pancakes
Exchanges:
Starch/Bread 2
Fat 2

Nutrient Content per Serving:

CAL	248	PRO	7 (gm)
FAT	12 (gm)	CHO	29 (gm)
Na	229 (mg)	K	183 (mg)
Fiber	2 (gm)	Chol	2 (mg)

Ingredients

½ CUP ALL-PURPOSE FLOUR
½ CUP WHOLE WHEAT FLOUR
½ TEASPOON BAKING SODA
¼ TEASPOON SALT
6 PACKETS SUGAR SUBSTITUTE (NOT ASPARTAME)
1 CUP COLD COOKED RICE
1 CUP LOW-FAT BUTTERMILK
½ CUP SKIM MILK
2 TABLESPOONS UNSALTED MARGARINE, MELTED
1 TEASPOON VANILLA EXTRACT
2 EGG WHITES, BEATEN STIFF
¾ CUP FRESH OR FROZEN BLUEBERRIES, COATED IN 1 TABLESPOON FLOUR

Maple Topping

    1/4 CUP UNSALTED MARGARINE, SOFTENED
    1/2 TEASPOON IMITATION MAPLE FLAVORING
    1/4 TEASPOON VANILLA EXTRACT
    1/4 TEASPOON HONEY
        NONSTICK VEGETABLE SPRAY

Method

1. Combine flours, baking soda, salt, and sugar substitute; mix well.
2. Add rice, buttermilk, skim milk, melted margarine, and vanilla extract; mix just until dry ingredients are moistened.
3. Fold in beaten egg whites, then blueberries.
4. Combine all ingredients for maple topping in small bowl.
5. Spray griddle or large frying pan with nonstick vegetable spray; heat until hot. Bake pancakes until brown and puffy on both sides; serve with maple topping.

Baked Lentils au Gratin* **

Yield: 4 servings†
Serving Size: 3/4 cup
Exchanges:
Starch/Bread   1
Meat, lean   1/2
Vegetable   2

Nutrient Content per Serving:
CAL 161   PRO   11 (gm)
FAT   2 (gm)   CHO 26 (gm)
Na   461 (mg)   K   451 (mg)
Fiber   5 (gm)   Chol   7 (mg)

Key Source Nutrients:
Vitamin A 4,087 (IU)

Ingredients

        NONSTICK VEGETABLE SPRAY
    1/4 CUP ONION, CHOPPED
    1/2 CUP CARROT, SHREDDED
      1 CLOVE GARLIC, MINCED
      2 CUPS COOKED LENTILS (1 CUP DRY)

   1 8-OUNCE CAN STEWED TOMATOES,
     UNDRAINED
   ¼ SMALL RED BELL PEPPER, CHOPPED
   ½ TEASPOON SALT
   ⅛ TEASPOON BLACK PEPPER
   ⅛ TEASPOON BASIL
   ⅛ TEASPOON OREGANO, CRUSHED
   ¼ CUP MONTEREY JACK CHEESE, SHREDDED

Method

1. Preheat oven to 375°F. Spray 2-quart casserole with nonstick vegetable spray.
2. Spray 8-inch skillet with nonstick vegetable spray. Sauté onion, carrot, and garlic until soft. Pour into prepared casserole.
3. Add remaining ingredients except cheese.
4. Cover and bake for 45 minutes.
5. Uncover and sprinkle with cheese; bake for 5–7 minutes or until cheese is melted.

Method–Microwave

1. Combine onion, carrot, and garlic in 2-quart microwave-safe casserole. Cover and cook for 5 minutes on high power, stirring once.
2. Stir in rest of ingredients except cheese. Cover and cook on medium-high power for 12–15 minutes, stirring once.
3. Uncover and top with cheese; cook for 50 seconds or until cheese melts.

   *400 milligrams or more of sodium per serving.
   **3 grams or more of fiber per serving.
   †To make 8 servings, double the recipe.

Eggs Florentine* **

Yield: 2 servings[†]	Nutrient Content per Serving:			
Serving Size: ½ recipe	CAL	142	PRO	10 (gm)
Exchanges:	FAT	7 (gm)	CHO	11 (gm)
Meat, medium-fat 1	Na	481 (mg)	K	397 (mg)
Vegetable 2	Fiber	3 (gm)	Chol	320 (mg)
Fat ½				

Ingredients

    4 TABLESPOONS LOW-CALORIE HOLLANDAISE
SAUCE (SEE PAGE 336)

    2 EGGS, POACHED

    ½ CAN (7¾ OUNCES) SPINACH, SQUEEZED AND
DRAINED

    ⅛ TEASPOON SALT
PINCH OF BLACK PEPPER
PINCH OF NUTMEG

  3½ OUNCES ARTICHOKE BOTTOMS, DRAINED

    ½ TEASPOON GRATED PARMESAN CHEESE

Method

1. Prepare hollandaise. Preheat broiler.
2. Poach eggs in nonstick skillet ⅔ full of water. Bring water to a simmer; break egg into saucer and slide into water. Spoon simmering water over each egg for 2–3 minutes or until done.
3. Mix spinach with salt, pepper, and nutmeg.
4. Trim bottoms of artichoke bottoms flat; place on baking sheet. Fill each bottom with 1 tablespoon spinach mixture. Top with egg, 2 tablespoons hollandaise, and ¼ teaspoon Parmesan.
5. Broil 2–3 minutes or until golden; serve immediately.

Method–Microwave

1. To poach each egg, measure 2 tablespoons water into 6-ounce custard cup. Cook on high power until water boils (30–40 seconds). Break eggs into cups. Cover and cook on medium power for 65–95 seconds for two eggs, rotating dishes half-way through cooking time.
2. Prepare and assemble Eggs Florentine according to directions given above.

Note: Use leftover artichokes and spinach in a salad. Use left-over hollandaise over hot vegetables.

   *400 milligrams or more of sodium per serving.
   **3 grams or more of fiber per serving.
   †Each serving consists of 1 artichoke bottom, 2 tablespoons spinach mixture, 1 egg, 2 tablespoons hollandaise, and ¼ teaspoon Parmesan. To make 4 servings, double the recipe.

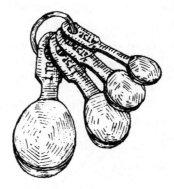

Baked Orange French Toast

Yield: 6 slices
Serving Size: 2 slices
Exchanges:
Starch/Bread   2

Nutrient Content per Serving:

CAL	176	PRO	7 (gm)
FAT	2 (gm)	CHO	33 (gm)
Na	338 (mg)	K	129 (mg)
Fiber	1 (gm)	Chol	0 (mg)

Ingredients

NONSTICK VEGETABLE SPRAY
¼ CUP ORANGE JUICE (PREFERABLY FRESH)
2 EGG WHITES
½ TEASPOON VANILLA EXTRACT
6 SLICES DAY-OLD FRENCH BREAD, CUT 1 INCH THICK
2 TABLESPOONS LOW-CALORIE RASPBERRY PRESERVES (NO SUGAR ADDED)

Method

1. Preheat oven to 350°F. Spray cookie sheet with nonstick vegetable spray.
2. Beat orange juice, egg whites, and vanilla extract together. Dip bread slices on both sides and place on prepared cookie sheet.
3. Bake for 15–17 minutes or until golden brown, turning over after 8 minutes. Serve with preserves.

Vegetables and Side Dishes

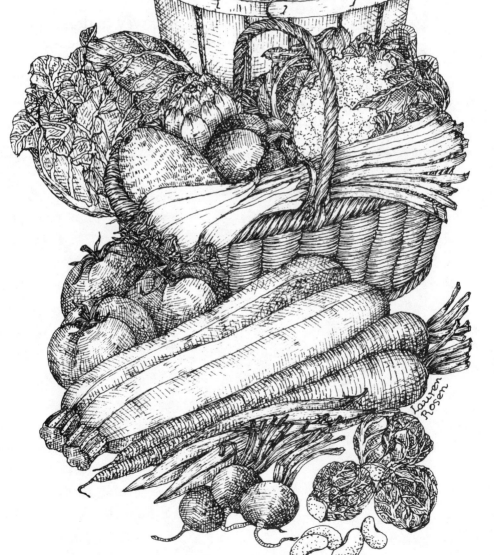

*V*egetables and side dishes are a great way to dress up a simple meal. Colorful, nutritious, and low in calories, they usually take little time to cook, and when properly chosen and combined can make the simplest meal a special one.

Noodle Kugel

Yield: 12 servings
Serving Size: ½ cup
Exchanges:
Starch/Bread 1½
Fat ½

Nutrient Content per Serving:
CAL 148   PRO 5 (gm)
FAT 6 (gm)   CHO 19 (gm)
Na 99 (mg)   K 110 (mg)
Fiber 1 (gm)   Chol 64 (mg)

Ingredients

NONSTICK VEGETABLE SPRAY
2 EGGS, BEATEN
½ CUP LOW-FAT COTTAGE CHEESE
1 TEASPOON CINNAMON
1 TEASPOON VANILLA EXTRACT
¼ TEASPOON BROWN SUGAR SUBSTITUTE
8 OUNCES (ABOUT 4 CUPS) BROAD EGG NOODLES, COOKED
1 LARGE TART APPLE, PEELED AND DICED INTO ¼-INCH PIECES
¼ CUP RAISINS, PLUMPED IN HOT WATER AND DRAINED
¼ CUP MARGARINE, MELTED

Method

1. Preheat oven to 350°F. Spray 2-quart baking dish with nonstick vegetable spray.
2. Combine eggs, cottage cheese, vanilla extract, and brown sugar substitute in large bowl. Stir in noodles, apple, and raisins.
3. Pour into prepared dish; pour margarine evenly over all ingredients.
4. Bake uncovered for 45–55 minutes or until lightly browned.

Method–Microwave

1. Follow mixing directions given above; pour noodle mixture into 2-quart microwave-safe baking dish.

2. Cover with waxed paper; cook on medium-high power for 8–10 minutes, rotating dish once halfway through cooking time.
3. Let stand for 10 minutes before serving.

Mock Mashed Potatoes*

Yield: 4 servings
Serving Size: ½ cup
Exchanges:
Vegetable   1
Fat   ½

Nutrient Content per Serving:

CAL	36	PRO	2 (gm)
FAT	2 (gm)	CHO	4 (gm)
Na	166 (mg)	K	281 (mg)
Fiber	3 (gm)	Chol	0 (mg)

Key Source Nutrients:
Ascorbic acid 57 (mg)

Ingredients

¼ CUP WATER
1 MEDIUM HEAD CAULIFLOWER (ABOUT 1¼ POUNDS), CUT INTO FLORETS
2 TEASPOONS MARGARINE
1 TEASPOON DEHYDRATED MINCED ONION
¼ TEASPOON SALT
⅛ TEASPOON WHITE PEPPER

Method

1. In 2-quart saucepan, bring about ¼ cup water to a boil. Place cauliflower in steamer basket and steam, covered, about 10 minutes or until tender; drain.
2. Purée in food processor or in batches in blender until smooth.
3. Stir in margarine and seasonings and serve.

Method–Microwave

1. Place cauliflower in 1½-quart microwave-safe casserole. Cover with plastic wrap; cook at high power for 6 minutes or until tender; drain.
2. Purée in food processor or in batches in blender until smooth.
3. Stir in margarine and seasonings and serve.

   *3 grams or more of fiber per serving.

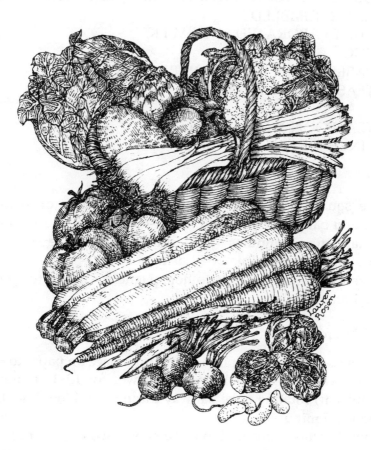

Spaghetti Squash Carbonara

Yield: 6 servings

Serving Size: ½ cup

Exchanges:

Vegetable   1

Fat   1

Nutrient Content per Serving:

CAL	86	PRO	4 (gm)
FAT	5 (gm)	CHO	7 (gm)
Na	235 (mg)	K	172 (mg)
Fiber	1 (gm)	Chol	51 (mg)

Ingredients

     2 POUNDS SPAGHETTI SQUASH
     4 OUNCES BACON, COOKED CRISP, DRAINED,
        AND CRUMBLED
   ¼ CUP EVAPORATED SKIM MILK
     1 EGG
     1 TABLESPOON GRATED PARMESAN CHEESE
     1 TEASPOON MARGARINE
   ¼ TEASPOON SALT
   ⅛ TEASPOON WHITE PEPPER
       PINCH OF NUTMEG

Method

1. Pierce squash in several places with fork. Place on cookie sheet and bake in 350°F oven for 50–60 minutes or until soft. Let stand for 5 minutes. Split squash lengthwise; remove seeds. Shred meat into a bowl using a fork.
2. Add remaining ingredients to hot spaghetti squash; toss and serve immediately.

Method–Microwave

1. Pierce squash in several places with fork. Place on paper towel in microwave oven. Cook on high power for 10–12 minutes or until soft, rotating once halfway through cooking time. Let stand for 5 minutes.
2. Follow directions given above. To cook bacon in microwave oven, place on microwave-safe roast rack; cover with paper towel. Cook on high power for 3–4 minutes or until crisp; drain.

Mediterranean Stuffed Zucchini

Yield: 6 servings
Serving Size: ½ zucchini

Nutrient Content per Serving:

CAL	109	PRO	3 (gm)
FAT	3 (gm)	CHO	18 (gm)
Na	267 (mg)	K	295 (mg)
Fiber	2 (gm)	Chol	0 (mg)

Exchanges:
Starch/Bread   ½
Vegetable   2
Fat   ½

Ingredients

      3 LARGE ZUCCHINI
        NONSTICK VEGETABLE SPRAY
      1 TABLESPOON OLIVE OIL
      1 TABLESPOON PINE NUTS
     ½ CUP ONION, CHOPPED
     ½ CUP TOMATO, FINELY CHOPPED
     ½ CUP RAW RICE
     ½ CUP PLUS ¾ CUP WATER
     ¼ CUP RAISINS
     ½ TEASPOON DRIED MINT
     ½ TEASPOON SALT
     ½ TEASPOON CINNAMON
     ½ TEASPOON DRIED ORANGE PEEL
        PINCH OF BLACK PEPPER
     ¼ CUP TOMATO PASTE

Method

1. Scrub zucchini and trim ends. Boil in water to cover, about 3 minutes or just until tender. Preheat oven to 350°F. Spray 8-inch baking dish with nonstick vegetable spray.
2. Split in half lengthwise; scoop out pulp. Chop pulp from one zucchini; reserve rest for another use (mixed vegetables, soup, or stew).
3. Heat olive oil in 8-inch skillet. Toast pine nuts; drain on paper towel. Sauté onion in remaining oil for 5 minutes.

4. Add tomato, zucchini pulp, rice, ¾ cup water, raisins, and seasonings. Bring to a boil; reduce heat. Cover; simmer for 15 minutes or until rice is almost tender. Stir in pine nuts; stuff mixture into hollowed zucchini. Place in prepared dish.
5. Combine tomato paste and ½ cup water; pour over and around zucchini.
6. Cover with foil; bake 30 minutes.

Method–Microwave

1. Prepare zucchini as directed above.
2. In 2-quart microwave-safe saucepan, cook pine nuts in oil on high power for 2 minutes, stirring once halfway through cooking time.
3. Set aside. Cook onion in remaining oil for 4 minutes on high power or until softened. Add tomato, zucchini pulp, rice, ¾ cup water, raisins, and seasonings.
4. Cover and cook on high power for 10–12 minutes, stirring once.
5. Stuff zucchini with mixture and arrange in 8-inch microwave-safe baking dish. Mix tomato paste with ½ cup water; pour over and around zucchini. Cover with plastic wrap. Cook for 10 minutes on high power. Let stand for 5 minutes before serving.

Swedish Potato Pancakes

Yield: 14 pancakes
Serving Size: 2 pancakes
Exchanges:
Starch/Bread   1½

Nutrient Content per Serving:

CAL	114	PRO	4 (gm)
FAT	0 (gm)	CHO	24 (gm)
Na	173 (mg)	K	195 (mg)
Fiber	2 (gm)	Chol	1 (mg)

Ingredients

- 1 CUP SKIM MILK
- 1 CUP ALL-PURPOSE FLOUR
- 2 CUPS RED POTATOES, PEELED, SHREDDED, AND PATTED DRY
- ¼ CUP ONION, GRATED
- ½ TEASPOON SALT
- ¼ TEASPOON BLACK PEPPER
- NONSTICK VEGETABLE SPRAY

Method

1. Combine milk and flour to make a fairly stiff batter. Stir in potatoes, onion, salt, and pepper.
2. Heat large skillet and spray well with nonstick vegetable spray. Drop 1 tablespoon batter per pancake into skillet; flatten with spoon. Fry until edges are brown, turn over, and continue to brown. Cook over medium heat for 15–20 minutes until brown and crisp.
3. Drain on paper towels. May need to cook in batches; spray skillet each time.
4. Serve with no-sugar-added apple sauce, low-fat sour cream, or plain yogurt.

Swiss Potato Cake

Yield: 4 servings

Serving Size: ¼ cake

Exchanges:

Starch/Bread   1

Fat   ½

Nutrient Content per Serving:

CAL	102	PRO	3 (gm)
FAT	4 (gm)	CHO	14 (gm)
Na	177 (mg)	K	232 (mg)
Fiber	1 (gm)	Chol	7 (mg)

Ingredients

NONSTICK VEGETABLE SPRAY

2 CUPS (1 LARGE OR 2 MEDIUM) BAKING POTATOES, PEELED AND THINLY SLICED

¼ TEASPOON SALT

⅛ TEASPOON BLACK PEPPER

2 TEASPOONS MARGARINE

1 OUNCE (¼ CUP) SWISS CHEESE, SHREDDED

Method

1. Preheat oven to 425°F. Coat 9- or 10-inch oven-proof skillet with nonstick vegetable spray.
2. Rinse and pat dry potatoes. Arrange half of potatoes in concentric overlapping rings in prepared skillet. Sprinkle with half of seasonings; dot with 1 teaspoon margarine. Repeat layers.
3. Cook on top of stove over medium heat for 8–10 minutes, pressing down with spatula.
4. Place in oven and bake for 20–25 minutes or until golden brown.
5. Top with cheese and bake for 4–5 minutes or until cheese is melted.

Minnesota Wild Rice Casserole* **

Yield: 8 servings

Serving Size: ½ cup

Exchanges:

Starch/Bread   1

Vegetable   1

Fat   ½

Nutrient Content per Serving:

CAL	128	PRO	7 (gm)
FAT	3 (gm)	CHO	18 (gm)
Na	500 (mg)	K	248 (mg)
Fiber	3 (gm)	Chol	1 (mg)

Ingredients

   1 CUP RAW WILD RICE
     NONSTICK VEGETABLE SPRAY
   1 CUP ONION, CHOPPED
  ½ CUP CELERY, CHOPPED
   2 TABLESPOONS GREEN PEPPER, CHOPPED
   1 CLOVE GARLIC, CHOPPED
  ¼ CUP PECANS, CHOPPED
 2½ CUPS CANNED CHICKEN BROTH†
  ¼ TEASPOON BLACK PEPPER

Method

1. To prepare rice, bring water to a boil (follow instructions on package for correct amount).
2. Turn off the heat, wash rice, and let stand in the water for 1 hour.
3. Preheat oven to 325°F. Spray 1½-quart casserole with nonstick vegetable spray.
4. Sauté all vegetables in sprayed skillet for 5 minutes or until soft. Add pecans; cook for 1 minute.
5. Drain rice and add to onion mixture. Add chicken broth and pepper. Pour into prepared casserole. Cover and bake for 1 hour; uncover and bake for 15 minutes.

*400 milligrams or more of sodium per serving.
**3 grams or more of fiber per serving.
†For reduced salt and fat, use homemade chicken broth.

Potatoes au Gratin*

Yield: 4 servings

Serving Size: ½ cup

Exchanges:

Starch/Bread 1½

Meat, medium-fat 1

Fat ½

Nutrient Content per Serving:

CAL	214	PRO	9 (gm)
FAT	9 (gm)	CHO	25 (gm)
Na	443 (mg)	K	401 (mg)
Fiber	2 (gm)	Chol	23 (mg)

Ingredients

- ½ CUP SKIM MILK
- 2 TABLESPOONS FLOUR
- ½ TEASPOON SALT
- ⅛ TEASPOON CELERY SEED
- ¾ CUP CHEDDAR CHEESE, SHREDDED
- 2 CUPS POTATOES, UNPEELED AND THINLY SLICED
- 2 TEASPOONS MARGARINE
- ¼ TEASPOON PAPRIKA

Method

1. Preheat oven to 350°F. Heat milk in saucepan for 3 minutes.
2. Combine flour, salt, celery seed, and cheddar cheese in small bowl.
3. Place half of the potatoes in an 8-by-8-inch pan. Sprinkle half of cheese over potatoes. Repeat layers. Pour hot milk over all. Dot with margarine. Sprinkle with paprika.
4. Cover with foil and bake for 15–20 minutes. Uncover and bake for 10 minutes longer or until potatoes are fork tender.

Method–Microwave

1. Heat milk in 1-cup measuring cup for 1 minute on high power.
2. Follow steps given above for layering mixture.
3. Microwave on high power for 8–10 minutes, rotating dish once during cooking time.

*400 milligrams or more of sodium per serving.

Baked Potato Skins

Yield: 2 servings
Serving Size: ½ baked
potato skin (with topping)
Exchanges:
Starch/Bread   1

	MARGARINE	MEXICAN STYLE	PIZZA STYLE	BACON AND SOUR CREAM
CAL	66	74	69	86
FAT (gm)	1	1	0	2
Na (mg)	17	28	67	51
Fiber (gm)	0	0	0	0
PRO (gm)	1	2	2	3
CHO (gm)	13	14	14	15
K (mg)	167	170	196	175
Chol (mg)	0	4	2	1

Ingredients

    1 POTATO, BAKED

Toppings

    MARGARINE
    ½ TEASPOON MARGARINE
        PINCH GARLIC POWDER

    MEXICAN STYLE
    1 TABLESPOON MEXICAN CHILES
    1 TABLESPOON CHEDDAR CHEESE, SHREDDED
        (Heat until cheese melts)

    PIZZA STYLE
    1 TABLESPOON PIZZA OR TOMATO SAUCE
    1 TABLESPOON MOZZARELLA CHEESE,
        SHREDDED

BACON AND SOUR CREAM
1 TEASPOON BACON BITS
2 TABLESPOONS REDUCED-CALORIE SOUR
    CREAM OR PLAIN YOGURT

Method

1. Bake potato for 1 hour or until soft. Split lengthwise and scoop out potato. Reserve for mashed potatoes.
2. Top with favorite topping, wrap in foil and heat; keep warm until lunch.

Method–Microwave

1. Bake potato for 4–5 minutes or until soft. Split lengthwise, scoop out potato, and proceed as directed above.
2. To reheat, place on paper plate and heat for 30–45 seconds on high power or until topping is melted and potato is hot. Wrap in foil to keep warm.

Variations: Scoop out potato, mash, replace in skin, and use desired toppings. If using all of potato, consider a half-potato as 1 serving; if using skin only, consider 1 whole potato as 1 serving.

Appetizer: Cut skins in quarters. Bake skin side up in oven at 375°F for 10–12 minutes or until crisp. Dip in guacamole, salsa, vegetable dip, or sour cream.

German Style Sauerkraut* **

Yield: 4 servings   Nutrient Content per Serving:
Serving Size: ½ cup
Exchanges:
Vegetable   2
Fruit   ½
Fat   ½

Ingredients

    1 MEDIUM ONION, THINLY SLICED
      NONSTICK VEGETABLE SPRAY
    1 POUND SAUERKRAUT, RINSED AND DRAINED
    2 SLICES BACON, COOKED CRISP AND CRUMBLED
    1 LARGE GOLDEN DELICIOUS APPLE, PEELED,
      CORED, AND DICED
  1/2 TEASPOON CARAWAY SEEDS
    2 CUPS BOILING WATER
  1/4 TEASPOON BROWN SUGAR SUBSTITUTE OR TO
      TASTE

Method

1. Sauté onion until brown in 2-quart saucepan well sprayed with nonstick vegetable spray.
2. Add sauerkraut; cook for 5 minutes. Stir in bacon, apple, and caraway seeds. Cover with boiling water. Cook uncovered for 15 minutes over low heat. Cook covered for 15–20 minutes over low heat. Stir in brown sugar substitute.

Method–Microwave

1. Place onion in 1-quart unsprayed microwave-safe casserole. Cook for 8–10 minutes on high power or until brown. Stir several times. Stir in sauerkraut, bacon, apples, and caraway seeds. Cover with 1½ cups boiling water. Cook covered for 8–10 minutes on high power or until apple is soft and liquid is slightly reduced. If necessary, uncover and cook on high power for 3–5 minutes or until liquid is reduced.
2. Stir in brown sugar substitute.

Note: Can be served with pork chops, sausages, or beef.

    *400 milligrams or more of sodium per serving.
    **3 grams or more of fiber per serving.

Brussels Sprouts au Gratin*

Yield: 4 servings** Nutrient Content per Serving:

Serving Size: ¼ of recipe	CAL 101	PRO	6 (gm)
Exchanges:	FAT 6 (gm)	CHO	9 (gm)
Vegetable 2	Na 178 (mg)	K	283 (mg)
Fat 1	Fiber 3 (gm)	Chol	8 (mg)

Ingredients

    1 10-OUNCE PACKAGE FROZEN BRUSSELS
      SPROUTS
    ½ CUP WHITE SAUCE
    ¼ CUP CHEDDAR CHEESE, GRATED
      PINCH OF PAPRIKA

White Sauce

    1 TABLESPOON MARGARINE
    1 TABLESPOON FLOUR
    ½ CUP SKIM MILK
    ⅛ TEASPOON SALT
      PINCH OF BLACK PEPPER
      PINCH OF NUTMEG

Method

1. Preheat oven to 350°F.
2. Cook brussels sprouts in boiling water for 5 minutes; drain.
3. Prepare white sauce. Melt margarine in saucepan. Whisk in flour. Slowly whisk in milk and cook, stirring constantly until sauce is thickened. Remove from heat. Stir in cheese until melted and add seasonings except paprika. Adjust for taste.
4. Put brussels sprouts in 2-quart au gratin dish or 2-quart baking dish. Pour sauce over sprouts. Sprinkle with paprika. Bake for 15–20 minutes or until sauce is bubbly.

Method–Microwave

1. Place frozen brussels sprouts in 2-quart microwave-safe baking dish. Cover with plastic wrap and cook for 5–10 minutes on high power or just until tender.
2. Prepare white sauce. Melt margarine in 2-cup glass measure. Whisk in flour. Heat milk for 2 minutes on high power. Slowly whisk milk into flour mixture. Cook 1½–3 minutes on medium-high power, or until sauce is thickened. Whisk once during cooking.
3. Pour sauce over brussels sprouts. Sprinkle with paprika. Cook for 1–2 minutes on high power, uncovered, or until sauce is bubbly.

Note: Any vegetable may be prepared in this manner, but the sprouts are especially delicious, even if they are not the family favorite.

*3 grams or more of fiber per serving.
**To make 8 servings, double the recipe.

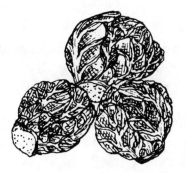

Carrot Purée*

Yield: 2 servings**
Serving Size: ½ of recipe
Exchanges:
Vegetable   2
Fat   ½

Nutrient Content per Serving:

CAL	69	PRO	1 (gm)
FAT	3 (gm)	CHO	10 (gm)
Na	364 (mg)	K	222 (mg)
Fiber	3 (gm)	Chol	0 (mg)

Key Source Nutrients:
Vitamin A   23,298 (IU)

Ingredients

   1 CUP WATER
   ½ POUND CARROTS, PEELED AND CUT INTO
     ½-INCH-LONG PIECES
 1½ TEASPOONS MARGARINE
   ¼ TEASPOON SALT
     PINCH OF NUTMEG
     PINCH OF WHITE PEPPER
   ½ TEASPOON DRIED DILL OR 1½ TEASPOONS
     FRESH DILL, CHOPPED
 1½ TEASPOONS SKIM MILK

Method

1. Bring water to a boil. Add carrots and blanch until tender, about 15–20 minutes. Drain.
2. Place carrots in food processor or food mill. Purée until smooth.
3. Add remaining ingredients. Process for 1 minute.
4. Put into individual serving dishes or 1 large bowl. Cover with foil and keep warm in oven at 150°F.

Method–Microwave

1. Slice carrots. Put into 1½-quart casserole. Add enough water to cover.
2. Cook covered for 7–8 minutes or until tender on high power.

3. Follow purée method given above.
4. May reheat carrot purée for 5–6 minutes on medium-high power.

*3 grams or more of fiber per serving.
**To make 4 servings, double the recipe.

Spinach Ring*

Yield: 4 servings**

Serving Size: ¼ of recipe

Exchanges:

		Nutrient Content per Serving:		
		CAL	82	PRO	5 (gm)
		FAT	5 (gm)	CHO	5 (gm)
Vegetable	1	Na	435 (mg)	K	267 (mg)
Fat	1	Fiber	1 (gm)	Chol	69 (mg)

Key Source Nutrients:
Vitamin A   4,502 (IU)

Ingredients

    NONSTICK VEGETABLE SPRAY
1 10-OUNCE PACKAGE FROZEN CHOPPED
    SPINACH, DEFROSTED AND DRAINED WELL
½ CUP CANNED CHICKEN BROTH†
¼ CUP SKIM MILK
1 WHOLE EGG
1 TABLESPOON WHOLE WHEAT FLOUR
1 TABLESPOON MARGARINE
¼ TEASPOON SALT
¼ TEASPOON NUTMEG
⅛ TEASPOON WHITE PEPPER

Method

1. Preheat oven to 350°F. Spray 1- or 1½-quart ring pan with nonstick vegetable spray.
2. Heat spinach in 1-quart saucepan for 4–5 minutes.
3. Combine rest of ingredients in food processor or blender. Blend until smooth. Add to spinach.

4. Pour into prepared ring pan.
5. Bake for 35–40 minutes or until toothpick inserted in ring comes out clean.

Method–Microwave

1. Place spinach in small microwave-safe casserole; cook for 3–4 minutes on high power.
2. Combine spinach with blended liquid.
3. Pour into a 1- or 1½-quart microwave-safe ring pan. Do not spray. Cover with waxed paper.
4. Cook for 6–8 minutes (10–12½ for eight servings) on medium power or preferably 60 percent power. Rotate dish once. Uncover and cook for 2–3 minutes on high power. Spinach ring should look dry and toothpick should come out clean when inserted in center.

*400 milligrams or more of sodium per serving.
**To make 8 servings, double the recipe.
†For reduced salt and fat, use homemade chicken broth.

Pineapple Glazed Yams

		Nutrient Content per Serving:		
Yield: 4 servings				
Serving Size: ¼ recipe		CAL 105	PRO	1 (gm)
Exchanges:		FAT 1 (gm)	CHO	24 (gm)
Starch/Bread	1	Na 149 (mg)	K	399 (mg)
Fruit	½	Fiber 2 (gm)	Chol	0 (mg)

Ingredients

    1 8-OUNCE CAN PINEAPPLE CHUNKS IN OWN
      JUICE, DRAINED (AND RESERVED)
    2 TEASPOONS CORNSTARCH
    1/4 TEASPOON SALT
    1/8 TEASPOON BLACK PEPPER
    1/8 TEASPOON CINNAMON
    1/2 POUND YAMS (2 SMALL), COOKED, PEELED,
      SLICED IN 1/4-INCH SLICES, WITH EACH SLICE
      HALVED
    1 TEASPOON MARGARINE

Method

1. Preheat oven to 350°F.
2. In 1¹/₂-quart saucepan, combine reserved pineapple juice mixed with cornstarch, salt, pepper, and cinnamon.
3. Cook until thickened, stirring constantly.
4. Combine yams and pineapple in 8-inch round casserole. Stir in sauce and coat well. Dot with margarine.
5. Cover with foil and bake for 10 minutes.

Method–Microwave

1. Pierce yams with fork in several places. Place on paper towel in microwave and cook for 3–5 minutes on high power. Cool, peel, and slice.
2. In 1-cup glass measure, combine reserved juice with cornstarch, salt, pepper, and cinnamon. Cook for 1–1¹/₂ minutes on high power or until sauce is thickened. Stir once.
3. Combine yams and pineapple in 1-quart round microwave-safe casserole. Coat with sauce and stir well. Dot with margarine. Cover with waxed paper.
4. Cook for 1–2 minutes on high power or until heated thoroughly. Stir once.

Indian Corn Pudding* **

Yield: 4 servings

Serving Size: ¼ of pudding

Exchanges:

Starch/Bread	1
Milk, skim	½
Fat	1

Nutrient Content per Serving:

CAL	173	PRO	9 (gm)
FAT	6 (gm)	CHO	23 (gm)
Na	640 (mg)	K	366 (mg)
Fiber	6 (gm)	Chol	138 (mg)

Ingredients

    NONSTICK VEGETABLE SPRAY
2 EGGS
½ TEASPOON SALT
⅛ TEASPOON WHITE PEPPER
¼ TEASPOON MACE
1 TABLESPOON ONION, GRATED
1 TABLESPOON MARGARINE
1½ CUPS SKIM MILK
1 16-OUNCE CAN WHOLE KERNEL CORN,
    DRAINED

Method

1. Preheat oven to 325°F. Spray 1½-quart casserole with non-stick vegetable spray.
2. Beat eggs with seasonings and onion.
3. Melt margarine in 1½-quart saucepan; stir in milk and heat for 5 minutes. Mix into egg mixture.
4. Stir in corn. Pour into prepared casserole. Bake for 1 hour or until set.

Method–Microwave

1. Melt margarine in 2-quart microwave-safe saucepan; stir in milk and heat for 2–2½ minutes on high power. Mix into egg mixture.
2. Stir in corn. Pour into unsprayed microwave-safe 1½-quart casserole. Cook on medium-high power for 13–15 minutes; rotate dish twice during cooking time. Cook for 2 minutes on high power. Let stand for 5 minutes before serving.

*400 milligrams or more of sodium per serving.
**3 grams or more of fiber per serving.

Summer Chutney

Yield: 3 cups (24 servings)	Nutrient Content per Serving:			
Serving Size: 2 tablespoons	CAL	28	PRO	0 (gm)
Exchanges:	FAT	0 (gm)	CHO	7 (gm)
Fruit ½	Na	3 (mg)	K	60 (mg)
	Fiber	2 (gm)	Chol	0 (mg)

Ingredients

  2 POUNDS FRESH OR FROZEN BLUEBERRIES (IF FROZEN, DEFROST AND DRAIN)
  ½ OUNCE FRESH GINGER, PEELED AND CHOPPED (1½ TABLESPOONS)
  1 MEDIUM ONION, CHOPPED
  ¾ CUP CIDER VINEGAR
  ¼ CUP GOLDEN RAISINS
 24 PACKETS SUGAR SUBSTITUTE (NOT ASPARTAME)
1½ TEASPOONS CINNAMON
  ½ TEASPOON DRY MUSTARD
  ½ TEASPOON GROUND CLOVES
  ¼ TEASPOON CAYENNE PEPPER
  ¼ TEASPOON CARDAMOM
  2 CUPS WATER

Method

1. Combine all ingredients in large noncorrosive saucepan. Bring to a boil over medium heat. Lower heat and boil gently uncovered for about 2 hours or until thick.
2. Store in sterilized jars and process in boiling water bath according to manufacturer's instructions, or freeze in separate air-tight containers for up to 6 months.

Note: Chutney is of Indian origin and is served like a relish with pork or poultry.

North African Couscous*

Yield: 4 servings
Serving Size: ½ cup

Exchanges:
Starch/Bread   2
Fat   ½

Nutrient Content per Serving:

CAL	186	PRO	8 (gm)
FAT	4 (gm)	CHO	31 (gm)
Na	441 (mg)	K	344 (mg)
Fiber	2 (gm)	Chol	1 (mg)

Ingredients

    1 TABLESPOON MARGARINE
    1 CUP COUSCOUS, QUICK COOKING
    1 CUP CANNED CHICKEN BROTH**
    ⅓ CUP CARROTS, PEELED AND THINLY SLICED
    ½ CUP ONIONS, THINLY SLICED
       NONSTICK VEGETABLE SPRAY
    ¼ CUP DARK SEEDLESS RAISINS
       PINCH OF CAYENNE PEPPER

Method

1. Melt margarine in medium saucepan. Add couscous and mix carefully, coating all grain with margarine. Bring chicken broth to a boil, add to the mixture, and cover. Remove from heat; let stand for 15 minutes.
2. Sauté carrots and onions in skillet well sprayed with nonstick vegetable spray. Cook for 5–6 minutes or until onions are soft. Stir onions, carrots, and raisins into couscous. Add cayenne pepper. Adjust to taste.

Note: Couscous is a semolina wheat pasta, usually served in stews or as a side dish in North African nations. Couscous can be found in Greek and Middle Eastern stores as well as the ethnic section in a grocery store. Use instead of rice or noodles. Serve with poultry or meat.

*400 milligrams or more of sodium per serving.
**For reduced salt and fat, use homemade chicken broth.

Sauces

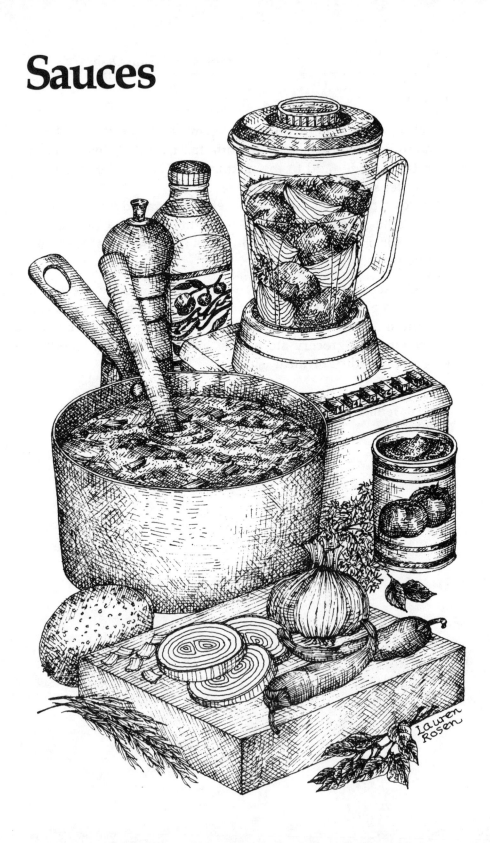

Lauren Rosen

Classic French cuisine developed more than 130 different sauces, divided into "mother" sauces and their variations. Here we present only five—small in number but important. Like the French, we think there's no easier way to transform and complement main dishes.

Use them all, from the mild, delicate Cucumber Sauce (excellent over fish) to Pesto Sauce, its polar opposite, so packed with flavor that just a bit fills up your whole mouth. Pesto is so good it's worth growing your own basil if you can't get fresh! Low-Calorie Hollandaise is as rich-tasting and lemony as its high-calorie, high-cholesterol counterpart—perfect on the season's first tender shoots of asparagus.

Cucumber Sauce

Yield: 1 cup (8 servings)
Serving Size: 2 tablespoons
Exchanges:
Free food

Nutrient Content per Serving:

CAL	12	PRO	1 (gm)
FAT	0 (gm)	CHO	2 (gm)
Na	285 (mg)	K	55 (mg)
Fiber	0 (gm)	Chol	1 (mg)

Ingredients

- 1 CUP CUCUMBER, SHREDDED, PEELED, AND SEEDED
- ½ CUP LOW-FAT PLAIN YOGURT
- 1 TABLESPOON FRESH LEMON JUICE
- 1 TEASPOON PREPARED YELLOW MUSTARD
- ½ TEASPOON DILL SEED OR FRESH DILL, CHOPPED
- ½ TEASPOON ONION POWDER
- ¼ TEASPOON SALT

Method

1. Squeeze cucumber dry.
2. Combine all ingredients; chill.
3. Serve with any poached, broiled, or grilled fish. Especially good with cold poached salmon or trout.

Pesto Sauce

Yield: ½ cup (8 servings)
Serving Size: 1 tablespoon
Exchanges:
Fat   1

Nutrient Content per Serving:

CAL	49	PRO	1 (gm)
FAT	5 (gm)	CHO	1 (gm)
Na	25 (mg)	K	32 (mg)
Fiber	0 (gm)	Chol	1 (mg)

Ingredients

- 1 CUP FRESH BASIL, LOOSELY PACKED, RINSED, AND PATTED DRY
- 1 CLOVE GARLIC
- 2 TABLESPOONS PINE NUTS
- 2 TABLESPOONS GRATED PARMESAN CHEESE
- ¼ TEASPOON BLACK PEPPER
- 2 TABLESPOONS OLIVE OR CORN OIL

Method

1. Combine basil, garlic, pine nuts, and Parmesan cheese in food processor or blender. Process until smooth.
2. In food processor, pour oil through feed tube with machine running slowly, and process until blended. In blender, pour oil into container and process until blended.
3. Serve as dressing for green salad or mozzarella and tomato salad, mix with chicken for chicken salad, or stir into pasta.

Bolognese Sauce*

Yield: 4 servings**
Serving Size: ¾ cup
Exchanges:
Meat, medium-fat 2
Vegetable 2

Nutrient Content per Serving:

CAL	200	PRO	16 (gm)
FAT	12 (gm)	CHO	8 (gm)
Na	650 (mg)	K	508 (mg)
Fiber	2 (gm)	Chol	53 (mg)

Ingredients

¾ POUND LEAN GROUND BEEF
½ CUP ONION, CHOPPED
1 CLOVE GARLIC, MINCED
¼ CUP CARROT, CHOPPED
1 16-OUNCE CAN TOMATOES, UNDRAINED
¼ CUP DRY RED WINE
¾ TEASPOON SALT
½ TEASPOON BASIL
½ TEASPOON OREGANO
⅛ TEASPOON BLACK PEPPER
1½ TEASPOONS TOMATO PASTE

Method

1. Brown ground beef with onion, garlic, and carrot; drain.
2. Add tomatoes, wine, and seasonings. Cover and simmer for 40–45 minutes, stirring occasionally.
3. Stir in tomato paste; uncover and boil until slightly thickened.
4. Serve over 1 cup cooked spaghetti for each serving, if desired.

Method–Microwave

1. Combine ground beef, onion, garlic, and carrot in 2- or 3-quart microwave-safe casserole.
2. Cover and cook at high power for 4 minutes or until beef is no longer pink; stir once. Drain.
3. Add tomatoes, wine, and seasonings; cover. Cook for 15–20 minutes at medium-high power.
4. Stir in tomato paste; uncover and cook for 8–10 minutes at high power or until thickened, stirring occasionally.

*400 milligrams or more of sodium per serving.
**To make 8 servings, double the recipe.

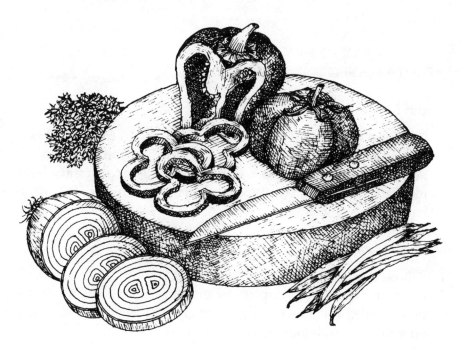

Low-Calorie Hollandaise

Yield: ¾ cup (6 servings)
Serving Size: 2 tablespoons
Exchanges:
Meat, lean   ½

Nutrient Content per Serving:

CAL	25	PRO	2 (gm)
FAT	1 (gm)	CHO	3 (gm)
Na	110 (mg)	K	43 (mg)
Fiber	0 (gm)	Chol	46 (mg)

Ingredients

- ½ CUP WATER
- 1 TABLESPOON CORNSTARCH
- 2 TABLESPOONS NONFAT DRY MILK SOLIDS
- 1 EGG YOLK
- ¼ TEASPOON SALT
- ⅛ TEASPOON DRY MUSTARD
- 2–3 TABLESPOONS LEMON JUICE

Method

1. Combine all ingredients except lemon juice in food processor or blender. Blend for 10 seconds or until smooth.
2. Pour mixture into 1-quart saucepan. Whisk constantly over medium heat until thickened, about 5–8 minutes. Whisk in lemon juice.

Method–Microwave

1. Follow directions given above in step 1.
2. Pour mixture into 2-cup glass measure. Cook on medium-high power for 1½–3 minutes or until thickened, whisking once. Whisk in lemon juice.

Washington State Apple Butter

Yield: 3 cups
Serving Size: 1 tablespoon
Exchanges:
Free food

Nutrient Content per Serving:

CAL	8	PRO	0 (gm)
FAT	0 (gm)	CHO	2 (gm)
Na	0 (mg)	K	16 (mg)
Fiber	0 (gm)	Chol	0 (mg)

Ingredients

2½ POUNDS GOLDEN DELICIOUS APPLES,
    WASHED, CORED, AND CUT INTO EIGHTHS
¾ CUP WATER
2 TABLESPOONS LEMON JUICE
¾ TEASPOON CINNAMON
⅛ TEASPOON GROUND CLOVES
⅛ TEASPOON MACE
¾ TEASPOON BROWN SUGAR SUBSTITUTE

Method

1. Combine apples, water, and lemon juice in 5-quart stock pot. Bring to boil over high heat. Cover and simmer for 30 minutes.
2. Put apples through a food mill or sieve. Return them to pot of water and add cinnamon, cloves, mace, and brown sugar substitute. Simmer uncovered until mixture thickens, about 45–60 minutes.
3. Pour into glass jars, cover, cool, and refrigerate. Keeps in the refrigerator for 1 week. Freeze for longer storage.

Note: Wonderful on French toast, waffles, muffins, or toast.

Desserts

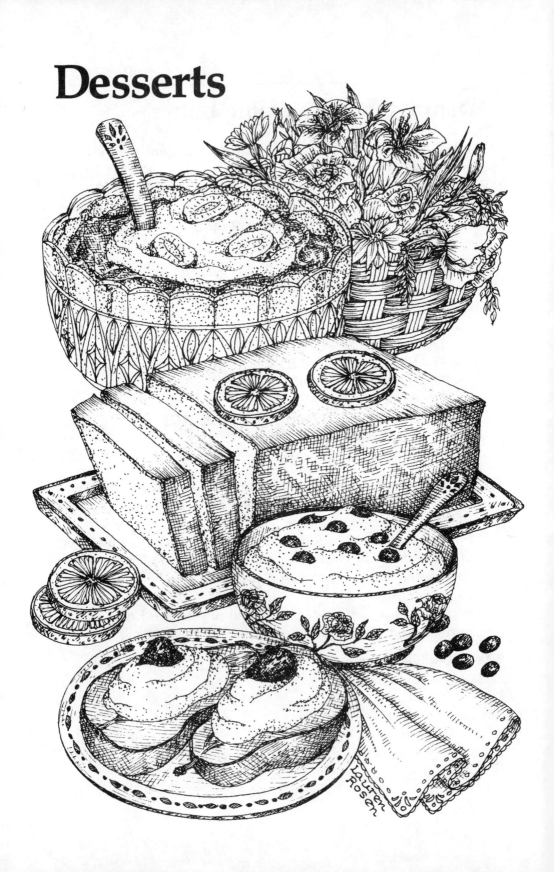

Lauren Rosen

*D*essert—it's the part of the meal that most of us wait for, so, fortunately, nearly any dessert will be greeted with glee. Remember, though, that most dessert recipes are higher in fat than other dishes. Take that into consideration in planning your meals. To get the very most out of your desserts, choose those that complement the rest of a meal. After a filling, fairly heavy meal, try a refreshing dessert like a fruit ice, while if your main dish has been simple and plain, treat everyone to a rich-tasting baked goody— all those you'll find on the following pages are far less calorie-laden than they taste!

Apricot–Almond Rice*

Yield: 4 servings**
Serving Size: ½ cup
Exchanges:
Starch/Bread 1
Fruit 1
Fat 1

Nutrient Content per Serving:
CAL	181	PRO	3 (gm)
FAT	5 (gm)	CHO	33 (gm)
Na	90 (mg)	K	306 (mg)
Fiber	4 (gm)	Chol	0 (mg)

Ingredients

      1 TEASPOON MARGARINE
   1½ CUPS HOT COOKED RICE
    ¼ CUP DRIED APRICOTS, CHOPPED
    ¼ CUP RAISINS
    ¼ CUP CELERY, CHOPPED
      2 TABLESPOONS ALMONDS, SLICED, BLANCHED,
        AND TOASTED
    ¼ TEASPOON CINNAMON
    ⅛ TEASPOON SALT

Method

1. Stir margarine into hot rice. Keep covered.
2. Soak apricots and raisins in boiling water for 10 minutes; drain.
3. Stir apricots, raisins, celery, almonds, cinnamon, and salt into rice.
4. Serve hot or at room temperature.

Method–Microwave

1. To make rice in the microwave, follow package instructions, but reduce water by ¼ cup. Put rice in 2-quart microwave-safe saucepan, add hot water, cover, and bring to a boil (about 6–10 minutes on high power, depending on beginning water temperature).
2. Let stand, covered, until all water is absorbed, about 10 minutes. If when ready to use, water is not absorbed, uncover and put back in microwave for 2–5 minutes on high power or until water is absorbed.

3. Follow directions given in steps 2–4 above.

Note: May add ⅛–¼ teaspoon curry powder.

*3 grams or more of fiber per serving.
**To make 8 servings, double the recipe.

Fruit Salad with Chocolate Cream*

Yield: 4 ½-cup servings
Serving Size: ½ cup
Exchanges:
Meat, lean   1
Fruit   1½

Nutrient Content per Serving:

CAL	139	PRO	7 (gm)
FAT	4 (gm)	CHO	22 (gm)
Na	79 (mg)	K	455 (mg)
Fiber	2 (gm)	Chol	138 (mg)

Key Source Nutrients:
Ascorbic acid   45 (mg)

Ingredients

        1 CUP EVAPORATED SKIM MILK
        2 EGG YOLKS
        1 TABLESPOON SUGAR
        1 TABLESPOON UNSWEETENED COCOA
        2 TEASPOONS VANILLA EXTRACT
        1 PINT STRAWBERRIES, HULLED AND HALVED
        1 SMALL BANANA, SLICED AND SPRINKLED WITH
           1 TEASPOON LEMON JUICE

Method

1. In 1½-quart saucepan, heat milk until simmering, but do not boil.
2. Beat egg yolks, sugar, cocoa, and vanilla extract. Stir some of the hot milk into egg mixture.
3. Stir egg mixture back into milk. Cook over medium heat, whisking constantly until sauce is thickened and coats the back of a spoon.
4. Chill over a bowl of ice or refrigerate for several hours.
5. Toss fruit together in serving bowl; serve with chocolate cream.

*This recipe has slightly more than ½ teaspoon of sugar per serving.

Pears Filled with Strawberry Cream Cheese*

		Nutrient Content per Serving:		
Yield: 2 servings				
Serving Size: ½ pear, 2		CAL 195	PRO	7 (gm)
ounces cream cheese		FAT 11 (gm)	CHO	23 (gm)
Exchanges:		Na 321 (mg)	K	254 (mg)
Fruit	1½	Fiber 4 (gm)	Chol	30 (mg)
Fat	2			

Ingredients

- 4 OUNCES CREAM CHEESE (LITE OR NUFCHATEL)
- 2 FRESH STRAWBERRIES, SLICED
- ¼ TEASPOON BROWN SUGAR SUBSTITUTE
- 1 LARGE PEAR, UNPEELED AND SLICED
- 1 TEASPOON LEMON JUICE

Method

1. Combine cream cheese, strawberries, and brown sugar substitute in food processor or blender. Blend until smooth.
2. Spread each pear slice with lemon juice, then ½ of the cheese mixture.

   *3 grams or more of fiber per serving.

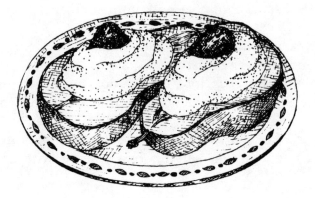

Strawberry and Rhubarb Compote

Yield: 8 servings*
Serving Size: ¼ cup
Exchanges:
Free food

Nutrient Content per Serving:

CAL	12	PRO	0 (gm)
FAT	0 (gm)	CHO	3 (gm)
Na	1 (mg)	K	113 (mg)
Fiber	1 (gm)	Chol	0 (mg)

Ingredients

- ½ POUND FRESH (TRIMMED) OR FROZEN (DEFROSTED) RHUBARB, CUT INTO ¼-INCH SLICES
- ¼ CUP WATER
- 1–3 PACKETS SUGAR SUBSTITUTE
- ¼ TEASPOON CINNAMON
- 1 CUP FRESH STRAWBERRIES, SLICED

Method

1. In 2-quart saucepan, combine rhubarb, water, sugar substitute, and cinnamon; cover. Cook over medium heat for 15 minutes or until soft.
2. Stir in strawberries; heat for 5 minutes.
3. Chill. May be served as a side dish with meat or poultry or with 2 tablespoons whipped topping as a dessert.

Method–Microwave

1. Combine rhubarb, water, sugar substitute, and cinnamon in 2-quart microwave-safe casserole. Cover; cook for 4–5 minutes on high power, stirring once.
2. Stir in strawberries and cook for 2–2½ minutes on high power. Let stand covered for 5 minutes; chill.

*To make 16 servings, double the recipe.

Pear/Cranberry Turnover*

Yield: 4 servings
Serving Size: ¼ turnover
Exchanges:
Starch/Bread   ½
Fruit   2
Fat   3

Nutrient Content per Serving:
CAL 289   PRO   4 (gm)
FAT   15 (gm)   CHO   36 (gm)
Na   276 (mg)   K   151 (mg)
Fiber   3 (gm)   Chol   0 (mg)

Ingredients

9-INCH PIE CRUST, READY-MADE OR
HOMEMADE
1 CUP (1 MEDIUM) PEAR, PEELED, CORED, AND
THINLY SLICED
¼ CUP CRANBERRIES, FRESH OR FROZEN,
UNSWEETENED
¼ CUP DARK SEEDLESS RAISINS
½ TEASPOON BROWN SUGAR SUBSTITUTE
1 TABLESPOON FLOUR
½ TEASPOON CINNAMON
1 TEASPOON LEMON JUICE
1 TEASPOON SKIM MILK
1 PACKET SUGAR SUBSTITUTE (NOT ASPARTAME)

Method

1. Preheat oven to 375°F. Place pie crust on ungreased cookie sheet.
2. In medium bowl, combine pear slices, cranberries, raisins, brown sugar substitute, flour, cinnamon, and lemon juice; blend well.
3. Spoon fruit mixture evenly on half of prepared crust, leaving ½-inch border. Fold remaining side over fruit; press edges to seal firmly. Flute edges; cut small slits in top of crust to allow steam to escape. Brush with milk; sprinkle with sugar substitute.
4. Bake for 30–40 minutes or until crust is golden.

*3 grams or more of fiber per serving.

Kichel

		Nutrient Content per Serving:		
Yield: 2 dozen				
Serving Size: 1 kichel		CAL 94	PRO	1 (gm)
Exchanges:		FAT 8 (gm)	CHO	4 (gm)
Starch/Bread	½	Na 13 (mg)	K	13 (mg)
Fat	1½	Fiber 0 (gm)	Chol	23 (mg)

Ingredients

> NONSTICK VEGETABLE SPRAY
> 2 EGGS
> 1 EGG WHITE
> PINCH OF SALT
> 3 PACKETS SUGAR SUBSTITUTE (NOT ASPARTAME)
> ¾ CUP VEGETABLE OIL
> 1 CUP ALL-PURPOSE FLOUR

Method

1. Preheat oven to 375°F. Lightly spray cookie sheet with nonstick vegetable spray.
2. In food processor or electric mixer, beat eggs with salt. Add 2 packets sugar substitute and oil; mix well. Add flour and blend just until flour is absorbed.
3. Drop dough by teaspoonfuls 1 inch apart. Sprinkle with remaining packet of sugar substitute. Bake at 375°F for 10 minutes; at 350°F for 10 minutes; and at 325°F for 15–20 minutes.

Note: Kichel are special cookies served on Jewish holidays.

Strawberry Banana Sorbet

Yield: 10 servings
Serving Size: ½ cup
Exchanges:
Fruit   1

Nutrient Content per Serving:

CAL	66	PRO	3 (gm)
FAT	1 (gm)	CHO	13 (gm)
Na	33 (mg)	K	264 (mg)
Fiber	1 (gm)	Chol	3 (mg)

Ingredients

- 1 POUND FROZEN UNSWEETENED STRAWBERRIES
- 2 RIPE BANANAS (6 OUNCES EACH), PEELED
- 1 16-OUNCE CONTAINER LOW-FAT PLAIN YOGURT
- ½ TEASPOON BROWN SUGAR SUBSTITUTE
- 2 PACKETS SUGAR SUBSTITUTE

Method

1. Purée strawberries and bananas in blender or food processor. Blend until smooth. Add yogurt, brown sugar substitute, and sugar substitute. Blend until smooth.
2. Pour into 8-by-8-inch pan. Freeze for 2–3 hours or until firm. Break frozen mixture into chunks and place in chilled mixer bowl.
3. Beat with electric mixer on medium speed until fluffy. Return to pan; cover and freeze for at least 6 hours or until firm.

Old-Fashioned Lemon Cake

Yield: 12 slices
Serving Size: ½-inch slice
Exchanges:
Starch/Bread   1
Fat   1

Nutrient Content per Serving:

CAL	138	PRO	3 (gm)
FAT	7 (gm)	CHO	16 (gm)
Na	54 (mg)	K	45 (mg)
Fiber	1 (gm)	Chol	46 (mg)

Ingredients

NONSTICK VEGETABLE SPRAY
6 TABLESPOONS MARGARINE
PINCH OF SALT
2 TABLESPOONS SUGAR
8 PACKETS SUGAR SUBSTITUTE (NOT ASPARTAME)
2 EGGS
1½ CUPS FLOUR
1 TEASPOON BAKING POWDER
RIND OF 1 LEMON, COARSELY CHOPPED
½ CUP SKIM MILK

Method

1. Preheat oven to 325°F. Spray 9-by-5-inch loaf pan with nonstick vegetable spray.
2. Cream margarine, salt, sugar, and sugar substitute. Add eggs; beat well. Add flour, baking powder, lemon rind, and milk; beat well.
3. Pour into prepared pan. Bake for 1 hour or until toothpick inserted in middle comes out clean. Cool on rack.

Note: This lemon cake is dense and moist like a pound cake.

Mock Shortbread Cookies

Yield: 2 dozen		Nutrient Content per Serving:		
Serving Size: 1 cookie		CAL 89	PRO	2 (gm)
Exchanges:		FAT 5 (gm)	CHO	9 (gm)
Starch/Bread	½	Na 23 (mg)	K	14 (mg)
Fat	1	Fiber 0 (gm)	Chol	11 (mg)

Ingredients

    NONSTICK VEGETABLE SPRAY
  2 CUPS ALL-PURPOSE FLOUR
  1½ TEASPOONS BAKING POWDER
  ½ CUP VEGETABLE OIL
  ¼ CUP WATER
  1 EGG
  2 PACKETS SUGAR SUBSTITUTE (NOT
    ASPARTAME)
  1 TEASPOON VANILLA EXTRACT

Method

1. Preheat oven to 350°F. Spray cookie sheet with nonstick vegetable spray.
2. Combine all ingredients to form a soft dough. Roll or pat out on floured board to ¼-inch thick.
3. Cut 2-inch rounds and place 1 inch apart on prepared cookie sheet. Bake for 15–20 minutes until edges are a light golden brown.

Sautéed Plantains

Yield: 2 servings*

Serving Size: ½ banana and sauce

Exchanges:

Fruit   2

Fat   ½

Nutrient Content per Serving:

CAL	121	PRO	1 (gm)
FAT	3 (gm)	CHO	27 (gm)
Na	24 (mg)	K	453 (mg)
Fiber	2 (gm)	Chol	0 (mg)

Ingredients

    1 TEASPOON MARGARINE
    ½ TEASPOON CINNAMON
    ¼ TEASPOON BROWN SUGAR SUBSTITUTE
    1 PLANTAIN OR LARGE BANANA, PEELED AND
      SLICED ¼ INCH THICK

Method

1. Melt margarine in 8-inch skillet.
2. Stir in cinnamon and brown sugar substitute.
3. Sauté plantain over medium-high heat for 3–5 minutes, stirring constantly to coat. Serve over ice milk, if desired.

    *To make 4 servings, double the recipe.

Frozen Blueberry Crème

Yield: 8 servings
Serving Size: ⅛ of recipe
Exchanges:
Milk, skim   ½

Nutrient Content per Serving:

CAL	53	PRO	5 (gm)
FAT	0 (gm)	CHO	9 (gm)
Na	58 (mg)	K	203 (mg)
Fiber	1 (gm)	Chol	2 (mg)

Ingredients

    1 PACKET UNFLAVORED GELATIN
    ¼ CUP COLD WATER
    1 CUP FRESH BLUEBERRIES, WASHED AND
      STEMMED
    1 CUP PLUS ½ CUP EVAPORATED SKIM MILK
    9 PACKETS SUGAR SUBSTITUTE
    1 TABLESPOON SUGAR
    3 TABLESPOONS LEMON JUICE

Method

1. Sprinkle gelatin over cold water in small saucepan.
2. Reserve a few blueberries for garnish. Purée remaining blueberries in food processor or blender with 1 cup evaporated skim milk, sugar substitute, and sugar.
3. Dissolve gelatin on low flame; stir in lemon juice. Stir gelatin into blueberry mixture.
4. Whip remaining ½ cup evaporated milk until thick but not stiff. Fold into blueberry mixture. Pour into 2-quart bowl. Freeze for several hours, stirring occasionally, until mushy.
5. Spoon into dessert dishes while still soft. Garnish with blueberries.

Fresh Fruit Trifle

Yield: 6 servings
Serving Size: ⅙ of recipe
Exchanges:
Starch/Bread   3
Milk, low-fat   1
Fat   3½

Nutrient Content per Serving:
CAL   520   PRO   8 (gm)
FAT   29 (gm)   CHO   57 (gm)
Na   384 (mg)   K   251 (mg)
Fiber   2 (gm)   Chol   46 (mg)

Ingredients

- 1 POUND CAKE, THINLY SLICED
- 2 TEASPOONS SHERRY EXTRACT OR 3 TABLESPOONS DRY SHERRY
- 1 PACKAGE INSTANT VANILLA LOW-CALORIE PUDDING
- 1 CUP STRAWBERRIES OR OTHER FRESH FRUIT, SLICED
- 1 PACKET WHIPPED TOPPING MADE WITH ½ CUP SKIM MILK AND ½ TEASPOON SHERRY EXTRACT OR 1 TABLESPOON DRY SHERRY

Method

1. Line a 6-cup glass bowl with cake slices (sides and bottom).
2. Sprinkle with sherry. Prepare pudding according to package directions, adding ½ teaspoon sherry extract or 1 tablespoon dry sherry, if desired.
3. Pour over cake slices; top with strawberries.
4. Spread whipped topping over all; chill for several hours.
5. Garnish with additional sliced strawberries, if desired.

Chilled Peach Soufflé

Yield: 8 servings
Serving Size: ⅛ of recipe
Exchanges:

Fruit	1
Fat	½

Nutrient Content per Serving:

CAL	75	PRO	2 (gm)
FAT	2 (gm)	CHO	12 (gm)
Na	20 (mg)	K	130 (mg)
Fiber	1 (gm)	Chol	34 (mg)

Ingredients

- 1 16-OUNCE CAN SLICED PEACHES IN OWN JUICE
- 1 PACKET UNFLAVORED GELATIN
- ¼ CUP BOILING WATER
- 3 PACKETS SUGAR SUBSTITUTE
- 1 EGG, SEPARATED
- ½ TEASPOON VANILLA EXTRACT
- 1½ TEASPOONS LEMON JUICE
- ¼ CUP ICE CUBES
- 1 PACKET WHIPPED TOPPING MIX
- ½ CUP SKIM MILK
- ½ TEASPOON VANILLA EXTRACT

Method

1. Drain peaches, saving juice; reserve ¼ cup juice. Place remaining juice in blender or food processor and add gelatin to soften for 1 minute. Pour boiling water into blender or food processor and whirl until frothy.
2. Add all but 4–5 peach slices (save for garnish), sugar substitute, egg yolk, vanilla extract, and lemon juice. Blend until smooth.
3. Add ice and blend until ice is melted. Pour mixture into bowl and refrigerate.
4. Beat egg white until stiff and gently fold into peach mixture.
5. Whip topping mix using skim milk and vanilla extract until stiff and gently fold into peach mixture.
6. Turn into 2-quart soufflé dish. Chill until firm.
7. At serving time, garnish with peach slices. Keep refrigerated until serving time.

Coeur à la Crème

Yield: 6 servings

Serving Size: ⅙ of recipe

Exchanges:

Milk, skim   ½

Fat   2

Nutrient Content per Serving:

CAL	142	PRO	7 (gm)
FAT	10 (gm)	CHO	9 (gm)
Na	333 (mg)	K	160 (mg)
Fiber	0 (gm)	Chol	30 (mg)

Ingredients

    12 OUNCES LOW-FAT CREAM CHEESE

    ½ TEASPOON LEMON JUICE

    ¼ CUP EVAPORATED SKIM MILK, COLD

    ½ TEASPOON MAPLE-FLAVORED EXTRACT

    ¼ TEASPOON BROWN SUGAR SUBSTITUTE

    ¼ CUP STRAWBERRY SAUCE PLUS ¾ CUP (SEE PAGE 359)

Method

1. In food processor or blender, purée cream cheese with lemon juice, evaporated skim milk, maple extract, and brown sugar substitute. Blend until smooth.
2. Place in strainer set into bowl. Drain and chill for 8 hours.
3. Turn out onto a platter and shape into a round ball. Surround with ¼ cup strawberry sauce. Pass remaining sauce.

Apple–Raspberry Crisp*

Yield: 4 servings

Serving Size: ¼ of crisp

Exchanges:

Starch/Bread	½
Fruit	1
Fat	2½

Nutrient Content per Serving:

CAL	208	PRO	2 (gm)
FAT	12 (gm)	CHO	24 (gm)
Na	134 (mg)	K	162 (mg)
Fiber	5 (gm)	Chol	0 (mg)

Ingredients

NONSTICK VEGETABLE SPRAY
¼ CUP MARGARINE
¼ CUP QUICK-COOKING OATS
¼ CUP FLOUR
¼ TEASPOON BROWN SUGAR SUBSTITUTE
½ PINT FRESH RASPBERRIES OR 1 10-OUNCE
PACKAGE FROZEN RASPBERRIES IN LIGHT
SYRUP, DEFROSTED AND DRAINED
1 LARGE TART COOKING APPLE, PEELED AND
CUT INTO ¼-INCH SLICES
2 TEASPOONS LEMON JUICE
½ TEASPOON CINNAMON
½ TEASPOON LEMON PEEL, GRATED
½ TEASPOON VANILLA

Method

1. Preheat oven to 400°F. Spray 8-inch round baking dish with nonstick vegetable spray.
2. Combine margarine, oats, flour, and brown sugar substitute in small bowl until crumbly; set aside.
3. Combine remaining ingredients, tossing to coat fruit. Pour into prepared dish. Top with oats mixture.
4. Bake for 15–20 minutes or until slightly browned.

Method–Microwave

1. Pour fruit mixture into unsprayed 8-inch microwave-safe dish. Top with oats mixture.
2. Cook on high power for 6–8 minutes, rotating dish halfway through cooking time. Let stand for 4–5 minutes before serving.

Note: Serve warm with low-calorie whipped topping, if desired.

*3 grams or more of fiber per serving.

New England Fried Apples

Yield: 4 servings
Serving Size: ½ apple
Exchanges:
Fruit 1
Fat 1

Nutrient Content per Serving:

CAL	111	PRO	3 (gm)
FAT	4 (gm)	CHO	17 (gm)
Na	26 (mg)	K	120 (mg)
Fiber	2 (gm)	Chol	0 (mg)

Ingredients

    3 TABLESPOONS FLOUR
    2 EGG WHITES
    3 PACKETS SUGAR SUBSTITUTE
    2 MEDIUM TART COOKING APPLES, CORED,
    PEELED, AND SLICED IN ¼-INCH RINGS
    NONSTICK VEGETABLE SPRAY
    1 TABLESPOON VEGETABLE OIL
    ½ TEASPOON CINNAMON

Method

1. Combine flour, egg whites, and sugar substitute in small flat bowl.
2. Dip apple slices lightly in batter.
3. Heat 10-inch skillet. Spray well with nonstick vegetable spray and add vegetable oil.
4. Fry apples in batches until golden on both sides, about 5 minutes.
5. Drain on paper towels; sprinkle with cinnamon. Serve warm.

Note: May be used as a side dish, breakfast accompaniment, or dessert.

Fresh Nectarine Mousse

Yield: 6 cups	Nutrient Content per Serving:			
Serving Size: ¾ cup	CAL	92	PRO	4 (gm)
Exchanges:	FAT	2 (gm)	CHO	17 (gm)
Meat, lean ½	Na	71 (mg)	K	361 (mg)
Fruit 1	Fiber	2 (gm)	Chol	2 (mg)

Ingredients

- 2 POUNDS FRESH NECTARINES PLUS ONE NECTARINE FOR GARNISH OR 2 POUNDS FROZEN PEACHES, DEFROSTED AND DRAINED (RESERVE SEVERAL SLICES FOR GARNISH)
- 2 PACKETS SUGAR SUBSTITUTE
- 1 TEASPOON VANILLA EXTRACT
- ⅛ TEASPOON SALT
- 1 ENVELOPE UNFLAVORED GELATIN
- 2 TABLESPOONS HOT WATER
- 1 CUP PLAIN LOW-FAT YOGURT
- 2 EGG WHITES, BEATEN STIFF NONSTICK VEGETABLE SPRAY
- 8 TABLESPOONS WHIPPED TOPPING

Method

1. Pit and purée nectarines.
2. Add sugar substitute, vanilla extract, and salt.
3. Sprinkle gelatin over hot water; let stand. Stir to dissolve (may need to heat until dissolved).
4. Fold yogurt and dissolved gelatin into purée; fold in egg whites.
5. Pour into individual dessert dishes sprayed with nonstick vegetable spray; chill for 6 hours or overnight. Serve each serving with 1 tablespoon whipped topping and garnish with reserved fruit.

Fresh Peach Sherbert Royale*

Yield: 2½ cups
Serving Size: ½ cup
Exchanges:
Fruit   1

Nutrient Content per Serving:

CAL	52	PRO	2 (gm)
FAT	0 (gm)	CHO	11 (gm)
Na	30 (mg)	K	167 (mg)
Fiber	1 (gm)	Chol	1 (mg)

Ingredients

2 MEDIUM OR 3 SMALL PEACHES, PEELED AND SLICED
⅔ CUP SKIM MILK
⅔ CUP DIET LEMON-LIME SODA
1½ TABLESPOONS PEACH SCHNAPPS
1 EGG WHITE
5 PACKETS SUGAR SUBSTITUTE

Method

1. Blend peaches, milk, and lemon-lime soda in blender (not food processor) until smooth.
2. Add peach schnapps, egg white, and sugar substitute; blend until smooth.
3. Freeze in metal bowl or pie plate until partially firm (1–1½ hours); break up with fork or purée. Cover and freeze until firm. (Or, freeze in ice cream freezer according to manufacturer's instructions.)

*Recipe from the Miami Valley Chapter, Ohio Affiliate of the American Diabetes Association.

Strawberry Sauce

Yield: 1 cup
Serving Size: 1 tablespoon
(as sauce)
Exchanges:
Free food

Nutrient Content per Serving:
CAL 5   PRO   0 (gm)
FAT 0 (gm)   CHO   1 (gm)
Na   0 (mg)   K   21 (mg)
Fiber 0 (gm)   Chol 0 (mg)

Serving Size: ⅓ cup
(as dessert)
Exchanges:
Fruit   ½

Nutrient Content per Serving:
CAL 27   PRO   0 (gm)
FAT 0 (gm)   CHO   7 (gm)
Na   2 (mg)   K   113 (mg)
Fiber 1 (gm)   Chol 0 (mg)

Ingredients

½ POUND FROZEN STRAWBERRIES,
  UNSWEETENED
½ TEASPOON LEMON JUICE
¼ TEASPOON BROWN SUGAR SUBSTITUTE
2 TABLESPOONS WATER

Method

1. Purée all ingredients in food processor or blender until smooth. Chill until ready to serve.
2. Serve with Coeur à la Crème (see page 353) or over ice cream or cake.

Bittersweet Chocolate Sauce*

Yield: 1 cup

Serving Size: 1 tablespoon

Exchanges:

Fruit	½		
Fat	½		

Nutrient Content per Serving:

CAL	49	PRO	1 (gm)
FAT	3 (gm)	CHO	7 (gm)
Na	6 (mg)	K	73 (mg)
Fiber	0 (gm)	Chol	0 (mg)

Ingredients

    3 1-OUNCE SQUARES UNSWEETENED
      CHOCOLATE, COARSELY CHOPPED
    ⅓ CUP EVAPORATED SKIM MILK
    ½ CUP UNSWEETENED PINEAPPLE JUICE
    1 TEASPOON VANILLA EXTRACT
    3 PACKETS SUGAR SUBSTITUTE
    ¼ CUP SUGAR
    1 TABLESPOON CORNSTARCH MIXED WITH 1
      TABLESPOON UNSWEETENED PINEAPPLE JUICE

Method

1. In double boiler over low heat, melt chocolate with evaporated skim milk.
2. Stir in pineapple juice, vanilla extract, sugar substitute, sugar, and cornstarch mixed with pineapple juice.
3. Stir constantly until sauce thickens and is smooth.
4. Serve warm. If sauce becomes too thick when cooled, reheat over double-boiler or in microwave about 30–45 seconds.

Note: Serve over ice cream, cake, cream puffs, fruit with crêpes, or dip well-dried strawberries halfway and allow to dry. Use to dip rice crackers.

*This recipe has more than ½ teaspoon of sugar per serving.

Beverages

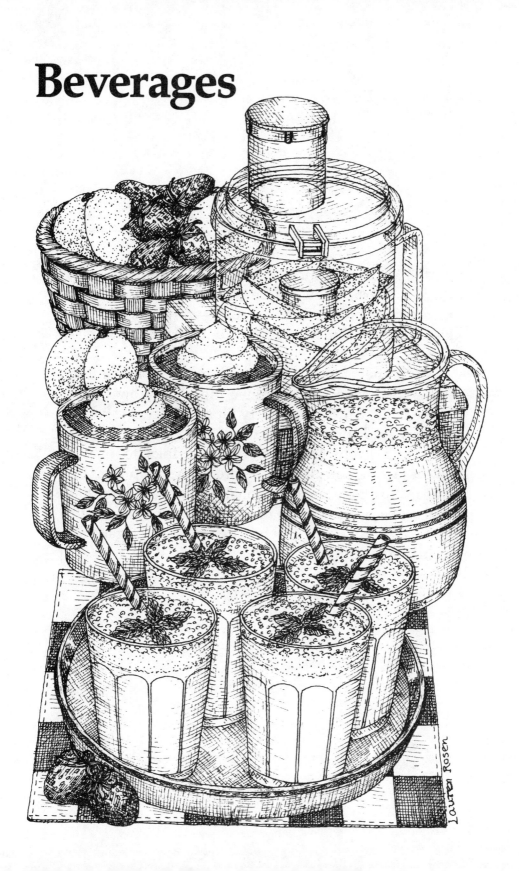

*D*rinks do a lot more than quench thirst. They refresh or warm, they can be snacks in themselves or accompaniments to a meal. And—witness the coffee klatch—they sometimes inspire friendly conversation.

All the beverages in this section can be made in a flash. Kids especially will love the Black Cow Drink or the fizzy, fruity Strawberry Slush or Georgia Peach Cooler. And they may find they prefer the real fruit taste and lively sparkle of these drinks to overly sweet-tasting soft drinks. Before dinner, sip the Hawaiian Sunrise Punch, a nonalcoholic beverage that tastes like a fruity rum drink. Afterward, top your meal off with a Hot Mocha Dream as an elegant alternative to coffee.

Hawaiian Sunrise Punch

Yield: 1 serving
Serving Size: 1 cup
Exchanges:
Fruit 1

Nutrient Content per Serving:

CAL	54	PRO	1 (gm)
FAT	0 (gm)	CHO	13 (gm)
Na	38 (mg)	K	180 (mg)
Fiber	0 (gm)	Chol	0 (mg)

Ingredients

¼ CUP UNSWEETENED ORANGE JUICE
2 TABLESPOONS UNSWEETENED PINEAPPLE JUICE
1 TABLESPOON LIME OR LEMON JUICE
1 TEASPOON RUM EXTRACT
⅓ CUP CLUB SODA
¼ TEASPOON GRENADINE SYRUP (OPTIONAL—SUNRISE)

Method

1. Combine all ingredients except for grenadine syrup in a tall glass. Add 4 ice cubes. Pour in grenadine syrup. Serve with ½ orange slice for garnish.

Black Cow Drink

Yield: 2 servings*

Serving Size: 1 cup

Exchanges:

Milk, skim   ½

Nutrient Content per Serving:

CAL	21	PRO	2 (gm)
FAT	0 (gm)	CHO	3 (gm)
Na	32 (mg)	K	102 (mg)
Fiber	0 (gm)	Chol	1 (mg)

Ingredients

    ½ CUP SKIM MILK
    6 OUNCES DIET ROOT BEER
    ¾ CUP ICE CUBES
    ½ TEASPOON VANILLA EXTRACT

Method

1. Place all ingredients in blender; blend until smooth.

    *To make 4 servings, double the recipe.

Georgia Peach Cooler

Yield: 3 servings

Serving Size: ½ cup

Exchanges:

Fruit   ½

Nutrient Content per Serving:

CAL	38	PRO	1 (gm)
FAT	0 (gm)	CHO	10 (gm)
Na	8 (mg)	K	174 (mg)
Fiber	1 (gm)	Chol	0 (mg)

Ingredients

    1 CUP FRESH PEACHES, PEELED AND CUBED, OR 1
      6-OUNCE CAN SLICED PEACHES IN JUICE,
      DRAINED
    ½ CUP CLUB SODA
    1 PACKET SUGAR SUBSTITUTE
    4 DASHES BITTERS
    ½ CUP ICE CUBES

Method

1. Purée peaches in blender.
2. Add remaining ingredients; blend until smooth.

Hot Mocha Dream

Yield: 2 servings*
Serving Size: 1 cup
Exchanges:
Milk, skim   ½

Nutrient Content per Serving:

CAL	53	PRO	5 (gm)
FAT	1 (gm)	CHO	8 (gm)
Na	67 (mg)	K	340 (mg)
Fiber	0 (gm)	Chol	2 (mg)

Ingredients

  1½ TEASPOONS INSTANT REGULAR OR DECAFFEINATED COFFEE
   1 PACKET SUGAR SUBSTITUTE
   1 TABLESPOON UNSWEETENED COCOA POWDER
  ½ CINNAMON STICK
   1 CUP HOT WATER
   1 CUP SKIM MILK
  1½ TEASPOONS VANILLA EXTRACT

Method

1. Combine coffee, sugar substitute, cocoa powder, cinnamon stick, and ¼ cup hot water. Bring to boil and boil for 1 minute.
2. Add remaining water and milk. Reheat to boiling and stir in vanilla extract.
3. Remove cinnamon stick before serving. Garnish with whipped topping if desired.

Method–Microwave

1. Combine coffee, sugar substitute, cocoa powder, cinnamon stick, and ¼ cup hot water in 2-quart microwave-safe saucepan. Bring to a boil for 5 minutes on high power.
2. Add remaining water and milk. Reheat to boiling for 3–5 minutes on high power. Stir in vanilla. Remove cinnamon stick before serving. Garnish with whipped topping, if desired.

*To make 4 servings, double the recipe.

Strawberry Slush

Yield: 4 servings
Serving Size: ½ cup
Exchanges:
Fruit   ½

Nutrient Content per Serving:

CAL	26	PRO	1 (gm)
FAT	0 (gm)	CHO	6 (gm)
Na	5 (mg)	K	140 (mg)
Fiber	2 (gm)	Chol	0 (mg)

Key Source Nutrients:
Ascorbic acid   46 (mg)

Ingredients

- 1 PINT FRESH STRAWBERRIES, HULLED AND WIPED CLEAN
- 1 OUNCE LEMON JUICE (PREFERABLY FRESH)
- 1 OUNCE LIME JUICE (PREFERABLY FRESH)
- 2 PACKETS SUGAR SUBSTITUTE
- ¼ CUP CLUB SODA
- ½–1 CUP ICE CUBES

Method

1. Purée strawberries in food processor or blender.
2. Add remaining ingredients. Blend well until smooth and foamy.
3. Garnish with fresh strawberry and a lime or lemon slice.

Mango Frappé

Yield: 3 cups
Serving Size: 1 cup
Exchanges:
Fruit   1

Nutrient Content per Serving:
CAL 68   PRO   1 (gm)
FAT   0 (gm)   CHO   18 (gm)
Na   27 (mg)   K   225 (mg)
Fiber 1 (gm)   Chol   0 (mg)

Ingredients

    1 WHOLE RIPE MANGO, PITTED AND PEELED*
    ¾ CUP ORANGE JUICE
    ¼ CUP LIME JUICE (2 LIMES)
    1½ CUPS CLUB SODA

Method

1. Purée mango in food processor or blender. Add orange and lime juice; process until smooth.
2. Add club soda; process just to blend (2 on/off pulses). Serve over ice in tall glasses.

    *If mangoes are not available, substitute ⅔ cup canned fruit nectar.

Lunch Box Treats

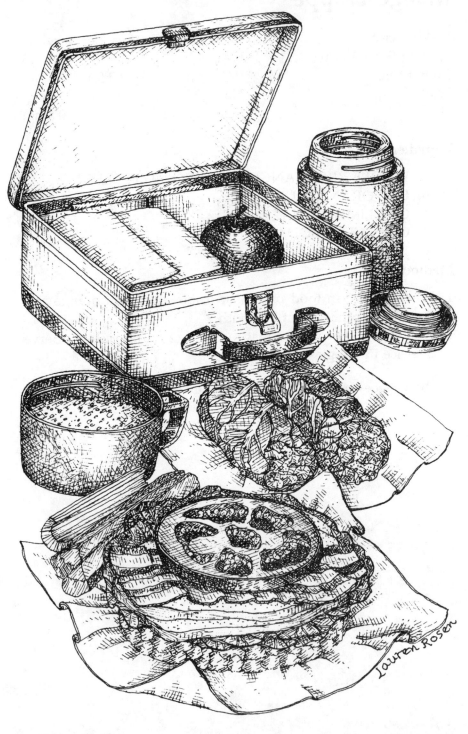

Lauren Rosen

*C*hildren are notoriously picky eaters, but these finger-food recipes might surprise you. They're different enough in taste and texture to prompt some experimenting, and the ingredients are tasty, although solidly nutritional. We can't guarantee success with a child, but for adult brown-baggers these lunch or snack recipes are well worth investigating.

Rice Cake Club Sandwich

Yield: 2 servings*
Serving Size: 1 cake plus
topping
Exchanges:
Starch/Bread   ½
Meat, lean   1½

Nutrient Content per Serving:

CAL	138	PRO	12 (gm)
FAT	6 (gm)	CHO	9 (gm)
Na	189 (mg)	K	168 (mg)
Fiber	0 (gm)	Chol	31 (mg)

Ingredients

- 2 RICE CAKES
- 2 TEASPOONS REDUCED-CALORIE MAYONNAISE
- 2 LEAVES LETTUCE
- 2 SLICES LARGE TOMATO
- 2 SLICES BACON, CRISPLY COOKED AND HALVED
- 2 THIN SLICES CHICKEN OR TURKEY BREAST
  (1 OUNCE EACH)

Method

1. Spread rice cakes with mayonnaise.
2. Top with lettuce, tomato, bacon, and chicken.

*To make 4 servings, double the recipe.

Chickpea Sandwich* **

Yield: 6 lettuce roll-ups
Serving Size: 2 lettuce roll-ups with ½ cup filling
Exchanges:
Starch/Bread 2
Fat 1½

Nutrient Content per Serving:
CAL 255 PRO 11 (gm)
FAT 9 (gm) CHO 36 (gm)
Na 461 (mg) K 577 (mg)
Fiber 9 (gm) Chol 8 (mg)

Key Source Nutrients:
Vitamin A 4,208 (IU)

Ingredients

    1 16-OUNCE CAN CHICKPEAS, RINSED AND DRAINED
    ⅓ CUP CELERY, THINLY SLICED
    ⅓ CUP CARROT, SHREDDED
    ¼ CUP REDUCED-CALORIE MAYONNAISE
    2 TABLESPOONS CHILE SAUCE
    1 TEASPOON DRIED MINCED ONION
    ¼ TEASPOON SALT
    ¼ TEASPOON GARLIC POWDER
    ⅛ TEASPOON GROUND BLACK PEPPER
    6 LARGE LETTUCE LEAVES

Method

1. Purée chickpeas in food processor or blender until smooth.
2. Combine chickpeas and remaining ingredients except lettuce leaves; mix well.
3. Place ½ cup mixture in center of each lettuce leaf; roll up.

Note: Chickpea mixture makes a great appetizer to be served with crackers or pita triangles.

*400 milligrams or more of sodium per serving.
**3 grams or more of fiber per serving.

8 ◇ HEALTHY ETHNIC EATING

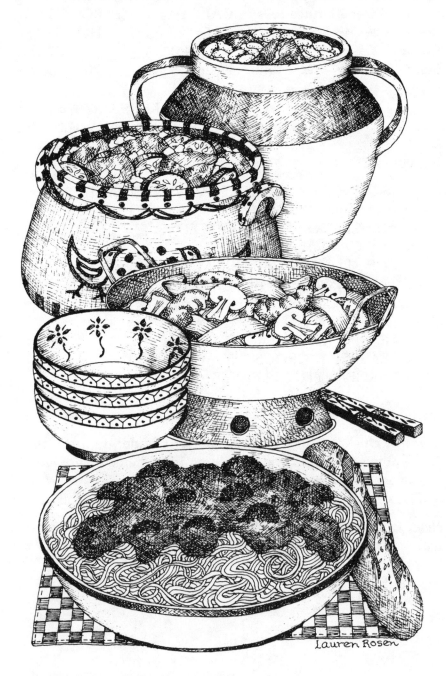

Lauren Rosen

If you think eating "ethnic" means eating "foreign," you're overlooking a whole range of regional cooking styles that have developed right here in America. "Domestic ethnic" cuisines are as exotic and interesting as the cooking of China or India; what's more, they make use of products and reflect a history that is distinctively American.

Family Cookbook, Volume II presented exchange values for some popular ethnic foods like gefilte fish, moo goo gai pan, and samosas—information that's useful when ordering in a restaurant or cooking a favorite recipe. Exchange values for Jewish, Oriental, southern United States, Native American, and Mexican American dishes can be found there.

This chapter focuses in much more depth on three U.S. cuisines: Mexican American cooking, Native American cooking of the northern Plains, and southern cooking. You'll find information not just on special foods but on typical, everyday eating: what advantages each cuisine offers someone with diabetes, and what to watch out for. In addition, there are:

- typical recipes for each cuisine
- exchanges
- guidance on how to modify recipes, seasonings, and cooking methods to make them more nutritionally sound
- a glossary of terms to enable you to find and use new ingredients

We have attempted to reduce the sugar, salt, and fat in these recipes while preserving their ethnic character. However, not all of these recipes meet the nutritional guidelines described in Chapter 1. You may want to consult with your doctor and dietitian when working these or your own regional and ethnic favorites into your meal plan.

What gives an ethnic cuisine its own unique flavor? Ethnic cooking goes beyond typical foods (pasta in Italian cooking, for example, or ginger and soy sauce in Oriental) to include cooking methods (a preference for broiled rather than stewed meats, for example) and methods of preservation (salting versus drying). Even textures and degree of doneness may be involved; Oriental cooks like vegetables crispy and underdone, while English and southern United States traditions call for soft, thoroughly cooked vegetables. Traditions such as these pervade the cooking of a region or group and often form the basis of both everyday fare and special traditional foods. Your own eating preferences probably relate to your ethnic origin.

MEXICAN AMERICAN COOKING

Mexican American cooking is rich in fiber and complex carbohydrate and is therefore generally appropriate for the diabetic diet. Some traditional dishes are high in fat, cholesterol, and calories, but they can be modified using the guidelines on pages 376–377.

Most of the dishes eaten in the typical Mexican American home are simpler than those served in restaurants. Tamales, enchiladas, and other mixed dishes that require added preparation time are eaten on Sundays, holidays, and on other special occasions. *Menudo* (tripe soup) is special for Saturday and Sunday breakfasts.

Everyday foods are much like those eaten by people of other cultures. Breakfast might be bacon and eggs, cooked or ready-to-eat cereal with fresh whole milk or evaporated milk, and coffee. *Pan dulce*, a sweet bread, is a breakfast favorite, although it is not a good choice for someone with diabetes because it contains both lard and sugar. *Churros*, thin, deep-fried yeast donuts sprinkled with sugar, are occasionally eaten at breakfast and should also be strictly limited or not eaten by people with diabetes.

Lunch, especially in large cities, might be burritos, tamales, tortas, or tacos purchased from a pushcart vendor. At home, soup (usually chicken stock and tomato based) is a popular midday meal.

Typical dinner dishes include stew *(caldo)* or a dish from meat, fish, or chicken; a rice or macaroni dish *(sopas)*; refried beans, bread, or *tortillas*; a lettuce and tomato salad; and a beverage. Vegetables characteristic of Mexican American cooking are *chayote* (squash), *nopales* (cactus), *calabazita* (squash), and *tomatil-los* (green tomatoes). See page 381 for exchange values.

A wide variety of tropical fruits is available for dessert, including the cherimoya, guava, cactus fruit, and coco plum (see page 381 for exchanges). Few sugary desserts are native to the Mexican American culture; however, chocolate seems to be a national favorite. Occasionally, carmelized sugar is served over chunks of coconut or pineapple; *flan* (custard) or *churros* are other special-occasion desserts.

Beans are a hallmark of Mexican American cooking. Often eaten more than once a day, beans are usually boiled until soft, then mashed and fried. These beans are called *frijoles refritos* (re-fried beans), and cheese is often added to them. Leftovers can be enjoyed for several meals in succession.

Tortillas made of cornmeal or wheat flour replace bread in the Mexican American diet. They are consumed in large quantities, up to six with a meal. (For families on a low or marginal income, tortillas and beans are staple foods.) Corn tortillas are preferable; they are higher in fiber and lower in lard than flour (wheat) tortillas.

Mexican American cooking derives flavor from chile peppers, citrus fruits, and a spicy tomato-based sauce called *salsa* (a combination of peppers, tomatoes, onions, garlic, salt, and other seasonings). *Salsa* is added to soups and stews, served cold as an accompaniment to meats or as a hot sauce over meat or eggs, or mixed into various dishes, including eggs, rice, potatoes, or other vegetables.

With its extensive use of beans and corn, its preference for fruit desserts rather than those high in concentrated carbohydrates, and its diverse flavoring agents, Mexican American cooking offers many healthy choices for the diabetic diet.

One drawback, nutritionally speaking, is that large amounts of fat are added during cooking. Mexican Americans prefer top-of-the-stove cooking (stewing or frying) over methods like baking or broiling, which tend to remove fat. Rice and pasta are fried in liberal amounts of oil before boiling broth is added to complete cooking. Lard is the customary fat in flour tortillas, and refried beans are commonly fried in lard or oil, often over and over again.

MODIFYING MEXICAN AMERICAN COOKING

Here are some suggestions for altering cooking methods and ingredients to make Mexican American cooking its healthiest.

Instead of: *frijoles refritos* (boiled, mashed beans fried in lard)
Try: *frijoles cocidos* (boiled, mashed beans with seasonings)
Advantage: less total fat, less saturated fat

Instead of: softening tortillas by frying
Try: softening by wrapping in foil, then heating in an oven, a microwave, or on a hotplate
Advantage: less fat

Instead of: packaged flour tortillas (they are made with lard)
Try: packaged corn tortillas (no lard) or homemade flour tortillas made with polyunsaturated margarine
Advantage: less saturated fat

Instead of: fried meats *(carnitas)*
Try: baked meats *(carne asada)* or boiled meats *(hervida)* or broiled meats
Advantage: less fat

Instead of: high-fat snack foods like *churros* or *chicharrones* (fried pork rinds)
Try: fruit
Advantage: less fat, more vitamins

Instead of: lard, coconut, or palm oils
Try: polyunsaturated vegetable oil or margarine
Advantage: less saturated fat

Instead of: *pan dulce*
Try: high-fiber cereal like oatmeal or whole wheat
    bread
Advantage: less sugar, less fat, more fiber, more
    nutrients

MEXICAN AMERICAN FOODS GLOSSARY

Albondigas: Meatballs made from ground beef or pork, eggs, and spices. Often used in soup.

Arroz: Rice.

Arroz con pollo: Browned rice with chicken, tomatoes, and spices.

Burrito: A soft flour tortilla filled with beans or ground or shredded beef or chicken. It is rolled and eaten plain, covered with an enchilada sauce, or deep fried.

Calabazita: Mexican squash that is similar in size and shape to the cucumber, except the skin is light green. Simmered with onion and spices and often combined with meat in a casserole dish.

Caldo: Soup or stew that is made with a clear broth.

Camotes: Sweet potato.

Carne: Meat.

Cassava: Yucca root (a starchy root) also called *manioc*. It has a bitter odor that disappears after cooking, so it is not eaten raw.

Chayote: A round, light-green squash.

Cherimoya: A fruit having a rough, green outer skin. When ripened and chilled, the flesh has a sherbet-like texture.

Chicharrones: Bacon rinds cut in strips that are usually fried and eaten as a snack. If used in a main dish, they are usually cooked with eggs or in a chile sauce.

Chile: Any variety of hot peppers, used raw or as an ingredient in sauces or dishes. (See "A note about chiles" at the end of this section.)

Chiles Rellenos: A green chile stuffed with cheese and fried in an egg batter.

Chorizo: A highly seasoned sausage of chopped beef or pork with sweet red peppers. The preparation is fried, mixed with scrambled eggs, and eaten in a taco, burrito, or tortilla.

Churros: Thin, deep-fried yeast donuts sprinkled with sugar.

Cilantro: The fresh leaves and stems of coriander, it imparts a distinctive flavor to salsa, meat dishes, and soups. Also known as Chinese parsley.

Elote: Corn on the cob.

Guava: A sweet, juicy fruit, ranging in color from green to yellow with red or yellow flesh.

Jicama: A crisp, refreshing root vegetable that is tan on the outside and white on the inside. It has a mild chestnut flavor and is always eaten raw. It's as familiar to Mexico as the potato is to the United States. (The recipe on page 164 of this cookbook gives an idea for preparing it.)

Masa: *Masa harina* is made from dried corn that has been soaked in lime water, cooked, and ground. Instant *masa* is commercially produced *masa harina* used for making corn tortillas and tamales. When wet, it will almost double in weight. Fresh *masa*, which contains water, must be used right away because it does not keep.

Menudo: Tripe soup.

Mole sauce: A chocolate sauce for chicken (uses very little unsweetened chocolate and sugar).

Nopales (cactus): The leaves or pods of the prickly pear cactus are used. They taste like crisp green beans. They are sliced in strips and cooked with onions and spices.

Pan dulce: Mexican sweet bread typically served for breakfast or snacks.

Pescado: Fish.

Plantain: Greenish-looking banana with rough skin and a number of blemishes. It is used as a starch rather than a fruit because it remains starchy even when fully ripe. Generally prepared by pan-frying. Never eaten raw.

Pollo: Chicken.

Puerco: Pork.

Rez: Beef.

Salsa: Chile sauce, especially hot sauce, usually served as an accompaniment.

Taco: *Taco* literally means snack. A corn tortilla is lightly fried in hot fat, folded in the middle, filled with seasoned ground beef, then fried on both sides until crisp. Grated cheese and shredded lettuce may be sprinkled over the beef filling.

Tamale: Spicy meat and sauce wrapped in cornmeal or *masa* dough that has been made with lard, salt, and water. The tamales are wrapped in corn husks and steamed until done. Usually consumed at parties and on special occasions.

Tomatillos: Small, green tomatoes that do not soften when ripe.

Torta: The Hispanic version of a sandwich. Fillings may vary, but generally include beef or pork.

Tortilla: A flat corn or wheat pancake.

A NOTE ABOUT CHILES

When handling hot chiles, keep your hands away from your face, especially your eyes. Wash hands thoroughly afterward. The hottest part of the chile is the seed. Normally seeds are discarded, except in hot sauce. For a hotter flavor, leave some of them in. Fresh chiles may be soaked for an hour or so in cold water and salt to remove some hotness.

To peel fresh chiles, wash them and pat dry. Rub with oil, then roast in 375°F oven for 15 minutes or until chiles become blistered. Place them in a paper bag or cover with a damp cloth and let stand for at least 15 minutes. Peel skin off, and make a small opening in the side of each chile. Brush seeds out (leave them in if you want a hotter taste). Green chiles prepared in this way are used for dishes such as Chiles Rellenos (stuffed chiles).

(The representative types of chiles listed below and on the next page are reprinted with permission of the publisher, from *A Taste of Mexico*, by Esther Gonzalez Davis. San Diego, CA: Rand Editions-Tofua Press, 1974.)

Ancho: A mild-flavored, 3-inch-long pepper that resembles the bell pepper, but is more pointed in shape and darker in color. Most often available dried, in the Mexican spice section of supermarkets; sometimes called "Mexican chiles." Dried anchos are dark red or black.

California: Also called "Anaheim" chile. The most commonly available chile, it is green when ripe and red when dried. It is 5–8 inches long and 1–1½ inches in diameter. This is the chile most often referred to as "fresh green chile" in recipes (as in Chiles Rellenos). Also available canned as "whole chiles" or "green chiles." If the can says "hot chiles," it contains jalapeño peppers.

Chile powder: Many variations are available; some are a blend of ground chiles and other spices, some are pure chile. They range from mild to very hot.

Jalapeños: Green tapered chiles, about 2 inches long. They are hot, probably the most widely available hot peppers. They come fresh, canned, and pickled.

Mulato: Larger than the ancho and a bit hotter, this chile is available dried and is often labeled "Mexican chiles." Combine with or substitute for the ancho or pasilla.

Pasilla: This long, thin pepper is dark green when immature and brown when ripe or dried. It is 6–10 inches long and 1 or 2 inches in diameter. Mild in flavor, it can be interchanged with the ancho or mulato.

Red peppers, dried: These can be of many different varieties, widely available in the spice section of markets. They are quite hot, so you may wish to soak them in boiling water for 30 minutes and drain them before using.

Serrano: Small green (red or yellow when ripe) tapered peppers about 1½ inches long. They are tasty and hot and most often found canned or pickled. If you can't find them, use jalapeños.

Yellow wax: These hot peppers come either fresh or pickled. There are several varieties, and they are interchangeable.

EXCHANGES OF COMMON FOODS AND STAPLES

STARCH/BREAD

Cassava	2 ounces uncooked weight
Hominy, yellow, canned	½ cup
Jicama	¼ cup or 2 ounces cooked weight
Plantain	⅓ of 11-inch plantain

(For corn or wheat tortillas—Mexican bread—taco shells, and tortilla chips, see *1986 Exchange Lists*.)

MEAT

Mexican style sausage (*chorizo*, beef, or pork)	1 ounce (1 high-fat meat)

VEGETABLE

Chayote	½ cup
Cactus leaf (nopales)	½ cup
Calabazita (Mexican squash)	½ cup
Tomatoes, small green	½ cup (1 small)

(For okra and hot chili pepper, see 1986 Exchange Lists.)

FRUIT

Cherimoya	⅛ of a 1¾-pound fruit
Guava	1 small (¾ cup)
Cactus fruit	1 medium
Coco plum	1 medium
Mamey	⅛ of a 3-pound fruit
Pummelo	¾-cup segments
Guava nectar	½ cup
Sapote	⅙ of ¾-pound fruit

(For mango and papaya, see 1986 Exchange Lists.)

FAT

Guacamole	2 tablespoons
Sofrito	2 teaspoons

(For avocado, see 1986 Exchange Lists.)

RECIPES

Mexican Rice* **

Yield: 6 cups
Serving Size: ¾ cup
Exchanges:
Starch/Bread   2½

Nutrient Content per Serving:

CAL	199	PRO	4 (gm)
FAT	3 (gm)	CHO	40 (gm)
Na	514 (mg)	K	173 (mg)
Fiber	4 (gm)	Chol	0 (mg)

Ingredients

   2 CUPS BROWN RICE, UNCOOKED
   1 TABLESPOON MARGARINE OR VEGETABLE OIL
1½ CUPS WATER
   2 CUPS CHICKEN BROTH[†]
   1 CUP TOMATO, CHOPPED
   ½ CUP ONION, CHOPPED
   ½ TEASPOON SALT

Method

1. Sauté rice in margarine in large saucepan for 5–8 minutes.
2. Add remaining ingredients; cover and simmer for 45–55 minutes or until rice has absorbed liquid.

*400 milligrams or more of sodium per serving.
**3 grams or more of fiber per serving.
†For reduced salt and fat, use homemade chicken broth.

Pork with Green Chile Sauce (Puerco con Salsa de Chile Verde)* **

Yield: 7 cups
Serving Size: 1 cup
Exchanges:
Meat, medium-fat 4
Vegetable   2
Fat   1

Nutrient Content per Serving:

CAL	390	PRO	33 (gm)
FAT	24 (gm)	CHO	9 (gm)
Na	407 (mg)	K	671 (mg)
Fiber	2 (gm)	Chol	127 (mg)

Key Source Nutrients:
Ascorbic acid   50 (mg)

Ingredients

- 3 POUNDS LEAN BONELESS PORK SHOULDER OR BUTT
- 1 TABLESPOON VEGETABLE OIL
- 1 LARGE ONION, CHOPPED
- 2 CLOVES GARLIC, MINCED
- 3 4-OUNCE CANS GREEN CHILES OR 1 10-OUNCE CAN JALEPEÑO PEPPERS, OR 6–7 LARGE FRESH ANAHEIM OR CALIFORNIA PEPPERS, SEEDED AND CHOPPED
- 3 MEDIUM TOMATOES, CHOPPED
- ½ CUP FRESH CILANTRO, CHOPPED, OR 2 TABLESPOONS GROUND CORIANDER
- ¼ CUP WATER
- 1 TABLESPOON WINE VINEGAR
- 1 TEASPOON SALT
- 1 TEASPOON OREGANO
- ½ TEASPOON CUMIN

Method

1. Trim fat from pork and cut into 1-inch pieces.
2. Brown in oil in small batches in large skillet or Dutch oven.
3. Remove each batch to bowl lined with paper towels. Sauté onion and garlic in pan until softened. Add pork and remaining ingredients.

4. Cover; simmer on top of range or in 325°F oven for 1½–2 hours or until tender. Skim any fat from surface. Serve with hot cooked rice or as a filling for tortillas.

> *Source:* Susan Algert, M.S., R.D.
> **400 milligrams or more of sodium per serving.

Spicy Salsa

Yield: 2⅔ cups
Serving Size: ⅓ cup
Exchanges:
Vegetable   1

Nutrient Content per Serving:

CAL	20	PRO	1 (gm)
FAT	0 (gm)	CHO	5 (gm)
Na	94 (mg)	K	165 (mg)
Fiber	1 (gm)	Chol	0 (mg)

Ingredients

    1 16-OUNCE CAN WHOLE TOMATOES, UNDRAINED
    1 SMALL GREEN BELL PEPPER, CHOPPED
    ⅓ CUP RADISHES, CHOPPED
    ⅓ CUP ONION, CHOPPED
    1 4-OUNCE CAN CHOPPED GREEN CHILES OR JALAPEÑO PEPPERS, DRAINED
    3 TABLESPOONS GREEN ONIONS, CHOPPED
    3 TABLESPOONS FRESH CILANTRO, CHOPPED
    ½–1 TEASPOON GARLIC POWDER

Method

1. Purée tomatoes and their liquid in blender or food processor.
2. Add remaining ingredients; mix well. May be stored in refrigerator up to 5 days.

Frijoles Cocidos*

Yield: 5½ cups

Serving Size: ½ cup

Exchanges:

Starch/Bread   2

Nutrient Content per Serving:

CAL	171	PRO	10 (gm)
FAT	2 (gm)	CHO	30 (gm)
Na	199 (mg)	K	471 (mg)
Fiber	9 (gm)	Chol	0 (mg)

Ingredients

- 1 POUND (2½ CUPS) PINTO BEANS, UNCOOKED
- 1 LARGE ONION, CHOPPED (1½ CUPS)
- 3 CLOVES GARLIC, MINCED
- 2 TEASPOONS CUMIN
- 1 TABLESPOON OLIVE OIL
- ½ CUP GREEN PEPPER, MINCED
- ½ TEASPOON GROUND CORIANDER
- 1 TEASPOON SALT
- ¼ TEASPOON BLACK PEPPER

Method

1. Soak beans in water to cover for 4 hours or overnight.
2. Drain beans; cover with fresh water in large saucepan. Bring to a boil; reduce heat. Cover; simmer for 1–1½ hours or until tender.
3. Sauté onion, garlic, and cumin in oil for 4 minutes. Add green pepper and continue sautéeing for 5–8 minutes or until tender.
4. Drain beans; reserve ½ cup liquid. Mash beans and reserved liquid; add sautéed vegetables and spices, mixing well.
5. Serve in tostadas or stuffed green peppers, or with steamed tortillas.

*3 grams or more of fiber per serving.

Chicken Caldo*

Yield: 3½ quarts (14 servings)
Serving Size: 1 cup
Exchanges:
Meat, lean   1
Vegetable   2

Nutrient Content per Serving:
CAL 108   PRO   12 (gm)
FAT   3 (gm)   CHO   10 (gm)
Na   353 (mg)   K   321 (mg)
Fiber   4 (gm)   Chol   27 (mg)

Ingredients

   1 WHOLE CHICKEN (3 POUNDS), SKINNED AND
     CUT UP
   1 LARGE ONION, CHOPPED
 2-3 CLOVES GARLIC, MINCED
   2 QUARTS WATER
   1 STALK CELERY, SLICED
   1 MEDIUM TURNIP, PEELED AND CUT INTO
     ½-INCH CUBES
   2 MEDIUM CARROTS, SLICED
   1 MEDIUM ZUCCHINI, SLICED
   1 15-OUNCE CAN (½ POUND) KIDNEY BEANS OR
     HOMINY, DRAINED
   1 SMALL HEAD CABBAGE, CHOPPED
   2 TEASPOONS SALT
  ¼ TEASPOON BLACK PEPPER

Method

1. Place chicken, onion, and garlic in large saucepan or Dutch
   oven.
2. Cover with water; bring to a boil. Reduce heat; simmer for
   50–60 minutes or until chicken is tender.**
3. Add remaining ingredients; simmer for 20–30 minutes or until vegetables are tender.

   *3 grams or more of fiber per serving.
   **At this point, chicken may be removed from broth and cooled.
Take meat from bones. Skim any fat from broth; return meat to pan.

Fillets Veracruz

Yield: 4 servings
Serving Size: ¼ pound fish
plus ¼ of sauce
Exchanges:
Meat, lean   3
Vegetable   2

Nutrient Content per Serving:

CAL	201	PRO	25 (gm)
FAT	7 (gm)	CHO	10 (gm)
Na	137 (mg)	K	880 (mg)
Fiber	2 (gm)	Chol	54 (mg)

Ingredients

- 1 POUND FISH FILLETS
- 2 16-OUNCE CANS TOMATOES, DRAINED AND CHOPPED, OR 3 LARGE FRESH TOMATOES, CHOPPED
- 1 SMALL ONION, CHOPPED
- 1 CLOVE GARLIC, MINCED
- 1 TEASPOON DILL WEED
- ¼ TEASPOON THYME
- 1 CUP WHITE WINE
- 2 TABLESPOONS FRESH CILANTRO, CHOPPED, OR 1 TEASPOON GROUND CORIANDER

Method

1. Preheat oven to 350°F.
2. Place fillets in shallow baking dish; cover with vegetables and seasonings. Pour wine over all.
3. Bake for 30–35 minutes or until fish flakes.

COOKING OF THE NORTHERN PLAINS

Many American cooking classics are of Native American origin. Barbecue, steamed lobster, succotash, popcorn, spoon bread, cranberry sauce, and mincemeat pie are inherited from the first Americans. Until the discovery of the Americas, the rest of the world knew nothing of such foods as avocados, sweet potatoes, white potatoes, pineapples, tomatoes, peppers, pumpkins, squashes, maple sugar, and, of course, corn.

As of 1984, there were more than 600 different tribes and/or village communities. Each is a cultural entity, sharing the same religion, language, traditions, and values. This discussion will be limited to the cooking traditions of the northern Plains tribes: Blackfeet, Sioux, Crow, and Cheyenne.

In this section you'll find recipes for some present-day specialties like Dried Corn Soup, Wild Berry Pudding, Fry Bread, and Pemmican on pages 391–394. Exchanges for common foods and staples are on page 390.

Historically, Plains tribes were large-game hunters. Elk, deer, antelope, and especially buffalo—among the lower-fat meats—formed the greatest part of their diet. Since the whole tribe migrated with the herds of wild game, cooking methods had to be simple. Typical cooking methods were boiling, roasting, and drying. The hot prairie sun and parching winds dried foods quickly, preserving them for later use. In addition, with water removed, food was 50 to 90 percent lighter and more concentrated in calories—ideal for a people always on the move.

The tribe dried game. Wild fruits such as chokecherries or Juneberries—a good source of fiber—were sun-dried whole or pounded into a paste and then dried. Prairie turnips were eaten raw or dried for soup.

Wasna or *pemmican* is a concentrated, high-energy food. Made of pulverized dried meat mixed with fat and dried crushed wild berries, it contains protein, fat, carbohydrate, and vitamins. Shaped into small patties or squares and allowed to harden, it somewhat resembles beef jerky.

The establishment of the reservation system, which meant tribes were no longer free to travel with herds of big game, brought major dietary changes, and foods provided by the federal government replaced the traditional fare. Salt pork, beef, flour, sugar, rice, beans, dried corn, and coffee entered the diet. Fry bread, one of the most popular foods today, was invented during the early reservation period.

Present-day Native Americans rely heavily on canned goods (chopped meats, vegetables, fruits) from local grocery stores or trading posts. Soups and stews are common meal-time fare. Fry bread is popular and hunting continues, although today it is more likely to be for small animals, fish, and deer.

Traditional Native American foods are served at feasts or ''give-aways'' honoring a person who died in the previous year or someone who has achieved special recognition. Buffalo meat, supplied through the National Park Service from a herd in the Black Hills of South Dakota, is sometimes available; *wasna* is always served at memorial feasts. *Wojopi*, a fruit pudding, is a traditional dessert.

MODIFYING NATIVE AMERICAN COOKING

Here are some suggestions for altering cooking methods and ingredients to make Native American cooking of the northern Plains its healthiest.

> **Instead of:** eating soups and stews immediately after cooking
> **Try:** refrigerating them for several hours; then spoon off the hard fat that rises to the top
> **Advantage:** less fat

> **Instead of:** cooking fry bread in shortening or lard
> **Try:** frying in polyunsaturated vegetable oil; make the oil hot, so the fry bread will absorb less fat
> **Advantage:** less fat

> **Instead of:** frying squash and potatoes
> **Try:** baking or boiling them
> **Advantage:** less fat

Instead of: adding salt to soups and stews made with canned commodity meats and vegetables
Try: leaving it out—since these ingredients already contain salt, you may not notice the difference
Advantage: less salt

Instead of: using commodity beef or pork as is
Try: removing the fat from the top and sides of the can before using
Advantage: less fat

Instead of: selecting white flour and white rice
Try: using whole wheat flour and brown rice
Advantage: more vitamins, more fiber

EXCHANGES OF COMMON FOODS AND STAPLES

STARCH/BREAD

Dried Indian corn	¼ cup
Wild rice	½ cup

MEAT

Buffalo	1 ounce
Oxtail	¼ cup (high-fat meat)
Powdered egg	2 tablespoons

VEGETABLE

Wild (prairie) turnips	½ cup

FRUIT

Chokecherries	1½ cups
Juneberries	1½ cups

RECIPES

Wojopi (Wild Berry Pudding)*

Yield: 1 serving
Serving Size: 1 cup
Exchanges:
Fruit   2

Nutrient Content per Serving:

CAL	135	PRO	2 (gm)
FAT	1 (gm)	CHO	31 (gm)
Na	0 (mg)	K	329 (mg)
Fiber	3 (gm)	Chol	0 (mg)

Ingredients

- 1 CUP UNSWEETENED WILD BERRIES, SUCH AS JUNEBERRIES, CHOKECHERRIES, SLICED STRAWBERRIES, PITTED CHERRIES, OR RASPBERRIES
- ½ CUP WATER
- 1 TABLESPOON CORNSTARCH DISSOLVED IN ¼ CUP WATER
- 1 PACKET SUGAR SUBSTITUTE

Method

1. Boil fruit with water until tender.
2. Add cornstarch mixture; boil and stir until thickened.
3. Remove from heat; add sweetener. Serve warm.

*3 grams or more of fiber per serving.

Wasna (Pemmican)* **

Yield: 8 servings

Serving Size: 1 square

Exchanges:

Meat, lean	1
Fruit	2
Fat	1

Nutrient Content per Serving:

CAL	225	PRO	9 (gm)
FAT	9 (gm)	CHO	28 (gm)
Na	952 (mg)	K	396 (mg)
Fiber	2 (gm)	Chol	26 (mg)

Ingredients

8 OUNCES DRIED MEAT
2 CUPS DRIED CHOKECHERRIES OR RAISINS
¼ CUP BEEF OR WILD GAME TALLOW OR
SHORTENING

Method

1. Combine all ingredients and put through a hand grinder until evenly mixed.
2. Pat out on wooden board and cut into 8 squares.

*400 milligrams or more of sodium per serving.
**This recipe contains saturated fat, which should be limited in the diet.

Fry Bread

Yield: 8 servings
Serving Size: 1 wedge
Exchanges:
Starch/Bread   2
Fat   ½

Nutrient Content per Serving:

CAL	191	PRO	5 (gm)
FAT	5 (gm)	CHO	30 (gm)
Na	369 (mg)	K	108 (mg)
Fiber	1 (gm)	Chol	1 (mg)

Ingredients

  2 CUPS FLOUR
½ CUP NONFAT DRY MILK POWDER
  1 TABLESPOON SUGAR
  2 TEASPOONS BAKING POWDER
  1 TEASPOON SALT
¾ CUP WATER
   VEGETABLE OIL FOR FRYING

Method

1. Sift together flour, milk powder, sugar, baking powder, and salt.
2. Stir in water to make a stiff dough.
3. Pat out two 6-inch circles of dough, each about ½ inch thick, on floured surface. Cut each circle into 4 wedges.
4. Drop each wedge into hot oil (350°F) 1½–2 inches deep in heavy skillet. Fry until golden brown, turning once. Drain on absorbent paper.

Dried Corn Soup* **

Yield: 8 servings
Serving Size: 1 cup
Exchanges:
Starch/Bread   1
Meat, medium-
     fat   ½
Fat   2

Nutrient Content per Serving:

CAL	214	PRO	9 (gm)
FAT	13 (gm)	CHO	19 (gm)
Na	805 (mg)	K	276 (mg)
Fiber	4 (gm)	Chol	28 (mg)

Ingredients

   1 EAR DRIED CORN OR 1 CUP DRIED CORN
     KERNELS
   7 CUPS PLUS 2 CUPS WATER
   ¼ POUND SALT PORK, DICED INTO ¼-INCH PIECES
   5 OUNCES DRIED MEAT
   ⅛ TEASPOON BLACK PEPPER

Method

1. Soak corn in 2 cups of water for 48 hours. Drain and rinse.
2. Place corn in large saucepan or Dutch oven; add 7 cups water
   and salt pork. Bring to a boil; cover and simmer for 4 hours
   or until corn is tender but not mushy.
3. Add dried meat and pepper; continue simmering for 10 minutes. Skim fat. Serve hot.

   *400 milligrams or more of sodium per serving.
   **3 grams or more of fiber per serving.

THE SOUL OF SOUTHERN COOKING

There's no single way to describe the cooking of the American South. From New Orleans to the Carolinas, the cuisines of the South's subregions differ from each other nearly as much as southern differs from northern cooking. One strong influence on southern cooking has been that of Black Americans. Sometimes called "soul food," this cooking style is now popular throughout the United States.

Many aspects of southern cooking fit well into a diabetic meal plan. Classic soul dishes such as Sweet Potato Pie, Hot Water Cornbread, and Mixed Greens (see recipes, pages 399–401) are high in fiber and complex carbohydrate. However, southern cooks tend to prefer highly salted food and often rely heavily on saturated fats (primarily pork products) for flavoring and frying. Fortunately, both can be modified.

Peas and beans have long been staples of southern cooking. "Field peas" (so named because they were planted around the borders of corn and cotton fields) were dried, soaked, and cooked with pieces of smoked or salted meat.

Today, favorite dishes include black-eyed peas, pinto beans, or pork and beans. Sweet potatoes and corn (including grits, hominy, and cornmeal) are popular. Meats, often fried, are served with gravy. More greens and cabbage are included in this cuisine than in others. Salted, smoked, or cured meats (salt pork, ham hocks, smoked neck bones, and jowl bacon), black and red peppers, and sage are widely used.

MODIFICATIONS OF SOUTHERN COOKING PRACTICES

Here are some suggestions for altering cooking methods and ingredients to make southern cooking its healthiest.

Instead of: seasoning vegetables and cornbread with cured meats (bacon, fatback, ham) that are high in salt and fat

Try: fresh, lean, well-trimmed pork, or cut seasoning meats in tiny cubes (¼ inch or less) and fry slowly until fat is rendered and cubes are light and dry. Drain off fat. Place cubes on paper towels to absorb remaining fat. Use cubes sparingly for flavor. They still contain salt, but less fat

Advantage: less saturated fat, less salt

Instead of: salt or fat used for flavoring

Try: hot sauce, Tabasco sauce, vinegar, fresh onion, garlic powder, hot peppers, spices, and herbs

Advantage: less fat and sodium

Instead of: canned baked beans

Try: dried beans

Advantage: less salt and sugar, lower cost

Instead of: frying

Try: oven frying (see recipe on page 403)

Advantage: less fat

SOUTHERN FOODS GLOSSARY

Chicory (dried): Root of the chicory plant, dried, roasted, and ground; originally used to "stretch" coffee, but it also adds body, aroma, and flavor.

Chicory (fresh): A green leafy vegetable used raw in salads or cooked as greens, especially in the southern part of the United States.

Chitterlings (chittlins, chiterlings, or chitlings): Intestine of the hog (a main dish). Usually seasoned and served with hot sauce and/or vinegar. They may be boiled, battered, and deep fried.

Corn pone: Bread made with cornmeal, salt, and water (sometimes flour), shaped into oval patties and fried on a griddle or in a skillet (sometimes called hot water cornbread).

Cracklings (cracklins): Small pieces of fresh pork fat that have been cooked until crisp and drained of lard, which may be eaten alone or added to cornbread.

Fatback: Fat with skin trimmed from the back portion of the hog; generally used in seasoning vegetables, or fried like bacon.

Ham hock (fresh): Lower end of ham shank, predominantly bone and skin, boiled and used as an entrée or seasoning.

Hog jowls: Cheek or tender jaw portion of the hog, boiled and served as a main dish; or cured and used as seasoning meat.

Hog maws: Stomach of the hog, boiled and used as a main dish.

Poke salad: Poke, an early spring green, is a coarse, perennial herb with a white flower and dark red berries. The roots are poisonous, but the young shoots, young tender leaves, and stems, can be eaten. The young leaves are parboiled, the water is discarded, and the leaves are simmered again in fresh water. The name "poke" is an abbreviation of pocan or pokeweed and is of American Indian origin. It is served as a hot vegetable.

Pot liquor (likker): The liquid that remains in the bottom of the pot after vegetables have been cooked. Traditionally it is soaked up with bits of cornbread and eaten at the end of the meal.

Salt pork: Salted pork fat from the loin area of the hog that is used for seasoning.

Seasoning meat: Cured, smoked, or salted pork products (ham hocks, fatback, salt pork, bacon, or bacon drippings) used to flavor foods.

EXCHANGES OF COMMON FOODS AND STAPLES

STARCH/BREAD

Hominy (canned)	½ cup

(For cornbread, biscuits, baked beans, and the dry legumes, such as black-eyed peas and pinto beans, see the 1986 Exchange Lists.)

MEAT

Chicken gizzard	1 ounce (lean meat)
Hog maw (stomach)	⅓ cup (lean meat)
Pig ear	1½ ounces (lean meat)
Neck bones (pork)	½ cup (medium-fat meat)
Oxtail	¼ cup (medium-fat meat)
Pig feet	6 ounces uncooked (high-fat meat)
Pig tail	1 ounce (high-fat meat)

(For pork ribs, see the 1986 Exchange Lists.)

VEGETABLES

Poke salad (pokeberry shoots)	½ cup, cooked

(For greens such as collard, mustard, and turnip, see the 1986 Exchange Lists.)

FATS

Chitterlings, fried	2 tablespoons
Crackling, pork	1½ teaspoons
Fatback	¾-inch cube

(For salt pork and simmered chitterlings, see the 1986 Exchange Lists.)

RECIPES

Sweet Potato Pie*

Yield: 8 servings
Serving Size: ⅛ wedge
Exchanges:
Starch/Bread   2
Fat   2

Nutrient Content per Serving:
CAL 263   PRO   6 (gm)
FAT   13 (gm)   CHO   32 (gm)
Na   296 (mg)   K   524 (mg)
Fiber   3 (gm)   Chol   34 (mg)

Ingredients

    3 TABLESPOONS MARGARINE
    ¼ CUP SUGAR
    ¼ TEASPOON SALT
    1 EGG YOLK
    3 TABLESPOONS LEMON JUICE
    1 TEASPOON LEMON PEEL (RIND FROM
       1 LEMON), GRATED
    ¼ TEASPOON CINNAMON
    3 LARGE SWEET POTATOES, COOKED AND
       MASHED (1½ POUNDS)
    1 CUP SKIM MILK
    3 EGG WHITES, BEATEN TO STIFF PEAKS
       9-INCH UNBAKED PIE SHELL**

Method

1. Heat oven to 350°F. Beat together margarine, sugar, and salt.
   Add egg yolk, lemon juice, lemon peel, and cinnamon. Stir
   in sweet potatoes and milk; mix well.
2. Fold in egg whites; pour into pie shell. Bake for 40–50 minutes or until knife inserted in center comes out clean.

   *3 grams or more of fiber per serving.
   **To reduce saturated fat, use a homemade pie shell made with
vegetable oil.

Hot Water Cornbread

Yield: 6 servings
Serving Size: ⅓ cup
Exchanges:
Starch/Bread   1
Fat   ½

Nutrient Content per Serving:

CAL	107	PRO	2 (gm)
FAT	3 (gm)	CHO	18 (gm)
Na	355 (mg)	K	28 (mg)
Fiber	2 (gm)	Chol	0 (mg)

Ingredients

    1 CUP YELLOW CORNMEAL
    1 TEASPOON SALT
 1½ CUPS SCALDING WATER
    1 TABLESPOON VEGETABLE OIL
      NONSTICK VEGETABLE SPRAY

Method

1. Combine cornmeal and salt; add water and oil. Mix well.
2. Fry ⅓ cup mixture on hot griddle or skillet coated with non-stick vegetable spray, pushing mixture into shape of a patty with back of spatula. Fry patties on both sides until golden brown, about 3 minutes per side. Serve hot.

Baked Sweet Potatoes*

Yield: 6 servings
Serving Size: 1 potato
(about 6 ounces)
Exchanges:
Starch/Bread   2

Nutrient Content per Serving:

CAL	137	PRO	2 (gm)
FAT	0 (gm)	CHO	32 (gm)
Na	14 (mg)	K	461 (mg)
Fiber	3 (gm)	Chol	0 (mg)

Key Source Nutrients:
Vitamin A   28,857 (IU)

Ingredients

    6 SWEET POTATOES (ABOUT 6 OUNCES EACH)
    2 TABLESPOONS VEGETABLE OIL

Method

1. Preheat oven to 375°F. Scrub potatoes; dry well.
2. Coat potatoes with vegetable oil. Cut cross in the top of each potato with fork; bake for 45 minutes.
3. Press on ends to fluff potato open.

   *3 grams or more of fiber per serving.

Mixed Greens

Yield: 6 servings
Serving Size: ½ cup greens
and ¼ cup liquid
Exchanges:
Vegetable   1

Nutrient Content per Serving:

CAL	20	PRO	2 (gm)
FAT	1 (gm)	CHO	3 (gm)
Na	388 (mg)	K	160 (mg)
Fiber	2 (gm)	Chol	1 (mg)

Ingredients

   1 POUND MUSTARD GREENS
   1 POUND TURNIP GREENS (OR ANY
     COMBINATION OF GREENS, SUCH AS KALE OR
     DANDELION)
   2 CUPS WATER
   1 SMALL RED HOT PEPPER, MINCED, OR ¼
     TEASPOON RED PEPPER FLAKES
   1 TEASPOON SALT
   1 SLICE BACON, CUT INTO STRIPS

Method

1. Wash greens well; cut off and discard tough stems. Slice greens; place in large saucepan or Dutch oven.
2. Add remaining ingredients; bring to a boil. Cover; simmer over low heat until wilted and cooked thoroughly, about 50 minutes.

Barbecued Spareribs*

Yield: 8 servings
Serving Size: ¼ pound ribs
plus 2 tablespoons sauce
Exchanges:
Starch/Bread   ½
Meat, medium-fat 2
Fat   1

Nutrient Content per Serving:

CAL	238	PRO	14 (gm)
FAT	15 (gm)	CHO	12 (gm)
Na	430 (mg)	K	284 (mg)
Fiber	0 (gm)	Chol	53 (mg)

Ingredients

    2 POUNDS SPARERIBS (PORK)
    1 TABLESPOON MARGARINE
    ½ MEDIUM ONION, MINCED
    1 SMALL CLOVE GARLIC, MINCED
    1 CUP KETCHUP OR CHILE SAUCE OR ½ CUP EACH
    2 TABLESPOONS BROWN SUGAR
    1 TEASPOON PREPARED MUSTARD
    1 TEASPOON WORCESTERSHIRE SAUCE
    6 DROPS TABASCO SAUCE
    ¼ TEASPOON PEPPER
    1 TEASPOON LEMON JUICE

Method

1. Cook ribs over low charcoals until well done (about 2 hours), basting frequently with water to keep moist.
2. Melt margarine in medium saucepan. Sauté onion and garlic in margarine until tender, about 5 minutes.
3. Add remaining ingredients except lemon juice. Simmer over low heat for 15–20 minutes or until thickened. Stir in lemon juice. Brush sauce on to ribs during last 5 minutes of cooking or serve with ribs for dipping.

    *400 milligrams or more of sodium per serving.

Oven-Fried Chicken*

Yield: 4 servings
Serving Size: ¼ chicken
(with skin)
Exchanges:
Starch/Bread   ½
Meat, medium-
   fat   4½

Nutrient Content per Serving:

CAL	397	PRO	41 (gm)
FAT	21 (gm)	CHO	10 (gm)
Na	433 (mg)	K	340 (mg)
Fiber	1 (gm)	Chol	127 (mg)

Serving Size: ¼ chicken
(without skin)
Exchanges:
Starch/Bread   ½
Meat, lean   4

Nutrient Content per Serving:

CAL	256	PRO	33 (gm)
FAT	9 (gm)	CHO	10 (gm)
Na	410 (mg)	K	276 (mg)
Fiber	½ (gm)	Chol	95 (mg)

Ingredients

   ¼ CUP FLOUR
   ¼ CUP CRACKER MEAL
   ½ TEASPOON PEPPER
   ½ TEASPOON SALT
   ¼ TEASPOON PAPRIKA
   ⅛ TEASPOON GARLIC POWDER
2½-POUND FRYING CHICKEN, CUT UP**
   NONSTICK VEGETABLE SPRAY

Method

1. Preheat oven to 350°F.
2. Combine all ingredients except chicken in plastic bag.
3. Wash chicken; shake in coating mixture and place on cookie sheet coated with nonstick vegetable spray.
4. Bake for 1 hour or until brown and crisp.

*400 milligrams or more of sodium per serving, either with or without skin.
**To reduce fat, remove the skin from the chicken.

REFERENCES AND RESOURCES

MEXICAN AMERICAN

Davis, E. G. 1974. *A Taste of Mexico (A Primer of Mexican Cooking)*. San Diego, CA: Tofua Press.

Franz, M. J. 1983. *Exchanges for All Occasions*. Minneapolis: International Diabetes Center.

General Clinical Research Center. 1986. *Cook This Book*. San Diego, CA: UCSD Medical Center.

Hall, T. A., K. Bertram, and S. B. Foerster. 1985. *Comer Bien Para Vivir Mejor* (Eat Well to Live Better). Sacramento: California Diabetes Control Program, Department of Health Services, State of California.

Institute of Nutrition of Central America and Panama and National Institutes of Health. 1961. *Food Composition Table for Use in Latin America*. Bethesda, MD: NIH.

NATIVE AMERICAN/NORTHERN PLAINS

American Indians. 1984. Washington, DC: Bureau of Indian Affairs, Department of the Interior.

Jackson, Y. J. 1986. Nutrition in American Indian health: past, present and future. *J. Am. Diet. Assn.* 86:1561.

Kavasch, B. 1979. *Native Harvests: Recipes and Botanicals of the American Indian*. New York: Random House.

Kimball, Y., and J. Anderson. 1965. *The Art of American Indian Cooking*. Garden City, NY: Doubleday & Co.

Lowie, R. H. 1982. *Indians of the Plains*. Nebraska: Bison Book.

Nutrition & Dietetic Branch, Indian Health Service. 1970. *Recipes to Build Strong Families*. Aberdeen, SD: IHS.

Plains Indian Diet Handbook. 1984. Prepared by Swanson Center for Nutrition, Inc., in cooperation with Indian Health Service Diabetes Control Program. Limited free copies available from the IHS Diabetes Program, Albuquerque, NM.

Toma, R. B., and M. L. Curry. 1980. North Dakota Indians' traditional foods. *J. Am. Diet. Assn.* 76:589.

Trapp, J. S. 1982. *Gifts of the Earth.* Boulder, CO: Pruett Publishing Co.

SOUTHERN REGIONAL

American Diabetes Association, Washington, DC Affiliate. 1987. *Black American Cookery.* May be obtained from the ADA, Washington, DC Affiliate, 1819 H Street, N.W., Suite 1200, Washington, DC 20006; (202) 331-8303.

Davidson, J. K., and M. P. Goldsmith. 1979. *Diabetes Guidebook: Diet Section,* 3rd ed. May be purchased from DAVI-CONE, Inc., 1075 Lullwater Rd., N.E., Atlanta, GA 30307.

Goldsmith, M. P., and J. K. Davidson. 1977. Southern ethnic food preferences and exchange values for the diabetic diet. *J. Am. Diet. Assn.* 70:61.

Appendix: Exchange Lists

The reason for dividing food into six different groups is that foods vary in their carbohydrate, protein, fat, and calorie content. Each Exchange List contains foods that are alike—each choice contains about the same amount of carbohydrate, protein, fat, and calories.

The following chart shows the amount of these nutrients in one serving from each Exchange List.

EXCHANGE LIST	CARBOHYDRATE (grams)	PROTEIN (grams)	FAT (grams)	CALORIES
Starch/Bread	15	3	trace	80
Meat				
Lean	—	7	3	55
Medium-Fat	—	7	5	75
High-Fat	—	7	8	100
Vegetable	5	2	—	25
Fruit	15	—	—	60
Milk				
Skim	12	8	trace	90
Low-Fat	12	8	5	120
Whole	12	8	8	150
Fat	—	—	5	45

As you read the Exchange Lists, you will notice that one choice often is a larger amount of food than another choice from the same list. Because foods are so different, each food is measured or weighed so the amounts of carbohydrate, protein, fat, and calories are the same in each choice.

You will notice footnotes on some foods in the exchange groups—for example, foods that are high in fiber (3 grams or more per normal serving). High-fiber foods are good for you so it is important to eat more of them.

Foods that are high in sodium (400 milligrams or more of sodium per normal serving) are also footnoted. It's a good idea to limit your intake of high-salt foods, especially if you have high blood pressure.

If you have a favorite food that is not included in any of these groups, ask your dietitian about it. That food can probably be worked into your meal plan, at least now and then.

1 STARCH/BREAD LIST

Each item in this list contains approximately 15 grams of carbohydrate, 3 grams of protein, a trace of fat, and 80 calories. Whole grain products average about 2 grams of fiber per serving. Some foods are higher in fiber. Foods that contain 3 grams or more of fiber per serving are footnoted.

You can choose your starch exchanges from any of the items on this list. If you want to eat a starch food that is not on this list, the general rule is that:

- ½ cup cereal, grain, or pasta is 1 serving
- 1 ounce bread product is 1 serving

Your dietitian can help you be more exact.

CEREALS/GRAINS/PASTA

Bran cereals*, concentrated (such as Bran Buds,® All Bran®)	⅓ cup
Bran cereals*, flaked	½ cup
Bulgur (cooked)	½ cup

*3 grams or more of fiber per serving.

CEREALS/GRAINS/PASTA (*continued*)

Cooked cereals	½ cup
Cornmeal (dry)	2½ tablespoons
Grape-nuts	3 tablespoons
Grits (cooked)	½ cup
Other ready-to-eat unsweetened cereals	¾ cup
Pasta (cooked)	½ cup
Puffed cereal	1½ cups
Rice, white or brown (cooked)	⅓ cup
Shredded wheat	½ cup
Wheat germ*	3 tablespoons

DRIED BEANS/PEAS/LENTILS

Baked beans*	¼ cup
Beans and peas* (cooked) (such as kidney, white, split, black-eye)	⅓ cup
Lentils* (cooked)	⅓ cup

STARCHY VEGETABLES

Corn*	½ cup
Corn on cob*, 6 inches long	1
Lima beans*	½ cup
Peas, green* (canned or frozen)	½ cup
Plantain*	½ cup
Potato, baked	1 small (3 ounces)
Potato, mashed	½ cup
Squash, winter (acorn, butternut)	¾ cup
Yam, sweet potato, plain	⅓ cup

*3 grams or more of fiber per serving.

BREAD

Bagel	½ (1 ounce)
Bread sticks, crisp, 4 inches long × ½ inch	2 (⅔ ounce)
Croutons, low-fat	1 cup
English muffin	½
Frankfurter or hamburger bun	½ (1 ounce)
Pita, 6 inches across	½
Plain roll, small	1 (1 ounce)
Raisin, unfrosted	1 slice (1 ounce)
Rye*, pumpernickel	1 slice (1 ounce)
Tortilla, 6 inches across	1
White (including French, Italian)	1 slice (1 ounce)
Whole wheat	1 slice (1 ounce)

CRACKERS/SNACKS

Animal crackers	8
Graham crackers, 2½ inches square	3
Matzoth	¾ ounce
Melba toast	5 slices
Oyster crackers	24
Popcorn (popped, no fat added)	3 cups
Pretzels	¾ ounce
Rye crisps, 2 inches × 3½ inches	4
Saltine-type crackers	6
Whole wheat crackers, no fat added (crisp breads, such as Finn®, Kavli®, Wasa®)	2–4 slices (¾ ounce)

*3 grams or more of fiber per serving.

STARCH FOODS PREPARED WITH FAT

(Count as 1 Starch/Bread serving, plus 1 Fat serving.)

Biscuit, 2½ inches across	1
Chow mein noodles	½ cup
Cornbread, 2-inch cube	1 (2 ounces)
Crackers, round, butter type	6
French fried potatoes, 2 inches to 3½ inches long	10 (1½ ounces)
Muffin, plain, small	1
Pancakes, 4 inches across	2
Stuffing, bread (prepared)	¼ cup
Taco shells, 6 inches across	2
Waffle, 4½ inches square	1
Whole wheat crackers, fat added (such as Triscuits®)	4–6 (1 ounce)

2 MEAT LIST

Each serving of meat and substitutes on this list contains about 7 grams of protein. The amount of fat and number of calories vary, depending on what kind of meat or substitute you choose. The list is divided into three parts based on the amount of fat and calories: lean meat, medium-fat meat, and high-fat meat. One ounce (1 meat exchange) of each of these includes:

	CARBOHYDRATE (grams)	PROTEIN (grams)	FAT (grams)	CALORIES
Lean	0	7	3	55
Medium-Fat	0	7	5	75
High-Fat	0	7	8	100

You are encouraged to use more lean and medium-fat meat, poultry, and fish in your meal plan. This will help decrease your fat intake, which may help decrease your risk of heart disease. The items from the high-fat group are high in saturated fat, cholesterol, and calories. Try to limit your choices from the high-fat group to three times per week. Meats and substitutes do not contribute any fiber to your meal plan. Meats and meat substitutes that have 400 milligrams or more of sodium per serving are footnoted. Following are some tips for cooking meat:

1. Bake, roast, broil, grill, or boil these foods rather than frying them with added fat.
2. Use a nonstick pan spray or a nonstick pan to brown or fry these foods.
3. Trim off visible fat before and after cooking.
4. Do not add flour, bread crumbs, coating mixes, or fat to these foods when preparing them.
5. Weigh meat after removing bones and fat, and after cooking. About 3 ounces of cooked meat equals 4 ounces of raw meat. Some examples of meat portions are:

   2 ounces meat (2 meat exchanges) =
      1 small chicken leg or thigh
      ½ cup cottage cheese or tuna

   3 ounces meat (3 meat exchanges) =
      1 medium pork chop
      1 small hamburger
      ½ of a whole chicken breast
      1 unbreaded fish fillet or
      cooked meat about the size of
      a deck of cards

6. Restaurants usually serve prime cuts of meat, which are high in fat and calories.

LEAN MEAT AND SUBSTITUTES

(One exchange is equal to any one of the following items.)

BEEF:	USDA Good or Choice grades of lean beef, such as round, sirloin, and flank steak; tenderloin; and chipped beef*	1 ounce
PORK:	Lean pork, such as fresh ham; canned, cured, or boiled ham*; Canadian bacon*; tenderloin	1 ounce
VEAL:	All cuts are lean except for veal cutlets (ground or cubed); examples of lean veal are chops and roasts	1 ounce
POULTRY:	Chicken, turkey, Cornish hen (without skin)	1 ounce
FISH:	All fresh and frozen fish	1 ounce
	Crab, lobster, scallops, shrimp, clams (fresh or canned in water*)	2 ounces
	Oysters	6 medium
	Tuna* (canned in water)	¼ cup
	Herring (uncreamed, smoked)	1 ounce
	Sardines (canned)	2 medium
WILD GAME:	Venison, rabbit, squirrel	1 ounce
	Pheasant, duck, goose (without skin)	1 ounce
CHEESE:	Any cottage cheese	¼ cup
	Grated Parmesan	2 tablespoons
	Diet cheeses* (with less than 55 calories per ounce)	1 ounce
OTHER:	95% fat-free luncheon meat	1 ounce
	Egg whites	3 whites
	Egg substitutes with less than 55 calories per ¼ cup	¼ cup

*400 milligrams or more of sodium per serving.

MEDIUM-FAT MEAT AND SUBSTITUTES

(One exchange is equal to any one of the following items.)

BEEF:	Most beef products fall into this category. Examples are all ground beef, roast (rib, chuck, rump), steak (cubed, Porterhouse, T-bone), and meatloaf	1 ounce
PORK:	Most pork products fall into this category. Examples are chops, loin roast, Boston butt, cutlets	1 ounce
LAMB:	Most lamb products fall into this category. Examples are chops, leg, and roast	1 ounce
VEAL:	Cutlet (ground or cubed, unbreaded)	1 ounce
POULTRY:	Chicken (with skin), domestic duck or goose (well-drained of fat), ground turkey	1 ounce
FISH:	Tuna* (canned in oil and drained)	¼ cup
	Salmon* (canned)	¼ cup
CHEESE:	Skim or part-skim milk cheeses, such as:	
	Ricotta	¼ cup
	Mozzarella	1 ounce
	Diet cheeses* (with 56–80 calories per ounce)	1 ounce
OTHER:	86% fat-free luncheon meat*	1 ounce
	Eggs (high in cholesterol, limit to 3 per week)	1
	Egg substitutes with 56–80 calories per ¼ cup	¼ cup
	Tofu (2½ inches × 2¾ inches × 1 inch)	4 ounces
	Liver, heart, kidney, sweetbreads (high in cholesterol)	1 ounce

*400 milligrams or more of sodium per serving.

HIGH-FAT MEAT AND SUBSTITUTES

Remember, these items are high in saturated fat, cholesterol, and calories, and should be used no more than three times per week.

(One exchange is equal to any one of the following items.)

BEEF:	Most USDA Prime cuts of beef, such as ribs, corned beef*	1 ounce
PORK:	Spareribs, ground pork, pork sausage* (patty or link)	1 ounce
LAMB:	Patties (ground lamb)	1 ounce
FISH:	Any fried fish product	1 ounce
CHEESE:	All regular cheeses*, such as American, Blue, Cheddar, Monterey, Swiss	1 ounce
OTHER:	Luncheon meat*, such as bologna, salami, pimento loaf	1 ounce
	Sausage*, such as Polish, Italian	1 ounce
	Knockwurst, smoked	1 ounce
	Bratwurst*	1 ounce
	Frankfurter* (turkey or chicken)	1 frank (¹/₁₀ pound)
	Peanut butter (contains unsaturated fat)	1 tablespoon

Count as 1 High-Fat Meat plus 1 Fat exchange:

	Frankfurter* (beef, pork, or combination)	1 frank (¹/₁₀ pound)

*400 milligrams or more of sodium per serving.

3 VEGETABLE LIST

Each vegetable serving on this list contains about 5 grams of carbohydrate, 2 grams of protein, and 25 calories. Vegetables contain 2–3 grams of dietary fiber. Vegetables that contain 400 milligrams or more of sodium per serving are footnoted.

Vegetables are a good source of vitamins and minerals. Fresh and frozen vegetables have more vitamins and less added salt. Rinsing canned vegetables will remove much of the salt.

Unless otherwise noted, the serving size for vegetables (1 vegetable exchange) is:

- ½ cup cooked vegetables or vegetable juice
- 1 cup raw vegetables

Artichoke (½ medium)	Mushrooms, cooked
Asparagus	Okra
Bean sprouts	Onions
Beans (green, wax, Italian)	Pea pods
Beets	Peppers (green)
Broccoli	Rutabaga
Brussels sprouts	Sauerkraut*
Cabbage, cooked	Spinach, cooked
Carrots	Summer squash (crookneck)
Cauliflower	Tomato (one large)
Eggplant	Tomato/vegetable juice*
Greens (collard, mustard, turnip)	Turnips
	Water chestnuts
Kohlrabi	Zucchini, cooked
Leeks	

Starchy vegetables such as corn, peas, and potatoes are found on the Starch/Bread List. For free vegetables, see Free Food List on pages 421–423.

*400 milligrams or more of sodium per serving.

4 FRUIT LIST

Each item on this list contains about 15 grams of carbohydrate and 60 calories. Fresh, frozen, and dry fruits have about 2 grams of fiber per serving. Fruits that have 3 or more grams of fiber per serving are footnoted. Fruit juices contain very little dietary fiber.

The carbohydrate and calorie contents for a fruit serving are based on the usual serving of the most commonly eaten fruits. Use fresh fruits or fruits frozen or canned without sugar added. Whole fruit is more filling than fruit juice and may be a better choice for those who are trying to lose weight. Unless otherwise noted, the serving size for 1 fruit serving is:

- ½ cup fresh fruit or fruit juice
- ¼ cup dried fruit

FRESH, FROZEN, AND UNSWEETENED CANNED FRUIT

Apple (raw, 2 inches across)	1 apple
Apple sauce (unsweetened)	½ cup
Apricots (canned)	½ cup, or 4 halves
Apricots (medium, raw)	4 apricots
Banana (9 inches long)	½ banana
Blackberries* (raw)	¾ cup
Blueberries* (raw)	¾ cup
Cantaloupe (cubes)	1 cup
Cantaloupe (5 inches across)	⅓ melon
Cherries (canned)	½ cup
Cherries (large, raw)	12 cherries
Figs (raw, 2 inches across)	2 figs
Fruit cocktail (canned)	½ cup
Grapefruit (medium)	½ grapefruit
Grapefruit (segments)	¾ cup

*3 grams or more of fiber per serving.

FRESH, FROZEN, AND UNSWEETENED CANNED FRUIT *(continued)*

Grapes (small)	15 grapes
Honeydew melon (cubes)	1 cup
Honeydew melon (medium)	1/8 melon
Kiwi (large)	1 kiwi
Mandarin oranges	3/4 cup
Mango (small)	1/2 mango
Nectarine* (1½ inches across)	1 nectarine
Orange (2½ inches across)	1 orange
Papaya	1 cup
Peach (2¾ inches across)	1 peach, or 3/4 cup
Peaches (canned)	1/2 cup, or 2 halves
Pear	1/2 large, or 1 small
Pears (canned)	1/2 cup, or 2 halves
Persimmons (medium, native)	2 persimmons
Pineapple (canned)	1/3 cup
Pineapple (raw)	3/4 cup
Plums (raw, 2 inches across)	2 plums
Pomegranate*	1/2 pomegranate
Raspberries* (raw)	1 cup
Strawberries* (raw, whole)	1¼ cups
Tangerines (2½ inches across)	2 tangerines
Watermelon (cubes)	1¼ cups

DRIED FRUIT

Apples*	4 rings
Apricots*	7 halves
Dates	2½ medium
Figs*	1½
Prunes*	3 medium
Raisins	2 tablespoons

*3 grams or more of fiber per serving.

FRUIT JUICE

Apple juice/cider	½ cup
Cranberry juice cocktail	⅓ cup
Grape juice	⅓ cup
Grapefruit juice	½ cup
Orange juice	½ cup
Pineapple juice	½ cup
Prune juice	⅓ cup

5 MILK LIST

Each serving of milk or milk products on this list contains about 12 grams of carbohydrate and 8 grams of protein. The amount of fat in milk is measured in percentage of butterfat. The calories vary, depending on what kind of milk you choose. The list is divided into three parts based on the amount of fat and calories: skim/very low-fat milk, low-fat milk, and whole milk. One serving (1 milk exchange) of each of these includes:

	CARBOHYDRATE (grams)	PROTEIN (grams)	FAT (grams)	CALORIES
Skim/Very Low-Fat	12	8	trace	90
Low-Fat	12	8	5	120
Whole	12	8	8	150

Milk is the body's main source of calcium, the mineral needed for growth and repair of bones. Yogurt is also a good source of calcium. Yogurt and many dry or powdered milk products have different amounts of fat. If you have questions about a particular item, read the label to find out the fat and calorie content.

Milk is good to drink, but it can also be added to cereal and to other foods. Many tasty dishes such as sugar-free pudding are made with milk (see the Combination Foods List). Add life to plain yogurt by adding one of your fruit servings to it.

SKIM AND VERY LOW-FAT MILK

Skim milk	1 cup
½% milk	1 cup
1% milk	1 cup
Low-fat buttermilk	1 cup
Evaporated skim milk	½ cup
Dry nonfat milk	⅓ cup
Plain nonfat yogurt	8 ounces

LOW-FAT MILK

2% milk	1 cup
Plain low-fat yogurt (with added nonfat milk solids)	8 ounces

WHOLE MILK

The whole milk group has much more fat per serving than the skim and low-fat groups. Whole milk has more than 3¼ percent butterfat. Try to limit your choices from the whole milk group as much as possible.

Whole milk	1 cup
Evaporated whole milk	½ cup
Whole plain yogurt	8 ounces

6 FAT LIST

Each serving on the fat list contains about 5 grams of fat and 45 calories. The foods on the fat list contain mostly fat, although some items may also contain a small amount of protein. All fats are high in calories and should be carefully measured. Everyone should modify fat intake by eating unsaturated fats instead of saturated fats. The sodium content of these foods varies widely. Check the label for sodium information.

UNSATURATED FATS

Avocado	⅛ medium
Margarine	1 teaspoon
Margarine*, diet	1 tablespoon
Mayonnaise	1 teaspoon
Mayonnaise*, reduced-calorie	1 tablespoon
Nuts and Seeds:	
Almonds, dry roasted	6 whole
Cashews, dry roasted	1 tablespoon
Other nuts	1 tablespoon
Peanuts	20 small or 10 large
Pecans	2 whole
Pine nuts, sunflower seeds (without shells)	1 tablespoon
Pumpkin seeds	2 teaspoons
Walnuts	2 whole
Oil (corn, cottonseed, olive, peanut, safflower, soybean, sunflower)	1 teaspoon
Olives*	10 small or 5 large
Salad dressing* (all varieties)	1 tablespoon

*If more than one or two servings are consumed, sodium levels will equal or exceed 400 milligrams.

UNSATURATED FATS *(continued)*

Salad dressing, mayonnaise-type	2 teaspoons
Salad dressing, mayonnaise-type, reduced-calorie	1 tablespoon
Salad dressing*, reduced-calorie	2 tablespoons

(Two tablespoons of low-calorie salad dressing is a free food.)

SATURATED FATS

Bacon**	1 slice
Butter	1 teaspoon
Chitterlings	½ ounce
Coconut, shredded	2 tablespoons
Coffee whitener, liquid	2 tablespoons
Coffee whitener, powder	4 teaspoons
Cream (light, coffee, table)	2 tablespoons
Cream (heavy, whipping)	1 tablespoon
Cream cheese	1 tablespoon
Cream, sour	2 tablespoons
Salt pork**	¼ ounce

FREE FOODS

A free food is any food or drink that contains fewer than 20 calories per serving. You can eat as much as you want of those items that have no serving size specified. You may eat two or three servings per day of those items that have a specific serving size. Be sure to spread them out through the day.

*400 milligrams or more of sodium per serving.
**If more than one or two servings are consumed, sodium levels will equal or exceed 400 milligrams.

DRINKS:
Bouillon* or broth without fat
Bouillon, low-sodium
Carbonated drinks, sugar-free
Carbonated water
Club soda
Cocoa powder, unsweetened (1 tablespoon)
Coffee/Tea
Drink mixes, sugar-free
Tonic water, sugar-free

NONSTICK PAN SPRAY

FRUIT:
Cranberries, unsweetened (½ cup)
Rhubarb, unsweetened (½ cup)

VEGETABLES: *(raw, 1 cup)*
Cabbage
Celery
Chinese cabbage**
Cucumber
Green onion
Hot peppers
Mushrooms
Radishes
Zucchini**

SALAD GREENS:
Endive
Escarole
Lettuce
Romaine
Spinach

*400 milligrams or more of sodium per serving.
**3 grams or more of fiber per serving.

SWEET SUBSTITUTES:
Candy, hard, sugar-free
Gelatin, sugar-free
Gum, sugar-free
Jam/Jelly, sugar-free (2 teaspoons)
Pancake syrup, sugar-free (1–2 tablespoons)
Sugar substitutes (saccharin, aspartame)
Whipped topping (2 tablespoons)

CONDIMENTS:
Horseradish
Ketchup (1 tablespoon)
Mustard
Pickles*, dill, unsweetened
Salad dressing, low-calorie (2 tablespoons)
Taco sauce (1 tablespoon)
Vinegar

Seasonings can be very helpful in making food taste better. Be careful of how much salt you use. Read the label, and choose those seasonings that do not contain sodium.

Basil (fresh)	Garlic	Oregano
Celery seeds	Garlic	Paprika
Chili powder	powder	Pepper
Chives	Herbs	Pimiento
Cinnamon	Hot pepper	Soy sauce*
Curry	sauce	Soy sauce,
Dill	Lemon	low-sodium
Flavoring	Lemon juice	("lite")
extracts	Lemon	Spices
(vanilla,	pepper	Wine, used in
almond,	Lime	cooking
walnut,	Lime juice	(¼ cup)
peppermint,	Mint	Worcestershire
butter,	Onion	sauce
lemon, etc.)	powder	

*400 milligrams or more of sodium per serving.

COMBINATION FOODS

Much of the food we eat is mixed together in various combinations. These combination foods do not fit into only one Exchange List. It can be quite hard to tell what is in a certain casserole dish or baked food item. This is a list of average values for some typical combination foods. This list will help you fit these foods into your meal plan. Ask your dietitian for information about any other foods you'd like to eat.

FOOD	AMOUNT	EXCHANGES
Casseroles, homemade	1 cup (8 ounces)	2 Starch, 2 Medium-Fat Meat, 1 Fat
Cheese pizza*, thin crust	¼ of 15 ounces (¼ of 10 inches)	2 Starch, 1 Medium-Fat Meat, 1 Fat
Chile with beans* ** (commercial)	1 cup	2 Starch, 2 Medium-Fat Meat, 2 Fat
Chow mein* ** (without noodles or rice)	2 cups	1 Starch, 2 Vegetable, 2 Lean Meat
Macaroni and cheese*	1 cup (8 ounces)	2 Starch, 1 Medium-Fat Meat, 2 Fat
Soup:		
Bean* **	1 cup	1 Starch, 1 Vegetable, 1 Lean Meat

*400 milligrams or more of sodium per serving.
**3 grams or more of fiber per serving.

FOOD	AMOUNT	EXCHANGES
Chunky, all varieties*	10¾-ounce can	1 Starch, 1 Vegetable, 1 Medium-Fat Meat
Cream* (made with water)	1 cup	1 Starch, 1 Fat
Vegetable* or broth-type*	1 cup	1 Starch
Spaghetti and meatballs* (canned)	1 cup	2 Starch, 1 Medium-Fat Meat, 1 Fat
Sugar-free pudding (made with skim milk)	½ cup	1 Starch

Beans as a meat substitute:

Dried beans**, peas**, lentils**	1 cup (cooked)	2 Starch, 1 Lean Meat

*400 milligrams or more of sodium per serving.
**3 grams or more of fiber per serving.

FOODS FOR OCCASIONAL USE

Moderate amounts of some foods can be used in your meal plan, in spite of their sugar or fat content, as long as you can maintain blood-glucose control. The following list includes average exchange values for some of these foods. Because they are concentrated sources of carbohydrate, you will notice that the portion sizes are very small. Check with your dietitian for advice on how often and when you can eat them.

FOOD	AMOUNT	EXCHANGES
Angel food cake	1/12 cake	2 Starch
Cake, no icing	1/12 cake, or a 3-inch square	2 Starch, 2 Fat
Cookies	2 small (1¾ inches across)	1 Starch, 1 Fat
Frozen fruit yogurt	⅓ cup	1 Starch
Gingersnaps	3	1 Starch
Granola	¼ cup	1 Starch, 1 Fat
Granola bars	1 small	1 Starch, 1 Fat
Ice cream, any flavor	½ cup	1 Starch, 2 Fat
Ice milk, any flavor	½ cup	1 Starch, 1 Fat
Sherbet, any flavor	¼ cup	1 Starch
Snack chips*, all varieties	1 ounce	1 Starch, 2 Fat
Vanilla wafers	6 small	1 Starch, 1 Fat

*If more than one serving is consumed, sodium levels will equal or exceed 400 milligrams.

Index